HEALTH CARE SYSTEM AND HOSPITAL ADMINISTRATION

4

EMERGING AND THRUST AREAS

HEALTH CARE SYSTEM AND HOSPITAL ADMINISTRATION

4

EMERGING AND THRUST AREAS

DR. S.L. GOEL

Professor of Public Administration (Retd.),
Panjab University, Chandigarh
Editor, Indian Journal of Public Administration, IIPA, New Delhi
Former Member, UGC, Former Member Distance Education Council
Former Member All India Board of Management, AICTE
Member, Executive Council, IIPA, New Delhi.
Former Vice-President, IIPA, New Delhi.
Emeritus Fellow, University Grants Commission
Former Director, State Bank of India (Local Board) Chandigarh
Former Director, National Horticulture Board, Ministry of Agriculture,
Government of India, New Delhi.

DEEP & DEEP PUBLICATIONS PVT. LTD.

F-159, Rajouri Garden, New Delhi-110027

HEALTH CARE SYSTEM AND HOSPITAL ADMINISTRATION
Vol. 4—Emerging and Thrust Areas

ISBN 978-81-8450-194-0 (Vol. 4)
ISBN 978-81-8450-198-8 (Set)

Typeset by S.S. COMPOSERS
3190, Mohindra Park, Shakur Basti, Delhi-110034.

Printed in India at MAYUR ENTERPRISES
WZ Plot No. 3, Gujjar Market, Tihar Village, New Delhi-110018.

Published by DEEP & DEEP PUBLICATIONS PVT. LTD.
F-159, Rajouri Garden, New Delhi-110027.
Phones: 25435369, 25440916
E-mail: ddpbooks@yahoo.co.in • ddpubs@gmail.com
Showroom:
2/13, Ansari Road, Daryaganj, New Delhi-110002 • Telefax: 23245122

Contents

Preface

Health affects and is affected by other sectors of Development. Therefore, there is a need to concentrate on other areas which are directly and indirectly beneficial to health. We must identify these areas and include them in the promotion of health.

Poor environmental sanitation in India is responsible for a number of diseases. We must ensure healthy environment for healthy living. Exposure to infection in India comes mainly from lack of safe water and sewerage disposal facilities in most of the areas. The condition in regard to these services is very serious. Safe water supply should normally include treated surface water and untreated but uncontaminated water from protected boreholes, springs and wells. Other sources of doubtful quality should be considered unsafe and not included in the estimate of coverage. Percentage figures of coverage are available, giving population served by completed water systems separately for urban and rural areas from the International Drinking Water Supply and Sanitation Decade (IDWSSD) which is very low. Facilities for hygienic waste disposal are considered adequate if they effectively prevent contact with or access to excreta by humans, animals and insects.

New developments are taking place in the area of health like Telemedicine, which should be harnessed to promote health in neglected areas. In addition, health education should be part and parcel of every health programme.

Health Education is the combination of planned social action and planned learning experiences designed to enable people to gain control over the determinants of health and of health behaviour and the social conditions that affect their health status and the health status of others.

Further development based on human ecology has been spelt out by WHO expert Committee—In recent years, however, a better understanding has developed of the processes that have a positive or negative influences on the harmonious functioning of a person, both as an individual and as a social being. This has prompted study of the role society plays in influencing the individual's health behaviour. It is now recognized that community's values and norms play a vital part in defining the general approach of people to illness and health as well as to treatment and prevention, and that the process of socialization is one of the most important mechanisms in transmitting certain values and norms from one generation to the next. This has resulted in the development of social intervention models of health education, in which the emphasis is placed in influencing social, instead of individual, factors associated with health and illness.

Health education is a 'process', which needs effective planning and implementation with appropriate consideration of ultimate goals and the best means for achieving them physical, mental and social health. The World Health Organisation expert committee on health education of the public (1954) has defined:

> "Health Education like general education is concerned with changes in knowledge, feelings and behaviour of people. In its most usual forms it concentrates on developing such health practices as are believed to "bring about the best state of possible well-being."

The International Union of Health Education (1988) defined:

> "Health Education is the combination of planned social action and planned learning experiences designed to enable people to gain control over the determinants of health, health behaviour and social conditions that affect their health status and health status of others.

The WHO Constitution specifically states that "informed opinion and active cooperation on the part of the public are of utmost importance in the improvement of the health of the people." Yet, a review of the WHO and country health education programmes did not reveal any impressive degree of progress. The chief reason identified for this was the approach which had been adopted. "Health Education", was synonymous with 'health knowledge', to be dispensed by experts to individuals who were assumed to have very limited ideas about health and illness, a classical top-down approach.

This was despite the fact that the WHO Expert Committee on Health Education, in 1954, had stated, "The aim of health education is to help people to achieve health by their own actions and efforts." The non-achievement of targets in programmes such as family planning, malaria eradication, diarrhoeal diseases control and others had led to a serious re-thinking of the concepts, scope, approaches and strategies of health education programmes.

A major challenge is how to harness the potential of science and technology to address current gaps and emerging problems in the health sector as India enters the 21st century. The building of the scientific capacities is an essential component of the international pursuit of health development. Over the next several decades the world and the Region will have to, through multisectoral research, respond to a number of new health problems, including those stemming from global environmental changes, political instabilities and social breakdown

One of the most substantial challenges to science and technology is to close the gaps that confront research -gaps in the research to be carried out, in the use of research results and in the need for new research methodologies. Depending on the nature of the gaps, priority might go to: (1) research to develop new interventions; (2) research into better use of existing interventions; (3) the development of new methodologies and general capacity strengthening researchers and policy-makers, need to interact around these variables, so that the options are seen and the opportunities and responsibilities are shared.

Innovative approaches aimed at responding to the socio-economic and political changes and epidemiological transitions that are taking place will be needed: How to sustain the commitment to PHC and HFA principles? How to reorient health systems (health care reform)? How to intensify efforts to increase managerial capabilities? What are the innovative measures needed to respond to the transition: moving from quantity to quality, health for the underserved or underprivileged, improving the shape of human resources for health, partnerships in health development, community actions for health, health system research?

Considering the vast numbers of people in India, the majority live in rural areas but with an expanding proportion in urban settings, the need for networks of health services developed as close as possible to these populations and adapted to their changing needs is a challenging priority.

Meanwhile, change will inevitably come in the way health services are planned, financed and managed, and new approaches to health care reform will be undertaken in various countries. Health sector reforms should take place as sustained process of fundamental change in the context of health policy and health institutional arrangements. They are not sequential, nor incremental processes. The main areas of reform are: (1) reorienting and restructuring of ministries of health, including publicly-financed and organized services; (2) broadening the health financing options; (3) improving the performance of civil service, including decentralization, and (4) expanding partnerships. Thus, it may be said that it is essential to develop a new framework for public health action to have a long-term perspective, and to strengthen national capabilities, infrastructure and technologies which can be sustained with available resources.

The role of education in health development, including family planning, cannot be overemphasized. The literacy rate, in particular the functional literacy rate of women, is crucial to health development. Health is so much in the hands of women that female literacy rate becomes crucial likewise, the education of children is important. As with growth, so with education, it is the length of time that improved rates of literacy have prevailed that makes a difference. The horizontal spread of primary education seems more critical for health development than the vertical spread of higher education to selected population segments. For example, the success of clean water and environmental sanitation is critically dependent upon education in the hygienic use of water and appropriate disposal of wastes.

In this volume, Emerging and Thrust Areas, we have divided the book into 19 chapters.

Chapter 1 deals with environmental health which is basic and most important in the new millennium for health promotion and development or even survival of human existence on this planet. Chapters 2 and 3 concentrate on the preventive health as 75 percent diseases are preventable and cost very little as compared to curative. However, it is very difficult to operate as it has been rightly said that it is easier to destroy the mountains than to change the minds of the people. Chapters 4 and 5 deal with health information system and telemedicine which are essential to lubricate the health system with right information at right time to take timely action. In addition, telemedicine can help to serve the patients and people in general living in difficult places as well as help in exchange of knowledge among specialists. Chapter 6 discusses about the issues of promotion of Medical tourism, its requirements, potentialities and problems. Chapter 7 examines Health and Travel, that is what health precautions may be kept during travel especially international travel. Chapter 8 deals with health and technology. In 21st century, technology for health has become complicated as new machines are coming very fast. This has made the medical treatment very costly and unaffordable to a large population. It has been suggested in this chapter as to how can we use appropriate technology and make the medical treatment simple. Chapter 9 concentrates on health and research. Research that is finding out new ways and innovative techniques to deal with diseases like heart transplant. Chapter 10 examines health and peace. Nuclear energy can help medical science to promote peace and happiness. Chapter 11 examines health and disaster that is how to provide health services during disaster which has become a frequent phenomenon. Chapter 12 examines health and stress and strain. Today's life has become complicated and is causing stress and strain inspite of physical progress. The chapter examine the methods to deal with stress and strain. Chapter 13 deals with health and housing as we know that there can be no good health without good housing. Chapter 14 discusses as how violence creates health problems. The need is to curb violence and if occurs, we can provide health to victims. Chapter 15 deals with the role of sports in health. Chapter 16 examines the role of healthy cities in promoting happiness and aesthetic values. Chapter 17 deals with the role of yoga in promoting holisitic health. Chapter 18 deals with health in urban areas to ensure healthy cities and the last Chapter 19 examines the impact of Population Explosion on Socio-Economic development of the country. There is a need of control of population on top priority.

Contemporary medicine faces a special challenge in India and other third world countires. We should, of course, embrace science and technology, else we will be left far behind. Yet, I believe, much greater emphasis must be placed on the preventive aspect of medicine. Far more money should be allocated to providng clear water, good nutrition, sanitation, housing, education with special emphsis on female education, population control and use of preventive vaccines, than to the purchase of glittering machines or to building five star hospitals in the urban centres of the country. An equitable distribution of the meager resources with a focused attention on the problems afflicting 70% of the population residing in the villages of India, may well be rewarded by greater benefit to a greater number of people.

The future world will witness new diseases and new infections. New diseases could result from changes in social or environmental conditions. Micro-organisms and in particular viruses can mutate for known and unknown reasons; and can produce diseases never before encountered in the history of man. HIV is an example of a virus which probably mutated several times before it struck our contemporary world.

What is needed is to lay emphasis on emerging and thrust areas to keep the medical science, knowledge and delivery of health services as per the needs of the people. It is hoped that this book on "Health Care System and Hospital Administration—Emerging and Thrust Areas" would make a modest contribution to the knowledge and existing literature on this expanding field. Besides, this would help the academicians, national health officials, public health administrations, medical research workers and the policy-maker and planners in the proper understanding of health care delivery system. I will consider my labour well rewarded if the findings of the study are translated to provide decent health care to the millions of people living in rural areas, urban slums and tribal areas. Comments and suggestions from the readers would always be welcome.

Chandigarh S.L. GOEL

CHAPTER 1

Environmental Health

A GOOD ENVIRONMENT IS THE KEY TO HEALTH AND DEVELOPMENT

Environment has been defined by Webster's New Collegiate Dictionary as "the aggregate of all the external conditions and influences affecting the life and development of an organism."

Shri T.N, Chaturvedi in his Editorial to *IJPA*, July-Sept. 1989 (Special Number on Environment and Administration) rightly sees the intimate relationship between human beings and nature since times immemorial. To quote: "Man, since his origin, has lived in harmony with Nature through the ages, holding Nature in awe and reverence. The Vedas, folklore and scriptures of different religions, faiths and beliefs also speak of the need for harmony with the universe, which is the habitat not only of man but also of all animals, birds, insects, plants and vegetation. The mutually supportive role of all living things is often mentioned as a crucial factor for a balanced social and harmonious existence. The ecological balance is inherent in the very process of creation. Everywhere, the seers, poets and thinkers, through the ages, have referred to the need for living in harmony with environment. In fact, the Taitariyopanishad looks at the relationship between man and his environment in its totality and stresses complete harmony and interdependence between them in order to attain real prosperity."[1]

Dr. Hiroshi Nakajima, Director-General of World Health Organisation, sounded a warning alarm about degradation of this planet in his Article, "A Wounded Planet."[2] He rightly visualises that it is now increasingly evident that more and more diseases stem from the degradation caused by man to his own environment. The potential harmful effects of industrial development on our global ecosystem are now better known. Ozone layer depletion, acid rain, climate change, chemical pollution are some examples of the man-made wounds to our planet.

Water and Sanitation

Water supply and sanitation are accepted as basic needs. Urban water supply and sanitation are areas critical to the quality of life, people's health and environmental protection. They affect the productivity in the towns and cities which contribute significantly to the national development. While water supply has received greater attention, sanitation has been comparatively neglected. Inadequate sanitation leads to degradation of environment and serious health problems of water-borne and vector-borne diseases. It is, therefore, necessary that both water supply and sanitation are treated together as issues in environmental health.

We are at a turning point; warnings of the damage to our health and quality of life are growing louder. An increasing number of people are acting to stop the degradation of our environment.

Sixty years of Indian Republic especially in the urban areas, are under great stress and strain. The degradation of our environment has to be arrested immediately otherwise it would have long-term impact on the quality of life of future generations. . . . We should also take this opportunity to educate our children regarding the importance of the preservation of our environment. Dr. Wilfried Kreisel also elaborates the aspects of environment which affect health of mankind.[3]

> "How can we make environmental health a more potent force to serve people faced with growing threats to their health? How can our improving environmental health technology be better used to foster positive health? I know of no country—developing or industrialized in which this issue is not urgent and important. I know of many countries in which it is critical."

The remarkably wide range of environmental concerns include the international problems of acid rain, the greenhouse effect, and depletion of the planet's ozone layer. It includes national concerns with medical wastes disposal, radioactive and toxic wastes control, transportation accidents, health aspects of urbanisation and traffic, occupational health and safety, and air and water pollution. It also includes local concerns over inadequate water supplies and sanitation facilities, water quality, clean air, solid wastes management and finding a balance between the economic incentives of development and a decent quality of life. In the report on Our Common Future, the World Commission on Environment and Development (sometimes called the Brundtland Commission) pointed out that the situation is getting increasingly critical.

WHO, South-East Asia Regional Office Declaration on 'Health and Development in the South-East Asia Region in the 21st Century mentions that significant differences exist between the environmental problems of rural and urban areas.[4] In rural areas, poverty, unsafe drinking water, inadequate excreta disposal, combined with contaminated food and illiteracy, are responsible for a majority of illnesses. Poor ventilation, coupled with the use of poorly-designed cooking stoves. causes severe indoor air pollution and health problems. particularly in children and infants. With the intensification of agricultural activities large quantities of pesticides and herbicides are being applied without taking adequate precautionary measures.

In urban areas, on the other hand, environmental problems are the result of rapid and massive population migration from rural to urban areas and of uncontrolled industrialization. Municipal services are unable to keep pace with the urban growth, like providing adequate water supplies, sewerage and sanitation. Overcrowding, inadequate housing with poor ventilation and absence of protection against rain, heat and cold add to the stresses and dangers of urban living. Industries are often located in and around urban areas with uncontrolled disposal of wastes. The Bhopal gas tragedy in India over a decade ago is an example.

Of course, there are other major environmental concerns such as deforestation, global warming, ozone depletion, cross-border movements of hazardous products and other forms of environmental degradation. Protection of the environment and of health endangered by environmental hazards comprises a very large and important international public policy agenda. In developing countries the problems are doubly difficult because of the immediacy of local environmental threats as well as the larger regional and global issues.

ENVIRONMENTAL ADMINISTRATION IN INDIA: GENESIS, GROWTH AND LEGAL FRAMEWORK

As stated in India 1999—A Reference Manual published by Ministry of Information and Broadcasting, in the beginning of the Fourth Five Year Plan, problems and issues centred around environment, "this resulted in the establishment of the National Council of Environmental Planning and Coordination in 1972 at The Department of Science and Technology. Another empowered Committee "as set-up in 1980 for reviewing the existing legislative measures and administrative machinery for ensuring environmental protection and for recommending ways to strengthen them. On the recommendations of this empowered committee, a separate Department of Environment was set-up in 1980 which was subsequently upgraded in a full-fledged Ministry of Environment and Forests in 1985 to serve as the focal point in the administrative structure of the Government of India for the planning, promotion and coordination of environmental and forestry programmes. The state department of environment, Central and State Pollution Control Boards, the Botanical and Zoological Survey of India, the Forest Survey of India, the National River Conservation Authority (formerly Central Ganga Authority), the National Afforestation and Eco-development Board, the Indian Council for Forestry Research and Education, the Wildlife Institute of India, the National Museum for Natural history, etc. are the Ministry's partners in carrying out environmental protection activities.

Prevention and Control of Pollution

The policy statement on Abatement of Pollution, adopted in 1992, provides instruments in the form of legislation and regulation. Fiscal incentives, voluntary agreements, educational programmes and information campaigns to prevent and control pollution of water. Air and land, since the adoption of the policy statement, the focus of activities has been on issues such as promotion of clean and low waste technologies, waste minimization, reuse/recycling, improvement of water quality, environment audit, natural resource accounting, development of mass-based standards, institutional and human resource development, etc. The whole issue of pollution prevention and control is dealt with by a combination of command and control methods as well as voluntary and regulatory, fiscal measures, promotion of awareness and involvement of public.

Central Pollution Control Board

The Central Pollution Control Board (CPCB) is the national apex body for assessment, monitoring and control of water and air pollution. The executive responsibilities for enforcement of the Acts for Prevention and Control of Pollution of Water (1974) and Air (1981) and also of the Water (Cess) Act, 1977 are carried out through the Board. The CPCB advises the Central Government on all matters concerning the prevention and control of air, water and noise pollution and provides technical services to the Ministry for implementing the provisions of the Environment (Protection) Act, 1986. Under the Act, effluent and emission standards in respect of 61 categories of industries have been notified.

Education, Awareness and Information

Priority is accorded by the Ministry of Environment and Forests to promote environmental education, create environmental awareness among various age-groups and to disseminate information through Environmental Information System (ENVIS) network to all concerned. Special emphasis is given to non-formal environmental education through seminars/symposia/ workshops, training programmes, eco-camps, audio-visual shows, etc. The Ministry has been organising a National Environment Awareness Campaign (NEAC) since July 1980. As a part of this campaign, 19 November to 18 December every year is observed as the National Environment Month. The main themes for the 1997-98 campaign were Pollution Prevention and Control, and Conservation and Plantation of Trees for Environmental Protection. A large number of organisations have been granted financial assistance by the Ministry to organise various activities for creating environmental awareness. The Ministry also provides financial support for setting up eco-clubs at schools and for production of films on environment.

A new scheme, Paryavaran Vahini, was launched in 1992-93 to create environmental awareness and to ensure active public participation by involving the local people in activities relating to environmental protection.

Paryavaran Vahinis are proposed to be constituted in 194 selected districts all over the country which have a high incidence of pollution and density of tribal and forest population. The Vahinis also play a watch-dog role by reporting instance of environmental pollution, deforestation, poaching, etc. They function under the charge of District Collectors, with the active cooperation of the State/Union Territory governments. This scheme is entirely financed by the Ministry of Environment and Forests.

International Cooperation

The Ministry of Environment and Forests functions as a nodal agency for United Nations Environment Programme (UNEP), South Asia Cooperation Environment Programme (SACEP) and International Centre for Integrated Mountain and Development (ICIMOD), International Union for Conservation of Nature and Natural Resources (IUCN) and various international agencies, regional bodies and multilateral institutions.

India is signatory to the following important international treaties/ agreements in the field of environment: (i) International Convention for the regulation of Whaling, (ii) International Plant Protection Convention, (iii) The Antarctic Treaty, (iv) Convention on Wetlands of international importance, (v) International Convention on International trade in endangered species of wild flora and fauna; (vi) Protocol of 1978 relating to the international convention for the prevention of pollution from ships, (vii) Vienna Convention for the protection of the ozone layer; (viii) Convention on Migratory Species; (ix) Basel Convention on trans-boundary movement of hazardous substances; (x) Framework convention of climate change; (xi) Convention on conservation of biodiversity; (xii) Montreal protocol on the substances that deplete the ozone layer; and (xiii) International Convention for Combating Desertification.

Environmental Legislation

Major legislations directly dealing with the protection of environment are the Wildlife (Protection) Act, 1972, the Forest (Conservation) Act, 1980, the Water (Prevention and Control of Pollution) Act, 1974, the Water (Cess) Act, 1977, the National Environment Appellate Authority Act, 1977, the Air (Prevention and Control of Pollution) Act, 1981, the Environment (Protection) Act, 1986, the Public Liability Insurance Act, 1991 and the National Environment Tribunal Act, 1995. The Constitution (Forty-Second Amendment Act of 1976) gave Parliament the power to enact laws on virtually any entry in the State list, and through Article 253 brought environmental regulation under the Concurrent List.

India has increasingly institutionalized its environment concern after the United Nations conference on Human Environment at Stockholm in 1972, to serve as a guideline to the governments, both Central and State. Article 148A was added to the Directive Principles of State Policy in 1976, which said, "The state shall endeavour to protect and improve environment and safeguard the forests and wildlife of the country." In a new chapter entitled 'Fundamental Duties', Article (51Ag) imposed a similar responsibility on every citizen to protect and improve the natural environment including forests, lakes, rivers and wildlife and to have compassion for living creatures. Supreme Court of India has held whenever a problem of ecology is brought before the Court, the Court is bound to bear in mind Art. 48A of the Constitution.

ENVIRONMENT *VIS-A-VIS* DEVELOPMENT

Nature and Scope of Environmental Health Programme

Meaning

Environmental health refers to the ecological balance that must exist between man and his environment in order to ensure his well-being. The deterioration of the human environment through the population explosion, pollution of air and water, and other disruptions of the ecological balance pose a major international health hazard and a serious challenge. Professor J. Logan, in a paper published in *American Journal of Tropical Medicine* in 1960, was able to show that environmentally transmitted diseases were responsible for the sufferings of 500 million people every year particularly among infants and children.[5] The UN Secretary-General's report on problem of the human environment sounds a similar ominous note: "If current trends continue, the failure of life on earth could be engendered and thus, it is urgent to focus world attention on these problems which threaten humanity in an environment that permits the realisation of the highest human aspirations."[6]

The close relationship that exists between an unhealthy Environment and the economic condition of a community was pinpointed by a panel of experts which met in 1971 to discuss the environmental problems of the developing countries. "Poverty and the very lack of development", these experts said, "constitute an essential environmental problem in the developing countries. They recommended an attack on the problems of inadequate water supply, poor housing, sanitation, nutrition and widespread disease as prime targets in an effort to improve the environment of millions of people, and to lay the groundwork for their economic betterment."[7]

Ninth Five Year Plan (Draft) also warns about the bad consequences of poor environment on Health. Environment can allot human health in many ways. Deficiency of iodine in soil, water and foodstuffs is the cause of iodine deficiency disorders. Excessive fluoride content in the water is the cause of fluorosis. Environmental degradation may affect air, land and water. Pollutants may enter the food chain. All these may enter human body through various portals and affect the health status. Rapidly growing population, urbanisation, changing agricultural, industrial and water resource management, increasing use of pesticides and fossil fuels have all resulted in a perceptible deterioration in the quality of environment and attendant adverse health consequences. Environment pollution due to developmental activities are increasingly becoming the focus of concern. The interactive interdependence of health, environment and sustainable development was accepted as the fulcrum of action under Agenda 21 at the Earth Summit in Brazil in 1992. Environmental health in its broader perspective would have to address the detection, prevention and management of:

(i) existing deficiencies or excesses of certain elements in natural environment;
(ii) macro-environmental contamination of air, land, water and food; and
(iii) disaster management,

Aspects of Environmental Health

The environment can be defined as an aggregate of all the external conditions and influences affecting the life and development of an organism. Human Environment means everything that is experienced by man and it is the total nature of this experience that determines the quality of life. According to Roggers, "the environment appears to possess two main avenues by which it may reach man and affect man health; it may act upon his body as a material agent or it may act upon his mind and emotions as non-material agent, although sooner or later this may very well produce a material effect.[8] The effect of both is the pollution of environment. Prof. Samuel Halter, Professor of Public Health at the University of Brussels defines pollution as "the presence in the ambient environment of chemical, physical or biological factors capable of inducing disturbances in the normal physiology and functioning of human organs.[9]

We can classify the environmental factors impinging on the health of the people as follows:

(a) Physical, Chemical and Biological factors.
(b) Social, Economic and Cultural factors.
(c) Ecological, Economic and Aesthetic factors.
(d) Individual human system.

All these agents in the environment interact with one another and produce the favourable or unfavourable impact on the health of the people.

MEANING AND ROLE OF ENVIRONMENTAL HEALTH ADMINISTRATION

Environmental Sanitation Administration is an activity of diagnosing and controlling the environmental factors which exercise or may exercise a deleterious and unhealthy effect on the physical, social, and mental life of the people. The Draft Five-Year Plan (1978-83) has rightly mentioned: "The essence of sound environmental growth lies in a happy blend of the realisation of the physical out limits to the exploitation of environmental resources and the inner limits to human needs and aspiration.[10] Environmental health administration is quite complex and complicated owing to the complexity and diversity of the socio-political and institutional arrangements in which the programmes are implemented and the complexity, multiplicity of the physical, biological, social and economic factors that they must take into account. The objective of the environmental sanitation administration is to plan thoroughly to change favourably the environment itself and modify the interaction of human beings with the environment so that the people can enjoy a good quality of life. The administration of environmental programme is not within the purview of any single discipline but presents a challenge to many disciplines. The administrators responsible for such programmes must plan to attack the unfavourable factors in concert with one another. We may mention some of the important areas which need the immediate attention of the planners, policy-makers and administrators to solve these impending problems, potable safe water supply and water pollution, solid wastes management, air pollution control, occupational health, food sanitation, urban planning and housing, slum clearance, soil erosion, noise pollution., etc. The administration must define in the geographical context the magnitude of each problem, its relationship with others and the benefits expected direct outputs, intermediate effects or impacts and the ultimate effects or benefits. Some of these have been indicated in the form of a table (see Table 1.1). The administration of environmental health programmes are very expensive and complicated. In order to translate the benefits of such programmes to the society, the administrators must ensure that the progmmme:

(a) receives acceptance and support;
(b) achieves the desired objectives and results;
(c) links its efforts with those of other health and socio-economic development programmes; and
(d) accomplishes its work economically, with a minimum waste of money and other scarce resources.[11]

We may now take up two important aspects of environment, i.e. water supply and sanitation which affect health development in a big way.

Environment Health Promotes Public Health which is defined as follows:

Public health is one of the efforts organized by society to protect, promote and restore people's health. It is the combination of services, skills and beliefs that are directed to the maintenance and improvement of the health of all people through collective or social actions. The programmes, services and institutions involved emphasize the prevention of disease and the health needs of the population as whole. Public health activities change with changing technology and social values, but the goals remain the same;

TABLE 1.1

Types of Output in Illustrative Environmental Health Programme

Programme	*Direct Outputs*	*Intermediate Effects or Impacts*	*Ultimate Effects or Benefits*
Water Supply	State water provide to households in adequate amounts and used efficiently	Reduced disease from water borne pathogens; support of hygiene, nutrition and economic activity	Longer survival
Water Pollution Control	Reduced contamination of (used water returned to) watercourses, seas, soil and food	Improved water resources for human use; reduced damage to marine life; improved aesthetics	Less disability, suffering impairement and pain
Solid Wastes management	Wastes confined, removed and disposed of (treated recycled)	Reduced disease from vectorborne pathogens and from pathogens and chemicals transferred to air, water and land; economic gains; improved aesthetics	More efficient personal and social performance
Air Pollution Control	Reduced introduction of toxic, irritant and nuisance elements into ambient air	Reduced death, disease and discomfort; reduced economic losses; improved aesthetics	Improved quality of life
Occupational Health	Reduced physical/ chemical hazards in work environment, through primary and secondary disease prevention services	Reduce illness trauma and poisoning; safer work environment, improved working condition and productivity	Socio-economic development
Food Sanitation	Food safeguarded against contamination in production, processing delivery, preparation, and consumption	Reduced disease and death from pathogens and toxins in food; enlarged markets; improved aesthetics	

Source: WHO: Public Health Paper No. 99, p. 113.

to reduce the amount of disease, premature death and disease produced discomfort and disability in the population. (J.M. Last, 1983)[12]

Water Supply and Sanitation

Safe water and improved sanitation are a necessary condition for better health. and there can be no lasting improvement of public health without them. There is no denying the fact that inadequacy of sate drinking water. improper disposal of human excreta. solid and liquid wastes leading to unfavourable environmental condition have been the causes of many killer diseases.

Water is variously considered as life giving, life sustaining, purifying, a vital nutrient and essential for life. However, it can also spread disease and kill. Predictions are that drinking water is becoming a scarcer commodity. With ground water being used faster than it can be recharged, shortage of drinking water is likely to become an important problem in the future. Fifty percent of infant deaths are attributed to waterborne diseases. An estimated 1.5 million under five deaths occur in India every year, due to water-related diseases, and approximately 1800 million person hours are lost annually in the country, due to same. It is estimated that poor quality and inadequate quantity of water accounts for about 10% of the total burden of disease in developing country situations, as in Karnataka state.[13]

M. Aktar has stated that inadequacy in the availability of safe drinking water, unfavourable environmental conditions and lack of personal hygiene have been the major causes of disease and disability among people. As per WHO statistics, 80 per cent of diseases in the developing countries are related to unsafe water supply and inadequate sanitation causing high child mortality, low life expectancy and poor quality of life. In India, more than one million children below 5 years die from dehydration caused by diarrhoea annually, while another 250 thousand are victims of tetanus. Poliomyelitis has been a cause of lameness among 170 thousand children per year. There is also a very high rate of occurrence of intestinal worms, particularly in West Bengal, Bihar, Orissa, Andhra Pradesh, Tamil Nadu, Kerala and Maharashtra. The national goal to reduce child mortality from 146 per thousand to 125 by 1995 and 70 per thousand by 2000 cannot possibly be achieved without a significant change in the existing mortality/morbidity-related to water and sanitation. Also important is to change the peoples' perception about the link between sanitation and health. According to a recent KAP survey in the country, 37 per cent people do not know/do not believe that exposed excreta can harm health. Outdoor defecation is not generally seen as a problem except in terms of inconvenience during rain, night or winter and to women.

Y.N. Nanjudiah has stated that majority of the rural people practice open air defecation as the coverage of sanitation facilities has reached only a negligible population. For want of awareness on health on the part of users quite a large number of latrines are out of use or misused. Further, open air defection generally enjoys social acceptability. It is considered

CHART 1.1

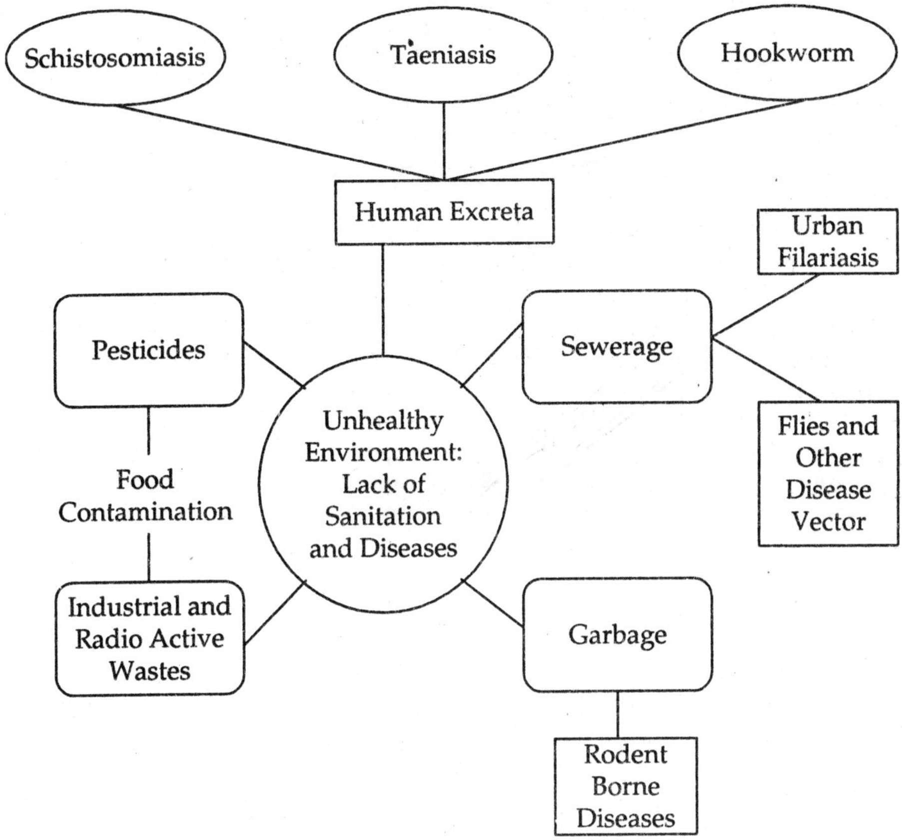

hygiene and wholesome and in tune with the nature and fresh air. At the same time toilet has a poor image. It is believed to be dirty and a breeding place for flies and mosquitoes. Social surveys carried out so far have highlighted that there is lack of knowledge regarding latrine, which can be summarised as under:

(a) Faecal-borne diseases can be prevented by using a latrine.
(b) Pathogenic microbes survive from days to years in the moist soil and may become wind borne.
(c) Social status and prestige can be attained by having a latrine.
(d) Constipation, particularly among rural women can be eliminated.
(e) Privacy can be achieved.
(f) Low cost sanitation options are available, and these can be maintained in an eco-friendly way.

Dr. H. Mahler, former WHO, Director-General, has rightly said that, "I am utterly convinced that the number of water taps per 1,000 population will be an infinitely more meaningful health indicator than the number of hospital beds per 1,000 population." Mr. Kurt Waldhelm, former UN Secretary-General also stressed that,* "the provision of safe water and sanitation does not merely mean happier, healthier citizens; it also means increased economic productivity." Nikolas P. Napulbow in his editorial "Water For All, a Human Right" has rightly said that, "water is a basic human need for health—indeed, for survival—and therefore it is not an exaggeration to call it one of the basic human rights. Without safe water and sanitation, there is no real development. A community ravaged by diarrheal diseases, dracunculiasis or schistosomiasis cannot look beyond its immediate problems towards social and economic welfare. Safe water is the doorway to health and health is the prerequisite for progress, social equity and human divinity."[14]

Infectious diseases resulting from water pollution can be classified into four groups, depending upon the ways in which their incidence can be lessened by improvements in water supply—

(1) "Water-borne" diseases are those in which infectious agent remains alive in drinking water e.g., typhoid, paratyphoid, gastroenterities, etc. The incidence of these diseases can be reduced by the purification of water.
(2) "Water-washed" diseases include infection of the outer body surface, e.g., trachoma, skin ulcers, scabies and typhus, bacillary and amoebic dysentery and gastro enterities. The incidence can be reduced by augmenting water quantity.
(3) "Water-based" infections, i.e., schistosomiasis, guinea worms. The infection occurs when the skin is in contact with water or through drinking water.
(4) "Water breeding" or water promixity diseases are caused by mosquitoes or flies living near aquatic conditions.

The group of disease, in (1) called the faecal oral group are transmitted from person to person through water or food via the oral route. Breaking the faecal-oral route forms the basis for public health intervention for disease control. This is through a combination of good personal hygiene, increased water quantity, improved water quality, food hygiene and provision of sanitary facilties.[15]

There is probably no single factor that has a greater effect on the health, well-being and development of a community than the provision of ample and convenient supply of wholesome and good quality water. In towns and cities water supply is recognised as a basic necessity for industrial and commercial purposes; it is vital for the maintenance of public health and the prevention of epidemics. Dame Barbara Ward, President of the International Institute for Environment and Development, rightly observes that, "Water is everywhere, the key to human health. . . .. clean water is a key to human comfort, health and even survival.[16] Martin Boyer, Adviser, Drinking Water Programme, UNICEF has observed that "The provision of ample supplies of safe water and the sanitary disposal of excreta have a direct and far-reaching effect upon the health and well-being of rural populations. Indeed, it is believed that no other single measure can make a comparable contribution to the improvement of their health and standard of living. The choice of an appropriate technology depends on local conditions."[17] To quote WHO: "One hospital bed out of four in the world is occupied by a patient who is ill because of polluted water Provisions of a safe and convenient water supply is the single most important activity that could be undertaken to improve the health of people living in rural areas of the developing world."

Kofi Annan, United Nations Secretary General says that the centrality of freshwater in our lives cannot be overestimated. Water has been a major factor in the rise and fall of civilizations. It has been a source of tensions and fierce competition between nations that could become even worse if present trends continue. Lack of access to water for meeting basic needs such as health, hygiene and food security undermines development and inflicts enormous hardship on more than a billion members of the human family. And its quality reveals everything, right or wrong, that we do in safeguarding the global environment.[18]

WHO estimates that as much as 80 percent of all diseases in the world are associated with water, Iain Guest (Geneva), a specialist in development topics submits that an astonishing number of people suffer from these water-related diseases at any time, 400 million with gastro enterities, 160 million with malaria, 30 million with river blindness, 200 million with Schistosomiasis.[19] At the 1969 World Health Assembly, a delegate from the region (SEA) estimated that water-borne diseases accounted for 40 percent of all morality, and 60 percent of all morbidity in his country.[20]

I.V. Rajeshwar, ex-Governor of West Bengal in his article, "Endemic Problems defying solution" in the *Daily Tribune,* dated January 16,2000 rightly says that Fifty-two years after independence even basic amenities like drinking water supply and unpolluted air are not available to most citizens. At present, water supply is available to 84.33% of urban population and 76.68% to rural population, However sanitation coverage is 49.91 in urban areas and 14.02 in rural areas.

Ninth Plan finds that the existing norms for rural water supply is 40 liters of drinking water per capita per day (LPCD) and a public stand post or a hand pump for 250 persons. Further, the sources of water supply should be within 1.6 km. horizontal distance in plains or 100 metres elevation distance in hills. For cattle in Desert and Drought Prone (DDP) areas, an additional 30 LPCD is recommended. Against this, the norm for urban water supply is 125 LPCD piped water supply with sewerage system, 70 LPCD without sewerage system and 40 LPCD in towns with spot sources. At least one source for 20 families within a maximum distance of 100 metres has been laid down.

As against these norms, the studies as on 1.4.1997 reveal that there were 61,724 habitations without any safe source of drinking water (called not covered habitation), 3.78 lakh habitations which were partially covered and 1.51 lakh habitations which had quality problems like excess fluoride, salinity, iron and arsenic, etc. Apart from the provision in the state plans for water supply, there are major Centrally Sponsored Schemes called the Accelerated Rural Water Supply Programme and the Urban Water Supply Programme for small towns with population of less than 20,000. In order to cover this backlog in rural drinking water supply, it has been estimated that approximately Rs. 40,000 crore will be required including the funds enquired for operations and maintenance and funds to tackle quality problems. Similarly, the estimates of investment required for full coverage of urban water supply is Rs. 30,734 crore.

Drinking water and sanitation improvements could reduce the overall incidence of infant and child diarrhoea by one quarter and cut total infant and child mortality by more than one-half. Country programmes are increasingly taking measures to improve water supply and sanitation within their primary health care programmes. Guinea worm disease can be effectively prevented by providing safe drinking water and its global eradication is clearly possible within the next few years. As for schistosomiasis, some 60% reduction could be achieved by improving water supplies. Building latrines, giving health education and introducing selected drug therapy could reduce the prevalence even more.[21]

A great surge in the population of India's big cities, poses hug problems for safeguarding water supplied.

We suggest here the methods of conserving water supply:

- Integration of water and waste water management, coupled with health education for cost-effectiveness and promotion of preventive measures for health;
- Prospecting for water resources through state of the art techniques of remote sensing and geophysical surveys;
- Protection of water sources against pollution;
- Decentralization of water supply matching the required quality and quantity through waste recycle and reuse;
- Maintenance of the water distribution system, which can prevent up to 50% of the purified waste water from being lost; and
- Application of mathematical programming techniques with exact fluid flow relationships in the design of water and waste water systems so as to ensure functionality and to conserve material and financial resources.

Lack of sanitation causes many diseases-related to human excreta,

CHART 1.2

Polluted Environment Resulting in Poor Quality of Human beings

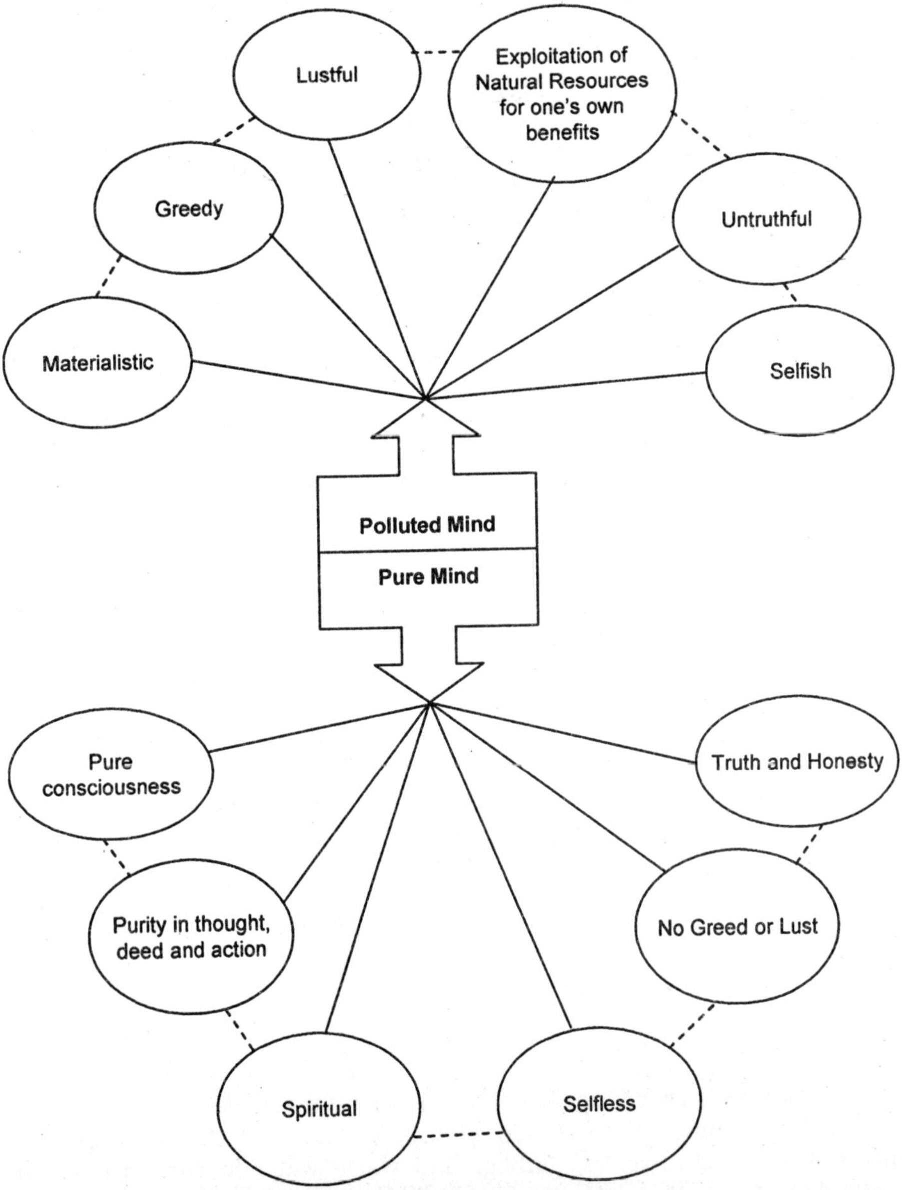

Pure Environment with Essential Necessities of Life Available to All Leading to Human Excellence

sewerage disposal. Garbage and the use of pesticides and the industrial and radio active wastes. (See Chart 1.2). Following the suspected plague outbreak in the country during 1994 the Planning Commission constituted a High Power Committee on Urban Solid Waste Management in India under the Chairmanship of Member (Health). This committee undertake a comprehensive review of current situation of urban solid waste management, specially in cities with one million or more inhabitants and made recommendations for safe methods for collection, transportation of waste and suitable cost-effective. environmentally friendly methods for disposal of these wastes. Pilot projects exploring the dimensions of the problem and aimed at seeking realistic solutions were initiated during the Eighth Plan period. During the Ninth Plan period it is expected that many more cities will initiate programmes for the efficient methods of management of wastes generated and improve environmental sanitation.

In the Johannesburg Earth Summit it has been agreed to halve, by the year 2015 the proportion of people who do not have access to basic sanitation, which would include action at all levels to develop and implement efficient household sanitation systems, improve sanitation in public institutions, especially schools, promote affordable and socially and culturally acceptable technologies and practices, promote safe hygiene practices and integrate sanitation into water resources management strategies.

Sanitation is a broad term that includes disposal of human excreta, wastewater, solid wastes, domestic and personal hygiene, etc. Human excreta is the cause of many enteric diseases such as cholera, diarrhea, dysentery, typhoid, infectious heptatitis, and those based on worm infestation, etc. Studies reveal that over 50 infections can be transmitted from diseased persons to healthy ones by various direct/indirect routes from human excreta that cause nearly 80% of sickness in developing countries.

The health implications of this state of affairs as said are appalling. Improved hygiene and sanitation help reduce sickness from diarrhea considerably. Intestinal worms infect about 10% of the population of developing countries that can be controlled through better sanitation, hygiene and water supply. As per the WHO report globally 200 million people are infected with schistosomiasis, of whom 20 million suffer seriously. Basic sanitation facilities reduce the disease by up to 77%. Sanitation facilities help check transmission of many feacal oral disease by preventing human excreta contamination of water and soil.[22]

So far, the major focus has been on communicable disease burden due to poor environmental sanitation in urban areas and due to improper disposal of human excreta, garbage and waste water in rural areas and methods to tackle these. These efforts will be intensified during the Ninth Plan. In addition, efforts to reduce pollution and related non-communicable disease burden will also be strengthened. Efforts will be made to document the extent of the problem of environmental pollution and its impact on health status of the population through linkages between existing environmental monitoring data and data on health status of population living in these areas. Prevention and management of health consequences of environmental deterioration will receive increasing attention.

The Expert Committee on Public Health System had noted that major developmental activities in any field such as agriculture, industries, urban and rural development may result in environment changes which could have adverse health implications and recommended that health impact assessment may become a part of environmental impact assessment of all large developmental projects. The feasibility of making appropriate provision for health care of people involved in developmental activities and prevention and management of health consequences of developmental activities on the population living in vicinity of the project as a part of the project budget will be explored.[23]

Brian Appleton in his article, 'Seven out of ten for Efforts" in the *World Health*, June 1988 clearly mentions that donors have agreed to collaborate globally and within individual developing countries, to ensure that water supply and sanitation programmes which receive external funding or technical assistance are based on the accepted Decade Approaches, namely:

- Complementary in developing water supply and sanitation;
- Strategies giving precedence to under-served rural and urban populations;
- Programmes promoting self-reliant, self-sustained actions;
- Community involvement in all stages of project implementation;
- Socially relevant systems that people can afford, using technologies appropriate to specific projects; and
- Association of water supply and sanitation with relevant programmes in other sectors, particularly with primary health care, concentrating on hygiene education, human resource development, and the strengthening of institutional performance.

Lori L. Heise in his article, 'Violence Against Women" in the *World Health*, Jan. 1993 clearly mentions that Seldom seen as a public health issue, violence against women is a significant cause of female morbidity and mortality around the globe. In the USA, for example, wife abuse is the leading cause of injury among women of reproductive age. Between 22% and 35% of women who visit United States emergency clinics are there for symptoms-related to on-going abuse. But women in the USA share the reality of violence with women in virtually every other culture in the world. Data from developing countries reveal that one-third to over half of women surveyed report being beaten by their partner. Not uncommonly, beatings are part of a pattern of emotional and physical abuse that escalates over time. In Papua New Guina, 18% of all urban wives surveyed had sought hospital treatment for injuries inflicted by their husbands. A survey of one Caribbean island revealed that one is three women had been sexually abused as a child.

Wife abuse also provides the primary context for many other health problems. Again, research from the USA indicates that battered women are four to five times more likely to require physchiatric treatment and five times more likely to attempt suicide than non-battered women. And they are at increased risk of alcohol abuse, drug dependence, chronic pain, and depression. In one US study of the use made of health care, a history of rape and/or assault was a stronger predictor of physician visits and outpatients costs than were a women's age or other health risks such as smoking. Along with physical injury and emotional trauma, rape survivors run the risk of becoming pregnant or contracting sexually transmitted diseases including AIDS.

Violence poses a powerful obstacle to achieving other goals that are high on the development agenda. During pregnancy, for example, it threatens the goal of "Safe motherhood" for all women. Battered women run twice the risk of miscarriage and four times the risk of having a low-birth-weight infant.

Occupational Health (see separate chapter)

WHO recently proposed a global plan of action on workers' health 2008-17. The plan envisages development of a comprehensive approach to workers' health. Workers' health is determined by numerous factors, e.g. physical, chemical and biochemical exposures within the work premises. There are other factors, such as social determinants of health (e.g. occupational status, employment conditions, income, inequalities in gender, race, age and residence). Individual behaviour (e.g. individual risk-taking behaviour, physical exercise, sedentary work, diet and nutrition and unhealthy habits such as smoking and alcohol) influence the health of workers. Besides the above mentioned factors, access to health services is also important.[24]

Climate Change and Human Health

Over the last 100 years, human activities, particularly related to burning of fossils fuels, have released sufficient quantities of carbon dioxide (CO_2) and other greenhouse gases to affect the global climate. The atmospheric concentration of CO_2 has increased by more than 30% since pre-industrial times, trapping more heat in the lower atmosphere.

As a follow-up of the 2005 Mukteshwar, India workshop, the Regional Office continued to create awareness and stress the urgent need to address climate change issues at various WHO-sponsored seminars and workshops attended by health professionals. It is recommending to:

- Assess the national health sector's response;
- Strengthen the response capacity of the health sector by preparing for medical emergency response;

- Strengthen public health systems aimed at controlling vector-borne and water-borne diseases;
- Set-up an early warning sub-system by coordinating disease surveillance and climate monitoring activities;
- Reduce the risks of vector-borne and water-borne diseases by engaging and empowering local communities to implement integrated pest and vector management and to safeguard drinking water sources; and
- Raise stakeholder engagement by advocating and creating awareness, notably at the level of local communities.

Food Safety

- The Health Department must review and revise the regulations and legislative measures governing food safety. Regulations must include all food serving facilities including street vending. They must check and prevent adulteration and contamination of foods at various stages of production, processing, storage, transport and distribution.
- The Health Department should develop guidelines for the health check-up and immunization of food handlers against typhoid fever and hepatitis A.
- Control measures recommended include, training and certification of food handlers in restaurants, hostels, hotels, etc.
- Personal hygiene, adequate cooking of food-this needs to be part of the health promotion package for children, women and public in general.[25]

Chemical Safety

The headlong expansion of science and technology is constantly providing human society and the environment with more and more new substances. Different molecules are being created, tested, discarded or commercialized according to their usefulness or economic advantage. But little or no attention is being paid to the consequent risks for human or environmental health.

It is neither practical not economically feasible to evaluate the short and long-term effects of the vast number of chemicals which are being invented and re-invented! The objectives of this dynamic creativity are usually beneficial: to protect crops, to increase food stocks, to simplify household chores, to protect our health and hygiene. But . . . are all those new chemicals really indispensable? Does mankind really need to be swamped by so many new chemical compounds?

What used to be "chemical development"—the production of highly useful pharmaceuticals, anilines, antiseptics and pesticides—turned into a "chemical revolution", and "is now", on the way to becoming "chemical chaos." Too many substances and compounds are entering our homes, our working place, our environment and our bodies without our really knowing their risks and benefits, without a true evaluation of their usefulness and—worse still—without complete studies of their harmlessness for other forms of life.

Examples of the poisonings and chemical disasters that have resulted are legion. It took many years to realize that industrial and domestic use of flurochlorocarbon propellants in aerosols were contributing to the depletion of the ozone layer, with all its environmental consequences, Prolonged use of asbestos fibers have caused malignant measotheliomas (tumours) in exposed workers, Clinical studies of patients who took high doses of analgesics shows that certain renal insufficiencies were due to those apparently innocuous pharmaceuticals, All too late did medicine link. The drug thalidomide was responsible for the birth of children with deformed arms and legs. And the indiscriminate use of pesticides is still causing a high toll of Morbidity and mortality in some rural areas of developing countries. Long-term "hidden" tragedies such as Mina-mata disease in Japan or explosive chemical disasters such as Bhopal in India are other examples where a large human group falls victim to uncontrolled chemicals.

In the intervening night of 2nd/3rd Dec. 1984, a lethal gas known as Methyl iso-Cyanate (MIC) stored in the tank of the Union Carbibe pesticide factory at Bhopal escaped suddenly into the atmosphere causing death and injury to a large number of people of the Bhopal City. The leakage of gas occurred between 12.45 a.m. to 1.30 p.m. By 6.30 a.m. the entire area was clear. But by then, massive damage and suffering had been inflicted. More than 800 persons died during the first three days of the incident. Subsequently, the casualty figure rose to more than 7000.

GUIDING PRINCIPLES FOR AVOIDING CHEMICALS POLLUTION

The guiding principles of responsible care are:

- To recognize and respond to community concerns about chemicals and the operations.
- To develop and produce chemicals that can be manufactures, transported, used and disposed of safely.
- To make health, safety and environmental consideration a priority in planning for all existing and new products and processes.
- To report promptly to officials, employees, customers and the public information on chemical-related health or environmental hazards and recommend protective measures.
- To counsel customers on the safe use, transportation and disposal of chemical products.
- To operate the plants and facilities in a manner that protects the environment health and safety of employees and public.

- To extend knowledge by conducting or supporting research of the health, safety environmental effects of the products, processes and waste materials.
- To work with others to rèsolve problems created by past handling and disposal of hazardous substances.
- To participate with government and other in creating responsible laws, regulations and standards to safeguard community, work place and environment.
- To promote the principles and practices of responsible care by sharing experience and offering assistance to others who produce, handly use, transport or dispose-off chemicals.

Among the measures to prevent acute and chronic poisoning and environment damage by pesticides that should urgently be taken by developing countries are:

- Good agricultural practice and integrated pest control;
- Manpower development in chemical safety—including training in clinical, occupational, analytical, experimental, predictive and regulatory toxicology;
- Risk assessment toxicological surveillance programmes;
- Reliable statistics system on mortality and morbidity data-related to pesticide poisoning;
- Monitoring analyses of pesticide residues in staple food, in the environment, and in human biological samples;
- Restricted use of highly toxic and persistent pesticides;
- Multi-level courses on safe use of pesticides;
- Certified operators, periodically, trained, and responsible for the acquisition and safe use of pesticides;
- Enforcement of the legislation;
- Intensive effort to reduce illiteracy among rural workers; and
- Establishment of an Interdisciplinary National Committee on Pesticides, acting as an advisory body to the Ministries of Health, Agriculture, Labour and Environment.[26]

Hospital Waste Management

Prof. K.J. Nath in his article Hospital wastes have always been considered as potentially hazardous. The major identified hazard was that of infection, because over millennia, communicable diseases had been the most common use of morbidity and mortality in the community and majority of persons receiving treatment in the hospitals were suffering from communicable diseases. Until the second half of the present century, there was due emphasis on safe collection, storage and disposal at site to minimize, if not eliminate, the health hazard associated with hospital waste. The advent of antibiotics led to complacency regarding infection control and safe disposal of hospital waste. This has resulted in increased risk of infection in health care setting both to the seekers and providers of health care. The rising prevalence of HBV and HIV infection in the community and among health care providers has led to an increasing awareness about the risks associated with this lackadaisical practice and the need to evolve and implement strategies for safe and sustainable methods of disposal of waste material generated at different sites in health care delivery system.

It is estimated that inpatients in India generate between 0.5 to 1 Kg of solid waste per person/day. Over 75% of hospital waste is non-hazardous. There is no well established system of segregating hazardous from non-hazardous waste in majority of the hospitals. This mixing of the various components results in increased quantity of hazardous wastes that require safe disposal. Very often the hospital wastes are dumped alongwith the municipal wastes. Sometimes the hospitals are provided with incinerators, but very often these are inappropriate in design, improperly operated or remain out of order.

CRITICAL ASSESSMENT AND SUGGESTIONS TO IMPROVE THE PROGRAMMES

The situation pertaining to environmental sanitation is horrifying at the global, regional and national levels. It has been admitted by various agencies responsible for it at all levels. Attainment of the global target of the UN Second Development Decade had not been feasible in most countries of the region. The Regional Director of the WHO in his Annual Report has warned the member-states:

> "In spite of the continuing efforts of governments and international and bilateral agencies, only the fringe of the problem has been tackled. . . there is an urgent need to mobilize further support from all available sources to solve this difficult problem. Investment in this field will be amply rewarded not only in terms of reduction in the incidence of communicable diseases, but also by substantially contributing towards an improvement in the standard of living."[27]

Dr. Abel Wolman, one of the "father-figures" of environmental health and Professor Emeritus of Sanitary Engineering at the Johns Hopkins School of Engineering, Baltimore, USA says while talking of the world health situation: "It always leads great conferences to pass resolutions to do something about providing water to impoverished people. Resolutions become opiates because they are gratifying substitutes for action."[28] He warns the policy-makers and administrators against complacence and says, "Viewed on a global basis, we have little to be sanguine about. The disease-consequences of poor and insufficient water, of living with human excreta, and of unhygienic personal habits, are disastrous—they have been familiar for so long a time that they no longer excite even the statistician or epidemiologist. People accept their devastation, as they so often abjectly bear their real and spiritual poverty. We speak of the toll of deaths, due to environmental deficiencies in a casual way, even though the figures mount to hundreds of millions. The communicable diseases, often the sequels of poor sanitation are maiming and killing men, women and children—not computer data."[29] It is beyond doubt that a lasting solution to many of the existing and future problems of public health require control on environment. The question arises as how to provide sanitary facilities to hundreds of millions of people still without even minimum sanitary facilities? How to tackle such programme? How to find the resources required for these programmes? What should be the administrative set-up to ensure speedy implementation? What are the responsibilities of planners and policy-makers to ensure integrated approach We shall discuss the facts and suggestions to provide good environment for the healthy growth of the people.

(1) Cooperation and Coordination among Allied Programmes

There is a close relationship between the environmental programmes and other programmes. In practice, this relationship is ignored by the planners and administrators of these programmes, e.g., a dam has to be constructed for irrigation and power purposes; its consequences on human health or soil salinity are ignored or underestimated. To remedy such unfortunate situations it is suggested that an 'integrated' approach may be adopted. It presumes an unprecedented, ungrudging cooperation between different services, as well as between various brands of natural scientists on the one hand and of social and human scientists on the other. We have to encourage such integrated approach to have full impact rather than piecemeal goals and approaches. It was mentioned in a WHO document that, "more effective administration requires that planners and managers take account of the full range of implications of their own programme goals and further, that they actively seek to participate as consultants and collaborators in the planning and execution of other community programmes that demonstratively or potentially interact with environmental health."[30]

UNESCO's MAB Programme (Man and the Biosphere Programme) coordinates various disciplines by mobilising applied research efforts all over the world on major man environment resources interactions. It relies on international cooperation among governments and the participation of all specialists. A major UNESCO research programme is closely studying the effects of human interventions in the environment and man himself in all the major socio-economic systems. We can get benefit out of such programmes.[31]

(2) Improve Administrative Capability and Competence

Environmental health programmes are administered by technically qualified people but such people lack administrative capability and capacity, i.e., the ability to achieve results. We have doctors, engineers, town planners, inspectors, nutritionists, geologists who are responsible for improving the environment. Every programme has its administrative component which is the heart and soul of that programme. It is suggested that the persons engaged on these programmes may be given suitable training in administration to enhance their competence.

(3) Deploy more Resources

The Environmental Health Improvement programmes require considerable financial investment. The World Bank and WHO reported to the Mar Del Plata Conference that $ 140,000 million would be needed to reach the target of clean water for all by 1990. Today, we need double this amount to cater to increased population. Where will it come from? External aid is limited. So, there is a need to exploit the resources available within each country. It is only a question of proper allocation of resources. Voluntary effort can be encouraged to accelerate the pace of development. With exploitation of local self-help, money can be generated. It is also a question of political will. This programme must be made an integral part of the community development programme. It should take the form of self-aided programme. The funds allocated should be used to achieve the aim of the policy and care should be taken that the funds are not diverted for other purposes. It was mentioned by Dr. B.H. Dieterich, Director, Division of Environmental Health, WHO that "Development planners confronted with meagre budgets are often forced to keep some projects in abeyance and give priority to others that may bring immediate economic benefit. It is now being increasingly realised that it is not a practicable or economically sound idea to defer environmental health projects. Planners are beginning to look at environmental health projects in the context of the ultimate socio-economic objectives of the development process."[32]

(4) Research to Meet the Requirements of Different Geographical Areas

There are many potential health hazards. We know much about some of these hazards and little about many of them. We must encourage research in the experimental laboratory and epidemiology to pin-point the areas of ignorance. Secondly, national institutes should carry out research to develop models for adapting measures to reduce costs. They may also find simple disinfection devices suited to rural needs. We may not adopt costly western models to supply safe water and sewerage disposal, e.g., the British Development Agency, Oxford has made a latrine which turns the human excreta into organic manure producing some 6,000,000 tons a year. In the Republic of Korea, human excreta is being exploited to produce methane gas. There is need to change the attitudes of experts so that they can design the machinery and equipment suitable and feasible in our country.

(5) Local Participation

Public Health administration is manned by and meant for human beings. It is therefore necessary to associate the people with the programmes of water supply and rural sanitary latrines. Sociologists, behavioural scientists and public relation experts should be associated with programmes to make the local involvement more effective.

Social mobilisation, People's participation and health and sanitation education are essential inputs into water supply and sanitation programmes. These help to make sure that the proposed activities fit into the targeted population's habits and socio-cultural environment where they do not suggest changes, it intends to ensure that the proposed water supply and sanitation technologies and activities are appropriate to men, women and children.

(6) Strong Political Will and Determination

It has been mentioned that the programmes of environmental health are deferred because of the lack of resources or the apathy on the part of the politicians. This assumption is totally wrong and baseless. "The major cause for delinquent action lies in the motivation of governments. Do they really mean what their resolutions say—militantly enough to go into action? Is only lip service the main response of Presidents, Prime Ministers, kings and ministers? The task for the future is difficult but possible. People should not be consigned to premature death simply because we are less than courageous and diligent. The pace must be accelerated."[33]

(7) Effective Maintenance

It is not only important to build the infrastructure for the environmental sanitation programmes but also to see that these projects function efficiently and regularly. We must ensure their competent construction, efficient and fool-proof operation and maintenance of completed supplies and effective surveillance on quality of drinking water. The maintenance is very poor in the developing countries. Even in the planned cities like Chandigarh, the headquarters of three governments—we are shocked to find germs, mosquitoes and flies coming in the tap water. Besides, the dirt is scattered in the whole of the city. Thus, there is a need to maintain the services once provided to the people through efficient and economical administration, involving the people.

(8) Guidance and Assistance from Bilateral and Multilateral Agencies

The capacity of the developing countries to solve the problem pertaining to environmental sanitation programmes are limited. International and bilateral agencies should be encouraged to increase their direct technical assistance to member-countries in the following ways:

(a) In making assessment studies;
(b) In the establishment of information systems and programme formulation, implementation and evaluation;

(c) In identifying and helping to meet specific needs for multilateral or bilateral assistance by way of expertise, equipment, materials and soft loans;
(d) In setting up research and training centers and collaborating laboratories;
(e) In assisting training programmes, including programmes for the production of manuals and training guides;
(f) In establishing health criteria and codes of practice; and
(g) In the local production of materials.

In addition to providing assistance itself, WHO should act in a coordinating capacity in respect of assistance received from these and other sources.[34]

(9) Civic Consciousness

Environmental sanitation cannot be achieved by the effort of the Government alone. It requires the active support and cooperation of the people. It was indicated to the writer by the authorities responsible for water supply that 25 per cent of the resources are being wasted because the people do not care to use the services only when in need. Most of the public and private taps remain working without any utility. Besides, the people lack civic consciousness and they do not cooperate in the maintenance of hygienic conditions. One is shocked to see the beautiful city of Chandigarh with heaps of debris all around. The difficult task of improving environmental sanitation is possible only if the people develop civic consciousness.

(10) Environmental Education

Dr. T. Sundaran in his Article from literacy to health in *Kurukshetra* (Oct. 1992). suggests Health Education and personal hygiene are necessary components of all such plans. Such education inputs may relate to:

(a) washing hands before collecting and carrying water, and pouring out water from a storage container without touching it or using a clean long handled dipper to take the water out;
(b) making sure that the water container, the cups and mugs used for drawing water are clean and that the water is kept covered at all times; and
(c) washing hands after defecation, before preparing and eating food, cutting of nails and other such basic measures;

Special care to ensure implementation of these measures in hotels and other public eating places is more difficult but essential to really checking diseases like typhoid.

The Stockholm Conference held in 1972 drew the urgency of tackling environmental problems through various efforts. One recommendation of this conference called for development of 'environmental education' as one of the most important steps to attack world's environmental crisis. The conference pleaded that "new environmental education must be broad-based and strongly related to the basic principles outlined in the United Nations Declaration on the New International Economic Order."

Environmental education has been defined as an educational process dealing with men's relationship with his natural and man-made surroundings, and encompass the relation of population, health, pollution, technology, urban and rural planning, housing, proper nutrition to the total human environment. The scope of environmental education is vast, touching every aspect of man and environment. The purpose of environmental education is to provide knowledge to the people so that they can adjust with the environment and enjoy decent environment. The goals of environmental education as discussed in the Inter-Governmental Conference on Environmental Education, organised by the UNESCO in cooperation with UNEP, at Tbilisi (USSR), from October 14-26, 1977, are mentioned below:

(a) To foster clear awareness of and concern about economic, social, political and ecological interdependence in urban and rural areas;
(b) To provide every person with opportunity to acquire the knowledge, value, attitudes, commitment and skills needed to protect and improve the environment; and
(c) To create new patterns of individuals, groups and society as a whole towards the environment.

The Secretary-General of the UN in his report on Population, Resources and Environment sums up the benefits of environmental improvement programmes. He mentions four social and economic benefits that would result from government action for environmental betterment in the poor countries besides the improvements in the people's health from control of infectious diseases—

(a) Employment of large number of poor people in public works projects;
(b) Reduction of food requirements and costs by lessening the mal-absorption caused by intestinal parasites. This might ultimately save $ 2,000 million per annum in India alone. This annual saving would be equal to the entire capital cost of needed water supply improvements in the whole of rural India;
(c) Increases in potential economic productivity through improved health of adults; and
(d) Greater receptivity of children at the early ages by improvements in health."[35]

(11) Appropriate Technology

A.S. Bal, A.N. Khan and P.R. Sarode in their Article, "Technological Options for Rural Sanitation" in *Kurukshetra* (October 1992), rightly suggest that high incidence of excreta-related diseases in the developing countries warrants that the sanitation programmes be designed with the primary objective of bringing about improvement in public health. This objective can be achieved through alternate sanitation technologies which are simpler and cheaper as also socially acceptable. An inter-disciplinary sanitation programme could prove to be more successful not only from the sanitation point of view but also from the point of view of problems faced by the local bodies by way of poor financial returns from provision of sewerage facilities in the low income areas. Selection of appropriate sanitation technology for a given community and its proper operation and maintenance after installation is ensured only when socio-cultural aspects are considered along with economic, financial, ecological and technical features in the planning process. The task of providing water and sanitation to the unserved population is so immense that it would be almost impossible to accomplish it without the development and application of low-cost technologies. Low-cost technologies are generally applied at the peripheral level, where construction, operation, maintenance and surveillance may vary greatly from one location to another, affected by the level of community motivation and participation.

Non-sewerage onsite sanitation facilities may be all that are needed when water supplies are limited, but if improvements result in greater water usage then eventually the need will escalate for sewers and offside disposal. In this case it can create a need for concentrated population to be controlled by treatment.

(12) Holistic Approach

Ninnta Deshpande, an eminent Gandhian has stressed the need to adopt holistic approach to sanitation, it is necessary to approach the problem in a holistic manner by linking sanitation with religion, culture, health, agriculture, environment and production of energy. The basic attitude that needs to be formed is to link it with Bhakti. It has to be stressed that cleanliness is godliness and unless cleanliness becomes a part of our lives, we cannot be true devotees of God. Construction of toilets, their proper use, maintenance and clean habits should form part of the psyche. The wrong notion that night soil is not to be touched has to go. Cleaning should become a part of daily practice. The linkage of cleanliness with health is also very important. It has to be impressed upon the minds of the people that this programme is essential for keeping good health and protecting the family and village from various diseases. With charts, slides, films, songs, cultural shows, this knowledge can be imparted. Imaginative and innovative methods have to be adopted to make people aware of health.

CONCLUSION

Dr. Zbigniew Bankowski,[36] spells out the code of ethics to protect the environment. It would be unrealistic, however, to suppose that the damage that has been done, and still continues to be done, can be arrested and undone in the short-term. Rather, long-term global policies must be envisaged and, if they are to be successful, they will require changes in our perceptions of man in nature. If our global physical environment is not to be further degraded, we must change our conceptual environment, our ways of thinking and behaving. Perhaps the worst environmental pollution is pollution of the mind, and the greatest need is for well thought out principles of environmental ethics.

All spheres of human conduct private and public, are subject to ethical principles or rules. When governments or other corporate bodies despoil the environment in the name of development or political dominance or national security, when government adopt *liaissez faire* policies that permit the exploitation of nature for narrow, short-term gains, they contravene the basic ethical principle of the greatest good for the greatest number of people.

Sh. M. Akhtar, Chief WESS/ICO UNICEF, New Delhi in his Article, "Strategies for rural sanitation (UNICEF Experience)" suggested the following based upon UNICEF experience to ensure fruitful application of strategies for safer water supply and sanitation. (*Kurukshetra*, October 1992).

1. If sanitation has to be a 'way of life' it should be treated as a package of facilities/services and not identified with latrines. All the low-cost sanitary facilities, both at domestic and community level, such as latrine, soak pit, garbage pit, smokeless chulha, bathing cubicle, drainage improvement, ground water sources and other community-based facilities should form a part of the package. A distinction may have to be made among 7 components of sanitation. These are: (i) Handling of drinking water; (ii) Disposal of waste water, (iii) Disposal of human excreta; (iv) Garbage disposal; (v) Home sanitation and food hygiene; (vi) Personal hygiene; and (vii) Sanitation in the community. This should be supported by a strong IEC back up to create awareness with regard to various sanitary practices including personal hygiene. It is necessary to modify the guidelines both at the Government of India and State Government levels to reflect the package deal and how to achieve the same.
2. In order that sanitation becomes a "peoples' movement", it is essential that their active involvement and participation receive due importance. In this regard subsidy can play only a limited role. Alternate financing mechanisms have to be developed to facilitate greater adaptability.

3. The low-cost sanitary facilities should have different technological options to suit different geohydrological conditions and also the varying socio-economic segments of the population. Such technologies should be affordable, acceptable and replicable. Identification and use of alternate materials should be a continuous process so as to keep the cost escalation under check.
4. Demand generation for sanitary facilities should get a high priority in Rural Sanitation Programme. For this purpose, a comprehensive and systematic communication strategy has to be developed and all possible methods and channels should be used to motivate people. In this regard inter-personal communication through village level motivators seems to be quite promising. Willing village level functionaries like Anganwadi workers, DWCRA group organisers. Traditional Birth Attendants, primary school teachers, Youth Club/Mahila Mandal office-bearers, etc. could be the core group of motivators. The panchayat members can also play an active role in this regard.
5. The demand generation strategy should be backed up by an efficient delivery system which need not be a part of the subsidy-oriented programme. At present, even if a person wants to have his/her own latrine in rural areas, it is not easy to find the required pan/trap/pit cover, etc. as adequate infrastructure has not developed as yet. Only in an area where government programme is under implementation, things are more readily available. It is, therefore, necessary to create alternate delivery channels/mechanism to have improved sanitation coverage.
6. Private initiative is a must to make the sanitation programme a success. The government-supported activity could at least be a stimulant. The results of the 44th Round on Sanitation Coverage is a pointer to this assumption. While figures from the government sources show a 3 percent coverage, the NSS survey reveals that more than one-tenth of the households were using latrines. The difference could be accounted for by the spread effect of the government programme. It is high time that a clear cut policy on how to encourage private initiative outside the subsidy-oriented approach is laid down. The policy should keep a flexible approach and suggest alternate social marketing strategies to promote sanitation through private initiative. Involvement of industrial houses/public sector units including the manufacturers of sanitary goods could form a part of it.
7. NGOs can play a very crucial role in promoting rural sanitation. They can very effectively be used to encourage private initiative because of their rapport with the community and can serve as an efficient channel for information dissemination, awareness

creation and motivation. Only those NGOs who have the required capacity to take up activities at a district level or at least for a group of blocks should be encouraged. The Government should come out with separate guidelines for involving NGO's in the Rural Sanitation Programme. The State Government should be well aware of such guidelines.

Dr. Martin Kaplan[37] has desired to look positively and is hopeful of solutions by mankind. He stated, "hazards to human health arising from environment factors are many and varied. We know much about some and little about many of them. We must therefore depend on future research both by the experimental laboratory and by epidemiology to clarify many of our areas of ignorance. The development of surveillance and monitoring mechanisms for changes in health status correlated with environmental components should provide the warnings necessary to avoid serious harm to present and future generations of the human race.

In reviewing all these environmental effects and their possible Dangers, we should not however reach too gloomy a conclusion. A comforting finding, which may be extended to many other aspects, is the recent discovery that fish caught in the last century and preserved in museums have been found to have similar mercury levels as those found in fish today. And after all, the human race with its great adaptability has survived the innumerable disasters and environmental hazards it has encountered for several million years. Modern life and times represent for man merely a new set of problems replacing old ones, and there is no reason to doubt that man's ingenuity and intelligence will prevail as far as environment problems are concerned."

Notes and References

1. T.N. Chaturvedi, Editorial, in *IJPA*, July-Sept., 1989.
2. Hiroshi Nakajima, "A Wounded Planet", in *World Health*, January- February, 1990, p. 3.
3. Dr Wilfried Kreisel, "Environmental Health in the 1990", in *World Health*, January-February 1990, p. 5.
4. WHO: SEARO, Declaration on Health Development in the South-East Asia Region in the 21st Century, New Delhi, 1997, pp. 17-18.
5. WHO, *World Health*, May, 1972, p. 28.
6. U. Thant quoted in Clellan, M.C. and S. Grant (ed.), Protecting our Environments (New York, 1970), p. 206.
7. WHO. *World Health*, May, 1972, p. 29.
8. Edwards S. Roggers, Human Ecology and Health Environment, Administrator, New York, 1960.
9. WHO Samuel Halter; "Man and his Environment," in *World Health*, July 1975, p. 18.
10. GOI, Planning Commission, Draft Five Year Plan (1978-83), p. 117.
11. WHO, *World Health Paper*, S-9, p. 12.

12. Karnataka towards Equity, Quality, and Integrity in Health, Final Report, Government of Karnataka, April, 2001, p. 52.
13. *Ibid.*, p. 56.
14. Nikolas P. Napulbow, Water For All: A human right, in *World Health*, July-Aug., 1992, p. 3.
15. Karnatka towards Equity, Quality, and Integrity in Health, Final Report, Government of Karnataka, April 2001, p. 52.
16. Barbara Ward, "The Key to Health" in *World Health*, January 1977, p. 3.
17. UNICEF, Assignment Children, 34, April-June 1976, p. II.
18. A Newsletter of Building Materials and Technology, Promotion Council, India, p. 13
19. WHO, *World Health*, January, 1979, p. 3.
20. UN, 1970, Report on the World Social Situation, New York, 1971, pp. 167-68.
21. *World Health*, July-August 1992, p. 7.
22. A Newsletter of Building Materials and Technology, Promotion Council, India, p. 22.
23. Purshotam Khanna and Bindo Koshy, "When City Growth Exceeds Supply" in *World Health*, July-August, 1992, p. II.
24. The Work of WHO in the South East Asia Region, Report of the Regional Director, 1 July 2006, WHO, pp. 47-48.
25. *Ibid.*, pp. 48-49.
26. Waldemar F. Ahmedia, The Dangers and the Precaution in *World Health*, Aug.-Sept. 1984, p. 12.
27. WHO, SEARO: Annual Report of the Regional Director, 1976-77, pp. xii-xiii.
28. WHO, *World Health*, January 1977, p. 17.
29. *Ibid.*
30. WHO, *Public Health Papers*, 59, p. 116.
31. Batisse Michel, "Man and Biosphere" in *World Health*, June 1978, p. 4.
32. WHO, *World Health*, May 1972, p. 29.
33. WHO, *World Health*, January 1977, p. 17.
34. WHO, SEA/RC27/p. 41.
35. UN, ST/ESAJSERA/S-7, New York, 1975, p. 101.
36. Zbigniew Bankowski, "A Code of Ethics" in *World Health*, January-February, 1990, p. 18.
37. Dr. Martin Kaplan, "Environmental Hazards for Human Health" in *World Health*, May 1972, p. II.

2

CHAPTER

Health Education

For thousands of years, disease and death have been accepted with resignation as normal ingredients of daily life-aspects of a tragic destiny, which strikes some and spares others without rhyme or reason. Today this resignation is unacceptable. We are aware that the dangers that threaten our health are often caused by imperfections in our social structures or in our own behaviour. We can afford to scoff at some of these threats, now that a correct application of new discoveries in medicine enables us to reduce them to reasonable proportions.

The task of education is to apprise people of their responsibilities, since diseases and accidents are so often linked with ignorance, carelessness, and inadequate precautions on the part of national authorities.

—*Etienne Berthet*

AIMS OF HEALTH EDUCATION

The most important aim of Health Education is to alter behaviour, which may have directly or indirectly influenced occurrence of spread of diseases in a given cultural setting. A culturally relevant health education programme can be planned only after understanding the behaviour in all its manifestations. One of the best definitions of Health Education was offered by Wood in 1926: "Health Education is the sum of experiences which favourably influences habits, attitudes and knowledge relating to individual, community, and racial health."[1]

Different authorities have differently viewed the aims of health education. According to one source:[2] "The aim of health education is to help people achieve health by their own actions and efforts. Health education begins therefore with the interest of people in improving their condition of living, and aims at developing a sense of responsibility for their own health betterment as individuals and as members of families, communities or government."[3]

Another source[4] highlights that, "Health education aims at promoting the greater possible fulfilment of inherited powers of the body and the mind and. the happy adjustment of individual to society. It is the educational approach to health problem and as such is concerned with practical measures for the promotion of health and the control and treatment of diseases.

Studies made in different countries of the world have shown that fluctuations in the toll of disease and death depend even more on the level of education than on the social and economic conditions in which people live. Ignorance can be just as much a killer as poverty, and these two often go hand in hand.[5]

An excellent examples of the success of health education can be cited from Egypt. Esmut Mansour in his article, "Egypt Tackles Polio", rightly suggests the role of health education in polio eradication. To quote: In fact, women in Egypt represent a considerable proportion of all private and public physicians and health service administrators. As in may other countries, the nursing staff are predominantly women and are therefore engaged in the front-line battle to eradicate polio. The nurse's role here is much broader than the one she plays during clinic hours, and her value to her community and its welfare should not be underestimated. Not only does she routinely give the polio vaccine, but she is the primary mechanism for dispensing health care information to each child's careers, thus increasing their awareness about the dangers of disease, the importance of vaccination, and any possible side-effects of the vaccine. Therefore, she acts as the first defence line against the disease, and her understanding of the early effects of polio and her ability to recognize the disease is essential.

Egyptian society is particularly blessed by a culture and history that produces strong family ties. So ultimately the success of our programme to eradicate polio must also credit the mothers who have listened to the information provided at the official level of health care and who have been convinced that the health of their children is worth all the expense and effort they make.

Egypt's Expanded Programme on Immunization is one of the most effective in the world. Reaching our goal of eradicating polio will be a worthy tribute to the hard work contributed by all of us-women and men together-to protect our children."[6]

MEANING OF HEALTH EDUCATION

"A term composed of two concepts, the first one denoting the content (health), and the second is the process (education)."[7]

James McCormick, defines health education: "The purpose of health education is not, as it is often seen to be the transmission of knowledge, but altered behaviour."[8]

CHART 2.1

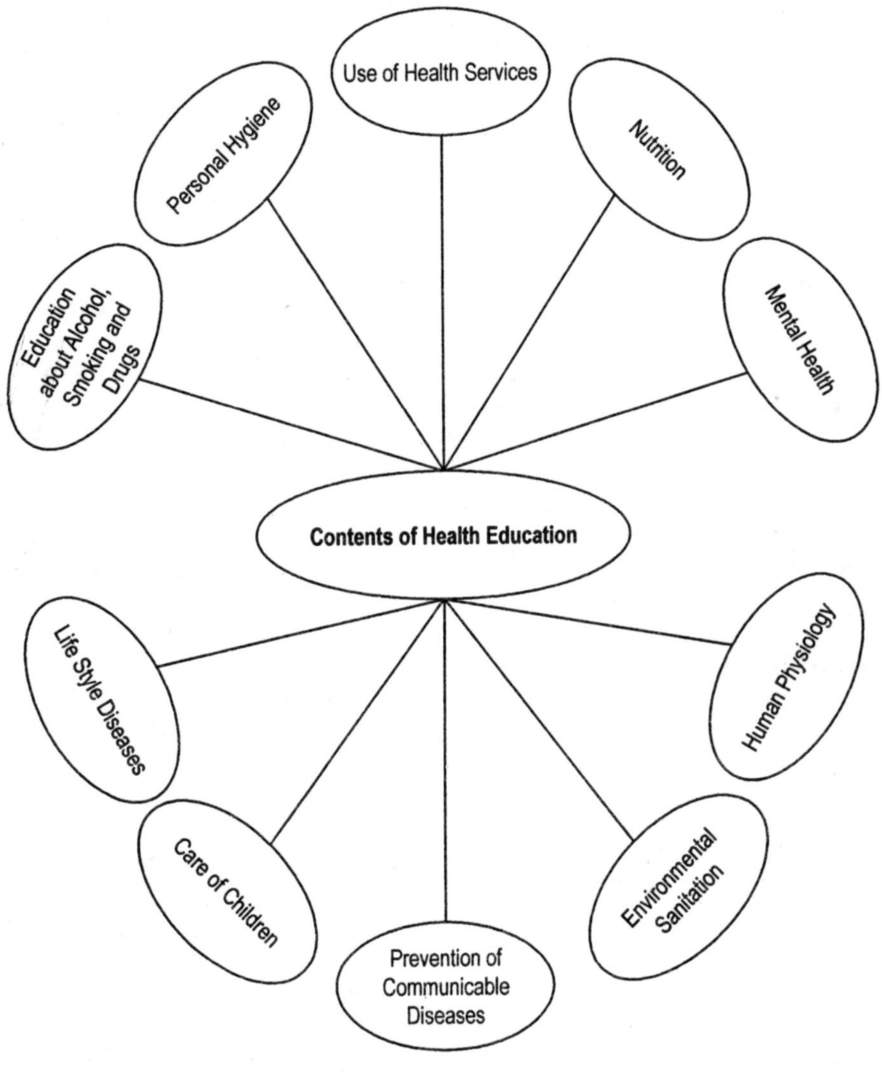

The Health Education Steering Committee of Association of School of Public Health (1966) defines health education as: "A process, which effects changes in the health practices of people and on the knowledge and attitudes related to such changes."[9] Sanjay Salooja in an article knowledge to action suggests the following top 7 "E"s to Motivate and Influence an Audience. Speak with "E"s. Be a speaker of influence—not control or guild. With the privilege of the platform comes the awesome responsibility of educationing, motivating and influencing your audience to feel/think/act differently.

1. Educate—provide your audience with extensive information on your topic. This will empower audience to feel competent and knowledgeable. Support your points with stories. Adults delineate their thoughts visually.
2. Entertain—give them the facts laced with a good dose of humour. Adults learn better when they are lightening up! Here's the place for some magic tricks, handwriting analysis or a song.
3. Experience—get the audience involved. When they interact, they "get it" better and retain it longer through. Group exercise, simple questions and answers, role plays.
4. Enthusiasm—vary your tone of voice, smile often, show passion for your subject matter. Make your body language reflect your comments.
5. Example—be the speaker/person who motivates the audience to admire and respect you. You have succeeded when people say "I want to be like him/her."
6. Encourage—be supportive to your audience—believe in them. Say "I did it . . . and so can you."
7. Excellence—hold yourself accountable for excellence. And then help your audience to be accountable and live up to its potential. Speakers need to give audience what they need, not what they want.

Hiroshi Nakajima in his article editorial, "The State of the World's Health" in *World Health*, March-April, 1995, stresses the need of the health education to control lifestyle and other diseases. To quote:

> Our future depends to a large extent on being adequately informed. The World Health Report, 1995 is a response of this more and more acutely felt need. Reliable health information is demanded not only by health professionals, politicians and business people who need it to meet the various responsibilities of their jobs, but by individuals and families in every walk of life. Their questions extend from universal concerns about what is happening in the world to very particular ones such as how to avoid diabetes, or how to look after a sick child, or how to ensure the safety of a blood transfusion. As the world's health authority, WHO is uniquely well placed to gather and publicize whatever information is available on such questions.[10]

Top 7 Insights to Effective Health Education

1. The most important objective of any Health worker is credibility and being knowledgeable about health education, i.e. speak to your audience as if you were having a conversation to have an impact.

2. Divert the audience's attention in the first few minutes with a question, starting comment, inspiring story, or funny experience about health education. This will help you connect immediately with everyone and reduce the tension. Stay away from jokes!
3. Feel confident and have faith as faith be gets faith.
4. Shift your focus from one to the other so that all persons remain attentive.
5. Use visual aids to increase audience retention of message. But NEVER become a master of ceremonies to overheads. Use case studies about health education.
6. Personal benefits from acquiring excellent speaking skills and knowledge of health education include: more self-confidence, becoming more persuasive and evolving into a magnetic or dynamic speaker.
7. Keep the people involved in the process of lecture—"Health education is not the same thing as health information. Correct information is certainly a basic part of health education; but health education must also address the other factors that effect health behaviour such as availability of resources, effectiveness of community leadership, social support from family members and levels of self-help skills. Health education, therefore, uses a variety of methods to help people understand their own situations and choose actions that will improve their health. Health education is incomplete unless it encourages involvement and choice by the people themselves. Merely telling people to follow good health behaviour is not health education."[11]

Baric, while describing relationship between behavioural sciences and health education maintains that health education can be defined in many ways based on the interest of the definers. He feels that whatever number of definitions one could find in the past are too general or cover all activities relating to health in to broadest sense of physical, mental and social well-being or have been operation definitions based on-the-job of health educators.[12]

The concept of health education defined by Wood in 1925 is one of the best-known and still applicable one. It withstood many pedagogical changes; and it also appears sounder today than when it was written. He defines health education—"represents the sum of experiences which favourably influence habits, attitudes; and knowledge relating to individual, community, and racial health."[13]

Unfortunately, the experts and development planners have failed to improve the lives of the people as they do not understand properly the science to communicate effectively with each other or with the people they are trying to help. Most of the people in authority today, who are guiding the people in this field, have not realized the urgency of such education and the benefit it can generate; consequently governments have not taken any substantial steps in this direction.

Health education does not mean merely removal of ignorance. On the contrary, it involves three important things:

(i) It provides a person with appropriate knowledge to enjoy decent health and also the knowledge about the occurrence and spread of disease thus enabling him to adopt relevant preventive measures;
(ii) It creates in him an interest for the health of other members of his family as well as of those living in his surrounding; and
(iii) It creates in him a desire to support health education programmes in his area.

Besides, Health Education should make the people understand the benefits that they can derive from modern medicine. K.S. Sanjive, Professor of Medicine has said:

> "It will not be an exaggeration to say that the paramount step in the effort to take modern medicine to every corner of the country and every citizen is health education. Health education in its widest sense of getting every one to understand what modern medicine can do to diminish disease and death and to be properly motivated to utilize this knowledge in their daily lives, requires the simple quality of sincerity more than highly specialized techniques."[14]

Neglect of health education is one of the main reasons why scientific medicine is not taking root in the country and people are steeped in ignorance and superstition.

ESSENTIALS OF HEALTH EDUCATION

Health education would be possible only if the health educator and the receiver are in constant dialogue with each other. It is not wholly correct that the purpose of health education is to manipulate the receiver. What might be more appropriate is a circular diagram in which the parties to the "Communication Contract". as it is sometimes called, function dually as senders and receivers.

This model would avoid the possibilities of misinterpretation. We know that even well planned campaigns can end in failures if there is no proper monitoring or feedback to make sure that the wrong effect is not being created by the communicator, however innocently.

In a democratic society, the dynamic power, which impels governments to action, is the voice and enlightenment of the people. People can only pressurize their executive or legislative machinery to undertake suitable health measures when they themselves are aware of the means of warding off disease and promotion of positive health. This knowledge (Health Education) is therefore a pre-condition and prerequisite to creating the demand for health and setting the pace of implementation of environmental sanitation and the total health policy.[15]

According to the World Health Organisation Expert Committee, health education serves three main general purposes.[16]

I. To make Health a Valued Community Asset

The value assigned to health by a particular organisation, the level of general education, the concern of the community for its members, the number and ability of its health workers, and financial resources of the people. High educational level of the community is important to enhance the value of health in a given culture. It also encourages people to join hands to find out many ways to solve public health problem. . . faced by them. It is recognized that the needs for education in health matters is intimately linked with other social, cultural, educational and economic problems, which have direct or indirect influence on determining health status of the people. A number of rural studies, mostly in developing countries resort that the first concern of the family is agriculture, housing, irrigation or "mere subsistence" but not health. Health Education, therefore, has a significant role to play to help people to come together and to achieve health through their own actions and efforts. It aims at developing a sense of individual as well as collective responsibility in the community for its own health betterment on which its intellectual, physical, mental, social and economic development depends.

2. To help individuals to become competent in and to perform those activities which they must undertake as individuals or in small groups, in order to realize fully the state of health as defined in the Constitution of the World Health Organisation.

In any community, many activities directed to achieve health development are initially launched by the government; but in the long-run, these activities need to be carried out by the individuals, families and community. In the health programmes such as childcare, feeding practices, food hygiene, first-aid, and many such programmes designed to educate the public about the health hazards caused primarily by the changing lifestyle of the individual; education of public is needed.

Health practices and values attached to health behaviour have roots in the social system of a given society or a group. These practices conflict with the improved or modern practices based on scientific findings. In such situation health education has a greater role to play to synthesize the old and new practices without modernizing the values attached to old practices by the community.

3. To Promote the Development and Proper use of Health Services

No matter how best health service delivery system exists and health services are offered to the people; their full utilization by the latter depends on their awareness of availability of services; their judgment of the value of the services; the distance between the health centre and the community; their confidence in effectiveness of services; attitude of health personnel toward. . . people, etc. In other words, the utilization of health services depends on predisposing, enabling and reinforcing factors. Here health education is necessary to prepare people to make adequate use of such services so that they can avoid economic loss incurred by wrong or inadequate use of services, which are often expensive.

PRINCIPLES OF HEALTH EDUCATION

Some of the most important principles underlying the practice of health education are:

1. Planning for health education should be an integral part of total health planning.
2. Since learning is a change in individual's ideas and practices, and since health education aims at changing people's ideas and practices, effective health education planning should be based upon the theories and principle of human learning.
3. People tend to accept change more readily when a change is directly relevant to their aspirations, needs and fulfilment of words, quick returns, personal goals. Therefore, health education should be in line with people's goals, needs, and interests.
4. Group norms and influences are the basic principles of individual behaviour, which also includes health. If a health norm is to change, it is desirable that such changes are compatible with group norms. Health education can succeed in changing individual health behaviour if it addresses itself to group's standards and norms.
5. An internalized change is a stable change. An individual learns better through his own action and effort. Health education, therefore, should aim at creating such a situation so that individual takes initiative for the change.
6. Belief in the dignity of man—Health education is based upon the conviction that individual has the right and ability to make his own decisions; and democratic change should always aim at stimulating the individual to decide his action by his own efforts.
7. Start where the people are if education efforts are not consonant with the level of understanding and needs of the people, people will not easily and promptly assimilate the ideas of change. Health education, therefore, aims to start where people are; and build from this base the necessary ingredients for better healthy life.

8. Plan with the people—Health education ideally is a catalytic process. It does not aim to force a manger by manipulating, forces without the involvement of the people. Therefore, involvement of the people is the most crucial factor in effective health education. Planning for health education is done with the people, and by the people.
9. Self-help—The concept of self-help for better health is one of the basic principles in health education. The objective of health education is not to provide temporarily a solution of people's problems but to develop the ability among them to identify problems, find solutions and practice it. Health education, therefore ultimately aims at developing the potentiality of self-help in a community.[17]

CONTROL OVER DETERMINATION OF HEALTH EDUCATION

Health Education is the combination of planned social action and planned learning experiences designed to enable people to gain control over the determinants of health and of health behaviour and the social conditions that affect their health status and the health status of others.[18]

Further development based on human ecology has been spelt out by WHO expert Committee—"In recent years, however, a better understanding has developed of the processes that have a positive or negative influences on the harmonious functioning of a person, both as an individual and as a social being. This has prompted study of the role society plays in influencing the individual's health behaviour. It is now recognized that a community's values and norms play a vital part in defining the general approach of people to illness and health as well as to treatment and prevention, and that the process of socialization is one of the most important mechanisms in transmitting certain values and norms from one generation to the next. This has resulted in the development of social intervention models of health education, in which the emphasis is placed in influencing social, instead of individual, factors associated with health and illness."[19]

Health education is a 'process', which needs effective planning and implementation with appropriate consideration of ultimate goals and the best means for achieving them physical, mental and social health. The World Health Organisation expert committee on health education of the public (1954) has defined health education as:

> "Health Education like general education is concerned with changes in knowledge, feelings and behaviour of people. In its most usual forms it concentrates on developing such health practices as are believed to "bring about the best state of possible well-being."

The International Union of Health Education (1988) defined: "Health

Education is the combination of planned social action and planned learning experiences designed to enable people to gain control over the determinants of health, health behaviour and social conditions that affect their health status and health status of others.[20]

HEALTH EDUCATION FOR QUALITY OF LIFE

1. The value placed on health by people depends mainly on social and cultural factors such as the needs, problems, social organisations, the standard of general education and the economic resources of the people for individual, family and community betterment. To enhance the importance of health in one's culture, education encourages people to come together to find ways of tackling the general problems of their community. The immediate problem concerning the community may not be. directly be related to health. This active participation being responsible for their own health is enhanced by insisting the people to find solution to the problems of immediate interest.

2. To help individuals to become competent in and carry on those health activities for themselves, as individuals or in small groups, in order to realize fully the state of health.

Health is not a commodity, which can be bought by individuals for their improvement. Individuals have to accept the scientific knowledge and health practices and act accordingly. Therefore, health education, aims to encourage the individual, family and community to take responsibility for their own health.

3. To promote the development and proper use of health services. The usefulness of any health service depends on the peoples' utilization of the services provided by the health agency. It depends upon the confidence of the people in the health personnel and the attitudes, which health workers have towards the people. By Educating the people one can avoid the economic loss incurred by wrong or inadequate use of services.

Health education begins with the people and leads them for broadly understanding the activities for better health. It translates the findings of the laboratory into language and activities understood and accepted by people. Health education is more showing and doing than mere telling. When health education is skillfully done, people continue with pride on what they themselves have accomplished. Health education should produce a cooperative relationship between the people and health personnel. Many workers in health profession are engaged in doing things for the people. They should understand and be able to apply the principles of the educational process in their contacts with people, as well as in their working relationships with others.

Health education is a basic function of all health workers and all the personnel of allied health organisations and agencies. Health education is an essential component of any programme to improve the health of a community, and it has a major role in promoting:

(a) good health practices—for example, sanitation, clean drinking water, good hygiene, breast feeding, infant weaning, and oral rehydration;
(b) the use of preventive services—for example, immunization, screening, antenatal and child health clinics;
(c) the correct use of medications and the pursuit of rehabilitation regimens—for example, in tuberculosis and leprosy respectively;
(d) the recognition of early symptoms of disease and promoting early referral; and
(e) community support for primary health care and government control measures.

Despite the potential benefits of health education, existing schemes are often inadequate and ineffective. The key decisions that form the basis for any planning are decisions over what the desired change should be, where the health education should take place, who should carry it out, and how it should be done.[21]

The following remarks of a working group on communications in family planning,[22] which summarizes the value of the mass approach in family planning, are of value in health education planning as well "Mass communications cannot replace fact-to-face approaches. Each has its definite and well-defined objectives. Mass communications can inform, help to create a favourable social climate, counter hostile propaganda, dispel rumours and clarify doubts and misunderstandings. They may motivate a relatively small section of the public to adopt contraceptive practices. But, for the large majority of the people, a sustained programme of education, persuasion and motivation, obviously in a face-to-face situation, is necessary ."[23]

However, education for health and training are both crucial to the successful implementation of a water supply and sanitation project, because they promote, on the one hand, favourable attitudes towards, and community participation in, the project, and on the other hand, provide the participants with a wide range of knowledge and skills contributing to a better standard of hygiene and health.

The Decade programme in the Philippines is moving towards its objectives, and there are many factors, which have contributed to its success so far. These include community participation, a primary health care approach, and increased emphasis on education for health; the financial help received on an international as well as a bilateral basis, and the technical support lent by WHO; the close cooperation between the various bodies concerned with carrying out the work, and with training administrators and primary-level workers. Finally, mention must be made of the importance of relying on appropriate technology and effective control measures carried out by the field staff in bringing the Programme's activities to a successful conclusion.[24]

CHART 2.2

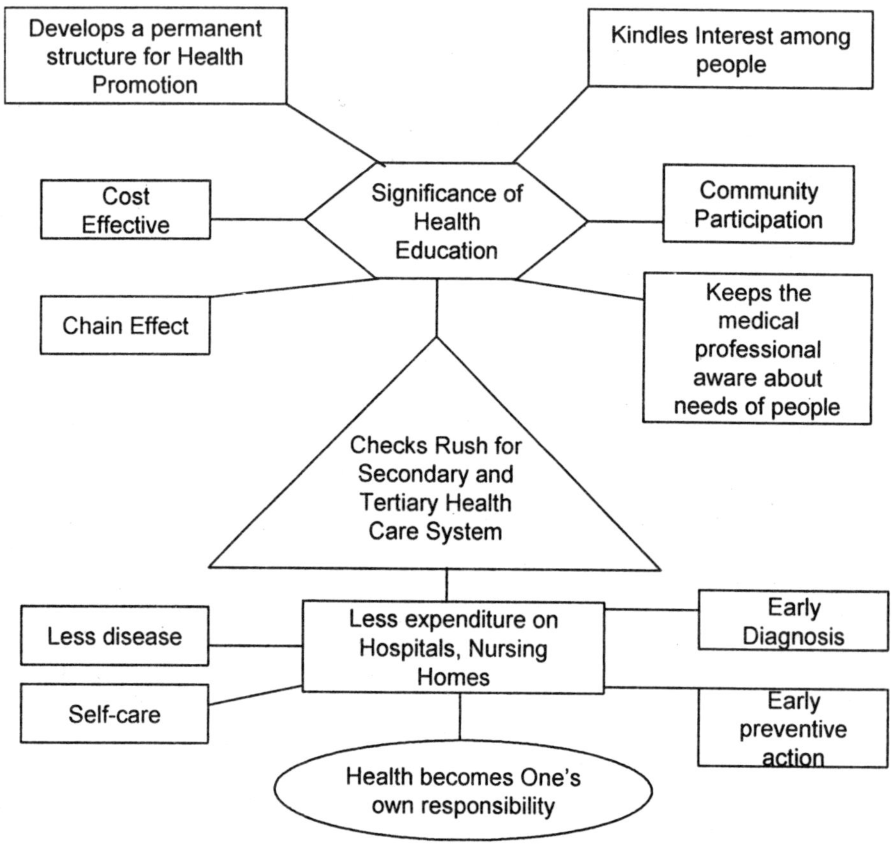

PROCESS OF HEALTH EDUCATION

Understanding Behaviour

The knowledge of the people's behaviour is essential before planning for health education. Understanding Behaviour is basic to influence through health education. Behaviour includes the following:

(a) Knowledge;
(b) Beliefs;
(c) Attitudes; and
(d) Values.

(a) Knowledge

Knowledge about health can be gained through personal experience or through teachers, elders, friends, reading material that is why, there has been a constant demand to include health education as subject so that students can get correct knowledge about health.

Knowledge is attained either through experience or reading books or the information provided by parents, teachers, elders. If we have some health problems and we have the knowledge for that, that in future we try to avoid this.

(b) Beliefs

Beliefs dominate our life as they pass on from generation to generation. People accept the belief since these have been handed down from their old traditions. Some of these may be good for health while others may be harmful. It is the duty of health educators to change these beliefs slowly keeping in view their sensitivity. If the people are too much attached to these beliefs, health educators may ignore them as co-operation of people may not be solicited.

(c) Attitudes

Attitudes are based upon our small experience or may be based upon the experience of others. Health educators must change the attitudes, which have taken roots wrongly and are harmful for health. It requires strenuous efforts on the part of health workers.

(d) Values

People in a community share some values, which they consider as important. What status we accord to women differ from community to community. The behaviour, beliefs, values when put together constitute culture, e.g. eating habits, marriage, etc. differ from community to community. Thus, there is a need to understand beliefs, behaviours, values of people or a community before introducing any health education, which can cause natural change or a planned change. Planned change is better, as the impact of health education would be lasting—

- Health educators can use health education successfully by:
- Talking to the people and listening to their problems;
- Thinking of the behaviour or action that could cause, cure, and prevent these problems.
- Finding reasons for people's behaviour (beliefs, friends' ideas, lack of money, and others).
- Helping people to see the reasons for their actions and health problems.
- Asking people to give their own ideas for solving the problems.
- Helping people to look at their ideas so that they could see which were the most useful and the simplest to put into practice.
- Encouraging people to choose the idea best suited to their circumstances.[25]

World Health Organisation defines Health Education as:

Health education does not replace other health services, but it is needed to promote the proper use of these services. One example of this is immunization: scientists have made many vaccines to prevent diseases, but is achievement is of no value unless people go to receive the Immunization. Similarly, incinerators for burning refuse are useless unless people will make the effort to put the refuse inside the incinerators.

Health education encourages behaviour that promotes health, prevents illness, cures disease, and facilitates rehabilitation. The needs and interests of individuals, families, groups, organisations, and communities are at the heart of health education programmes. Thus, there are many opportunities for practicing health education.[26]

Health Education is a part and parcel of every health activity and the health professional who ignores health education cannot be successful in any health programme.

Function of Health Education Programme

No health education programme can function in isolation. A health Education programme has to be an integral part of various other development programmes. Functionally, a health education programme would aim at bringing about the following changes as shown in Chart 2.2.

A Change In Knowledge

The most important need which health education programme can serve is to provide appropriate knowledge about health and diseases to the people. This knowledge should be provided in such a way that the recipients do not find it hard to accept it. How to provide this knowledge in an acceptable way? This is the first challenge faced by a health educator, meaningful responses are relatively easier to learn than the meaningless ones. The health educator can do a lot better by making his demands on the response of receivers, which are meaningful. For instance, the health educator who gives a big lecture to the mother on the value of practicing family planning without indicating its benefits to her as an individual would be showing inadequate understanding of this principle, for she has to look into her own benefits first. Vigorous efforts would be required to proliferate suggestions that are realistic and meaningful.[27]

Education for Family Health (An Example)

Although the basic conditions of organisation of services for family health are necessary, the attainment of true family health depends upon the education both of members of families (nearly every member of the general public is a member of a family) and of health workers of all categories. (See Table 2.1). This education and training will be effective only when behaviour is altered and decisions are made with new knowledge and different attitudes as the family member understands more of family dynamics and relationships, and as the health worker sees beyond the

TABLE 2.1

Areas of Family Functioning

Biological	*Psychological*	*Socio-Cultural*	*Economic*	*Educational*
(i) Reproduction of the species	(i) Emotional Security of member	(i) The transfer of values relating to behaviour, tradition, language and mores	(i) Acquisition of resources to fulfil other functions	(i) Inculcation of skills, attitudes and knowledge relating to other functions
(ii) Rearing of Children	(ii) Sense of Identity for members	(ii) Socialization of children	(ii) Distribution of resources, expenditure, saving	(ii) Preparation for adult life
(iii) Nutirtion of family members	(iii) Maturation of personality	(iii) The formulation of norms of behaviour for all stages in development and adult life	(iii) Economic buffering of members of family	(iii) Fulfilment of adult role
(iv) Proteciton of health of family members at all ages	(iv) Psychological protection			
(v) Recreation for family and its members	(v) Ability to make relationships outside the family			

Source: WHO: *World Health*, August-September, 1975.

individual into the family. This is manifestly easier said than done. For instance, the idea that the family itself is the greatest potential contributor to family health is not new, but the incorporation of education for family members at different ages as integral parts of health and educational services is far from being realized in practice. The education of health workers in family health, getting them to see the family as a group of interrelated persons, would also be a radical departure from almost every type of traditional training.

Thus, medical and health training for primary health care would once again be shared between community and hospital, the "normal" family and its dynamics would be understood as a background to the "abnormal" just as "physiology" and "anatomy" can be integrated with "pathology." Teaching and learning would then be related to the social context of the region in which the teaching organisation was situated, and the hospital would act as an institution within society rather than the centre of society as it seems to appear to so many medical teachers. In all health care there is a large element of education yet generally speaking health workers are relatively ineffective as educators. The reasons for this are complex; one is because most of their training is still directed to the alleviation of symptoms or of episodes of illness or disability, and does not lead or compel them to think through the symptoms of illness to its prevention in the future or to consider the long-term prevention of disease by changing patterns of individual or family behaviour. No one pretends it is easy to change such set patterns of human behaviour but it is regrettable that most training schemes for health workers do not even make the student aware of the problem, let alone give them any grasp of the techniques by which changes can be accomplished.

The delivery of health care will vary from one society to another and, as it does, so too will the roles of the various categories of health workers. Yet ultimately the effectiveness of all health workers depends upon their awareness of their own role in society and their attitude towards and understanding of the society in which they work. Understanding of society in its turn begins with understanding of family, so that an awareness of family dynamics and family health should form an integral part of the training and later of the practice of every health worker whatever their role or category.

The organisation of primary care service to provide family health care with the family as a health unit would require an educational set-up very different from that, which obtains today. Our submission is that at whatever level of development it could be applied, beginning with maternal and child health and family planning and progressing to a full primary care health team, such a set-up would give a better return for expenditure, Say a better foundation for health and provide a scheme for continuous development of family care and family health. The primary problem is to change the outlook, attitude and education of the health workers thernselves.[28]

A Change in Attitude

A change in attitude is possible only when the new knowledge that is offered is acceptable to the recipients. Its utility should also be well known to them. Normally, provision of appropriate knowledge should lead to formation of positive attitudes not only towards a person's own health but also towards the health of other members of the community.[29]

Ann Goerdt in an article, "Disability Prevention and rehabilitation", observes that Reduction of handicaps requires a great effort on the part of all sectors to promote changes in beliefs and attitudes which limits the activities of people with disabilities.[30]

Health educators should see to it that they put an abrupt end to that type of health education, which was concerned with telling people how to act. They should instead put the emphasis on understanding all those social forces, anywhere in the world, that cause people to act as they do.

Recently there has been a rediscovery of the contribution that lay people can make to health care. Say self-care is a fact. It has been, a fact ever since people were born. Today however it is realized that, far from reflecting mistrust in the health services or disappointment with their effectiveness, lay self-care offers a real potential for improving health status and decreasing health costs. Such care, however, must be applied intelligently and this is why health education is essential for ensuring appropriate self-care.

In the area of educational technology, health education needs to develop the educational technology most appropriate to promote individual and community involvement and self-reliance.

Next, health education needs to strengthen its multisectoral approach, and to increase the coordination of health education efforts through appropriate technology.[31]

A Change In Behaviour

Once positive attitudes are formed, these must reflect in the behaviour of the recipients. They should not only become mindful of their past behaviour but should also avoid doing things which can in any way influence occurrence or spread of diseases.[32]

A central point in the definition of McCormick is that health education is directed to change the behaviour of an individual so as to adopt advocated health practices. The change in the behaviour of an individual depends on individual decision (in the case of adult) in response to a number of factors; and knowledge, and awareness of risk of health hazard is one. Elaborating more of altered behaviour, the individual has to conform to the prevailing norms of the group and society in which he lives. Accepted norms by the family and society have equal influence in changing the behaviour as that of knowledge of risk. Behaviour of an individual has to be seen in the context of existing values and norms, which have greater influence; thus the efforts to change a behaviour needs to be gradual and slow. Behaviour is not arbitrary. It is the outward manifestation of values, which are deep-rooted and which can only be changed by an alteration in the individual's perception of him/her. For example, to stop smoking, the individual must perceive himself as a non-smoker and he must begin to dislike himself as a smoker and ultimately finds it intolerable to continue. McCormick believes that 'a form to non-directive counselling is much more like to facilitate behavioral change than didactic advice'.[33]

Abdulmoneim Aly in an Article: "Health Education through Religion", Achieving Health for all requires much more than just setting up a health centre in every high standard of medical care within easy reach of everyone.

A key element in the primary health care approach to Health for all is health education, which seeks to bring about a change in behaviour patterns by making essential health information available to all people in a simple, direct and effective manner. It is hoped that people will thus be motivated to evaluate their habits and practices, and will modify them according to the requirements of health protection and promotion.

Behvioural change, however, is too complex a process to be initiated simply by providing a set of facts. The motivation to break a habit must be much stronger than the force of habits or the pleasure derived from a certain practice. The spiritual dimension can be highly influential in this process of behavioural change.[34]

A Change In Habit

The change in the behaviour of the recipients must lead to habit formation. A habit can be formed only when the behaviour becomes repetitive. If proper habits are formed, not only the individual's concerned but the whole community will be benefited. Habit formation, however, is a slow process and it has been well said, that 'habits die hard'. The persuasive communication or health educator should be interested both in the long-range effects of his messages and in their initial effects.

As a matter of fact, he should be interested in turning the learned responses into habitual ones. What are the other principles that guide the establishment of a response? First, the probability of response will increase with the increase in the number of rewarded repetitions. As long as the stimulus with reinforcement following each correct response is not adequately repeated, it will not become a habitual response. Many messages are short-lived because of lack of reinforcement and are likely to become extinct. Second, in order to establish habit patterns, it would be necessary to have a shorter interval between response and reward. Third, habit formation is easier when stimuli are presented in isolation. A nutrition message when unaccompanied by another message such as sanitation message facilitates habit formation. Fourthly, timely increase in reinforcement will further strengthen habit formation. Fifth, receiver's original level of motivation will also influence her habit formation. The mother having a better level of motivation from the beginning will find habit formation much easier. Sixth, providing timely information about receiver performance, would lead to further improvement in performance. Providing selective information to a mother on the positive aspects of her performance will also improve her performance. Thus, communication of health ideas can yield the desired result if the above principles are followed religiously.

A Change in Customs

Acquisition of positive attitudes leading to appropriate habit formation must sooner or later, evolve into customs. Only when a substantial number of people in a given cultural setting start behaving in a customary manner, one can say that behaviour has become a part of their customs.

Don Palmer in his article, "Social Health: A True Story, Culture and Tradition as Medicine" in the *Daily Tribune*, dated 26th January 2000, rightly stresses the need of health education. Modern urban life, devoid of the goodness of social health, can be particularly tough for young indigenous inhabitants of developed countries. Some kill themselves, while many more drift into drugs, alcohol and crime. Now a prison programme is helping in rehabilitation of aboriginal offenders by reintroducing them to their cultural traditions.

Contents

It needs to be re-emphasized that health education is a slow process and that it proceeds gradually a part of the process may get established without any problem but additional efforts may be required to complete the whole process. This process may be directed towards the following important programmes:

(a) Personal hygiene;
(b) Knowledge of modern medicine, i.e., use of health services;
(c) Nutrition;
(d) Mental health;
(e) Prevention of communicable diseases;
(f) Care of children;
(g) Environmental sanitation;
(h) Human physiology;
(i) Lifestyle diseases; and
(j) Education about Alcohol and Drugs.

Health education must be imparted keeping in mind latest developments in the field of health. Life is changing fast and the individuals must be educated in the new technology-its role and limitations. Mr. V. Tatochenko, a member of the WHO Expert Panel on Maternal and Child Health in his article on "Education for Health" said, "Rapid changes in lifestyles and the evolution of views on health and disease call for new departures in health education. A quick glance of health education material of even one generation ago will show how fast it tends to get out of date. Medical facts, it has been estimated, get outdated within a decade or so. Effective health education, therefore, requires a continuous stream of knowledge, development of the people's ability to absorb it, and decisions taken on the basis of a constantly changing body of information.[35]

Let us give some studies to support our thesis:

Children become volunteers to change Asia's biggest slum. Using children as volunteer health educators is one of the methods being employed in an extensive programme taking place in Dharavi, an area of Bombay that is Asia's largest slum.

Four hundred thousand people live in one square mile, and 50,000 of them are the target of a primary health care project directed by Professor Gopa Kothari of the Lok Manya Tilak Municipal Medical College and General Hospital.

The aim is to improve the health and nutritional status of all the people, particularly children under five and women aged from 15 to 45.

The project began in 1981, with an extensive survey of behaviour and beliefs. The results were used to develop health education activities and a community-based health care programme with three main compliments-medical, welfare, and social activities. Three doctors, three medical social workers, a nurse, and 14 community health workers from the staff, with the active participation of local residents.

Training programmes were designed for health workers, traditional birth attendants, child volunteers, and other groups, Immunization, oral rehydration therapy, good nutrition, and personal and community hygiene were major elements in the training, with the young volunteers, aged from eight to 14, carrying the messages home to mothers and grandmothers, as well as to other children.

Opening a dialogue with community leaders helped to bring informal health committees into being, and adult literacy schemes were launched, as well as ideas on how to generate income by selling vegetables or making articles for sale.

Competitions were also held for different groups. Educational aids such as posters, flannelgraphs and slide shows were prepared locally, and used in-group meetings and at exhibitions. Experience has shown that the most successful health education activities have been the training programme, demonstrations of oral rehydration therapy, the production of flannelgraphs, and the establishment of a printing unit to produce posters. Cookery demonstrations and the provision of small feeding centres have also been successful. Evaluation shows that, since the programme began, breast-feeding has increased from 60 per cent to 90 per cent, and immunization rates have increased to 100 per cent, except for measles, which has risen to 60 per cent from a low base. A 68 per cent improvement in personal hygiene has been noted.

> "Well-planned communication makes an individual health-conscious, provides with knowledge on health matters, and promotes the requisite desire and motivation to avail of health services and stay healthy," says Dr. Kothari. "It also encourages measures at both the individual and community level to prevent sickness."

Rural Water Schemes Need Women if they are to Achieve Success

"As the International Drinking Water Supply and Sanitation Decade was nearing its end, enough evidence has accumulated to show that community involvement and responsibility are essential if rural supply and sanitation programmes are to be successfully introduced and sustained." Reports over the decade have clearly established the need for safe water supplies and sanitation, with million 'of preventable deaths each year. The vast majority of rural populations do not have access to such supplies, nor adequate facilities for disposing of excreta. And knowledge of basic hygiene practices is low.

Hygiene education programmes must become an integral part of all community partnership programmes and must be planned, designed and initiated before, during and from five to ten years after the construction of facilities. The primary purpose is to create a desire in the community to use facilities, and to keep them functioning. Community preparation and hygiene education constitute a support programme which appears to be vital to the development of effective community management, and to the success of the community management, and to the success of the community partnership approach advocated by WHO. In order to create a strong enough demand, materials used to convey messages about the benefits of safe water, adequate sanitation and hygienic, practices must be realistic, believable, and acceptable to the target population. This is why village groups should be organized, and particularly groups of women, since this tends to ensure that the information conveyed is sensitive to the socio-cultural characteristics of the people.

Educational materials based entirely on the 'germ theory concept' are not always acceptable to rural people, nor are they always particularly effective, because it is hard to give a meaning to invisible organisms. To suggest that people are drinking water, which contains the fasces of their friends and neighbours can be considerably more effective. Religious beliefs, superstitions and taboos all contain some positive elements, which can be used. In Papua New Guinea, for example, most people do not mind drinking from surface water sources (even though they may be contaminated), but are careful to avoid sources, which enemies might use to poison them.

Many religious and supernatural beliefs are concerned with water quality, sanitation, and proper hygienic practices, and can be used as a means of communicating positive messages. When developing educational materials, this type of information should always be considered.

Whether people feel the need to maintain and repair the systems, and maintain acceptable levels of sanitation and hygiene because of fear of 'germs' or fear of 'enemy poisons' is irrelevant, as long as they, manage, and maintain their programmes effectively.

A planned programme is the basis of the community partnership approach, with a national plan being established, and refined according to the circumstances of local communities.

National specialists, such as sociologists, anthropologists, health educators and community development personnel should be seconded to work with women's groups, and other organized groups in the project area. The aim should be to identify the most effective methods of implementing a programme through mass media techniques. Education and preparation should come before any facilities are constructed at community level. After educational materials have been developed, and an educational programme has begun in a project area, the materials should be refined to fit community requirements. Women and community leaders should be recruited and trained to organize, promote, and implement the programme.

Community hygiene education sessions should take place at least once a quarter, and no less than once every six months. Village caretakers should be trained in the operation, maintenance and repair of water supply and sanitation facilities, and latrine construction. They should work with women's groups and project personnel to advise on latrine construction in villages. The health and hygiene curricula of rural primary and secondary schools should be reviewed by the expert group, who should develop teaching materials. They should also develop practical exercises to involve students in building latrine slabs, making shallow wells, and installing hand pumps. The curriculum should include practical training in the operation, maintenance and repair of community facilities.

This schools programme should be launched not later than a year after the introduction of a community hygiene programme. But it is women who hold the key to success, since they are responsible for most water collection and use. They should be asked to advise on the acceptability of hygiene education materials, technologies, the location of facilities, and so on. Women should be trained by national project staff to promote programmes, construct systems, and operate them.

Only when a community has been prepared, and hygiene education programmes successfully run, should facilities be constructed. The link between community water supply, sanitation, and health education is well established. With the promotion of the community partnership approach, even closer collaboration between these two fields will be necessary of design and implement successfully programmes which will enhance the quality of life, and the maintenance of life, in the rural populations of the world.[36]

Methods of Health Education

Health education are set-up to promote positive health. A good health education must establish environmental linkages-points of interactions with the environment. These can be classified into four categories: enabling, functional, normative and diffused. The enabling linkage ensures and protects the organisational authority to operate, its access to resources and its power to achieve results. Functional linkage is to link the programme with the task environment. Normative linkages try to modify the behaviour of the people into the existing value system of the society. Diffused linkages imply reaching the clients through public relation (health education).

Sociologists have categorized diffusion process, which leads to a widespread acceptance of the programme into five critical stages: awareness (the individuals first introduction to a new idea or practice), interest (the stage at which he actively seeks further information and background data), trail (a limited phase of experiment), and finally acceptance or adoption. These processes have been occurring for centuries. The need of the present day health administration is to accelerate adoption of the health programmes and to control diffusion process in a short span of time to achieve effective implementation of health programmes.

Changes in knowledge, attitudes, behaviour, habits and customs can be brought about by 'personal' as well as 'impersonal' methods of health education. These methods have certain advantages and disadvantages. While personal methods involve face-to-face interaction, the impersonal methods do not require such a personal contact. Personal methods are indeed more convincing and generally more successful. However, the success of personal methods greatly depends on the establishment of a good rapport between the health educator and his recipients. The impersonal methods are relatively simpler and even less time-consuming. The radio, the newspapers, the posters and the pamphlets, etc. can all play an important role in imparting health education. Experience with personal and impersonal methods of health education have revealed that if both the methods are used simultaneously one can obtain better results than simply using one or the other method. The most important aspect in the adoption of the programme is the use of interpersonal relationships. Alastair Metheson, Deputy Director of UNICEF's division remarks on the basis of his research that:

> "To get people to act in ways that conform to new values almost always requires that mass communications need to be reinforced by personal influence."[37]

Thus, we see that communication, i.e., dissemination of information is only an important element in health education. The adoption or acceptance may not take place simply by communicating health information. A study conducted by United States Public Health services has revealed that, "Unfortunately knowledge alone does not motivate a person to act in accordance with it. He may well know the correct answers to questions without really believing and accepting such information as the basis for his own action."

Dr. Gisela Gastrin, a Finnish physician mentions in his article, "How Education Helps", "People can be motivated to adjust their outlook towards health and disease, but before this can happen their negative attitudes have to be countered with factual information. . . . Education needs to be a part of a comprehensive programme in which responsibilities involving the health authorities and others are clearly delineated and resources allocated."[38]

For effective health education, people's involvement is essential. Eric R. Ram[39] in his article, "Information is Power" in World Health rightly says that making people aware of their rights and responsibilities helps them to determine their own health priorities and take part in solving their own health problems, a step so essential in the process of empowerment of the people. We have to employ all credible channels of communication, including the traditional methods of story telling and drama, in order to reach all people. Films, radio and television whenever available can be useful, but we have to recognize their limitations; they are useful in creating awareness among people in their communities, but to bring about a real change in health practices, people have to decide for themselves and take responsibility for their own health.

It was mentioned by Dr. E. Berthat in his article, "A New Role for Teachers" that besides information and motivation, action is indispensable. He said that "information and motivation are not enough; it remains for governments to ensure that a good health infrastructure is available to all the people. Health education has to convince the men and women who are responsible for taking decisions that health is a basic raw-material for their country's eventual social and economic development."[40]

A health educator, as a persuasive communicator can make the best possible use of the personal methods of health education. But he has to see that the messages, which he is delivering, get mentally registered with his recipients. Actually, he can present his message and then wait until he gets the requisite response from his recipients. D.F. Skinner has distinguished between two types of approaches to the learning situation, as 'operant behaviour' and 'respondent behaviour'. The two situations have also been described as involving instrumental learning and conditional learning. In 'instrumental learning situation', which involves 'operant behaviour', the health educator will present his message and then wait for the receiver to make a correct response. When the receiver makes this response, the health educator will attempt to fix the response by the appropriate award or reinforcement. On the other hand, in 'conditioned learning situation' which involves 'respondent behaviour', the health educator presents his message in such a way that he elicits the response that he wants from his recipients and thus the stimulus that originally served to elicit the response becomes the reinforcing or rewarding element in conditioning. Undoubtedly, conditioning is much more efficient than instrumental learning. It is, however, necessary for the health educator to be aware of both kinds of situation since the condition for using 'respondent behaviour' may not be present in the persuasive situation. The health educator has to be aware that the recipients of his messages differ in the ways in which they learn a given response. They may give different responses essentially in the same situation because of certain specific reasons.[41]

COMMUNICATION IN HEALTH EDUCATION

1. "Health Education, like general education is concerned with changes in knowledge, feeling and behaviour of people." This definition implies that health education has knowledge, attitude and behaviour components.
2. "Health Education is translation of what is known about health into desirable individual, family and community behaviour patterns by means of educational process." This Statement implies that health education aims at individual, family and community behaviour and their interaction patterns.

3. "Health Education is a process, leading to programme planning, utilizing available resources, modifying health behaviour, breaking down barriers of ignorance, prejudice and misconceptions after the intelligent and thoughtful consideration of relevant health knowledge. . ." This statement means that health education is a process involving a series of steps and efforts by people and is not a single procedure.
4. Health education provides situations in which people educate themselves. This statement means that learning takes place through the efforts of learner and that the health educator provides the circumstances in which this learning takes place.

The principal objective of Health Education is to help people to achieve health by their own action and efforts. Its general purposes are:

1. To make health a valued community asset,
2. To help individuals to become competent in and to carry out the activities, and
3. To promote the development and proper use of health services.[42]

CONCLUSION AND RECOMMENDATIONS

Without evaluating the impact of health education programmes on the bulk of the people, one cannot possibly identify positive as well as negative aspects of the programme. An objective evaluation of the health education programme alone can help one improve the guidelines for future action. 'Cost-benefit' analysis should be an integral part of this evaluation, so that one may assess how available resources have been utilized. Through objective evaluation; one may also be able to curtail mass production of ritualistic health education material as produced by various health education bureaus. The amount thus saved can be effectively utilized for a more purposeful and meaningful health education programme. Health education is the most difficult task as habits, usages and customs are deeply entrenched. But health administration would fail in its purpose if it could not produce social change through health education. That is why it has been said that "it is easier to destroy mountains than to change our customs."[43] Professional training helps the health experts to deal with the health changes effectively. Their pharmacopoeia in both fields must be strong in order to translate the findings of biological investigations into social application. So over and above each technical act; there is a corresponding education function which doubles the value of the act, increases its efficiency and endows it with real human and social value.[44] G. Borkar in his book, "Health in Independent India" writes that all progress in public health depends ultimately on the willing assent and cooperation of the people and their active participation in measures intended for individual and community health protection, considering how much of illness is the result of ignorance of simple hygienic laws or indifference to their application. In practice, no single measure is productive of greater returns to outlay than health education.[45] Thus, health education can influence the lives of people for many generations. WHO conducted an interview of a Mongolian Feldsher. He stated that "conducting continuous health education is my first duty, prevention is our basic principle. Every effort is made to raise the health knowledge of the people. Child Care, correct feeding and vaccinations are among the most important topics for health education."[46]

In order to improve the functioning of the administration of health education at the Union and State levels in India, the following facts and suggestions may be taken into consideration:[47]

1. Effective Role for Hospitals in Health Education as Patients are Amendable to their Advice

Hospitals within the country are not serving as agencies of health education. Health education can be imparted to mothers when they come to hospitals with their babies. During their stay in the hospital, mothers can be taught how to care for their children during sickness and how to feed them correctly. The mental field is also full of promise. Hospital physicians can do much in this direction by their own attitude to patients, give them simple instructions and, above all, treat them as persons rather than cases.

2. Modernize Health Education Institutes

Those very institutions responsible for imparting health education courses are lacking in standards for sanitary facilities. It is difficult to see how the concepts of sanitation can be effectively imparted among trainees, under such conditions. The curricula and contents of health education need careful planning. The educational methods for health education used in a country or community should be regularly evaluated and revised in line with socio-economic development. Health education should be oriented to health consciousness and not disease consciousness.

3. Constant Research and Evaluation

There is the necessity of research in behavioural sciences for the improvement of health education. Dr. B.S. Sehgal, former Director, CHEB, New Delhi, said, "It was essential to conduct research on the behavioural sciences, in order to build up a body of knowledge for meeting the challenges posed by the health programmes."[48]

4. Special Attention to Training of Trainers

Training for trainers needs re-orientation and re-examination. We should supplement classroom-based academically-oriented training strategy in health education with the actual practice based on models of social change. The emphasis should be on learning by doing and not by listening alone. To quote a UNICEF/WHO study:

"Efforts in health education have often been limited to giving information dogmatically, as if this alone would bring about a transformation. Inevitably, the outcome has been disappointing. The pattern of existing resources-economic, human and cultural-has been forgotten and this too has contributed to health education's failure."[49]

5. Creation of Women's Club as in Democratic Republic of Korea (DRK)

Women can be effectively approached only by women workers. The experiment of mother's club has been sufficiently rewarding and useful in the People's Democratic Republic of Korea as agencies of socio-economic development. The process of social and economic development is a process of human development for people are the target as well as essential variable in development. Communication being a two-way process provides for participation at whatever stage of enlightenment the individuals composing a society find themselves. Mother clubs if established in India in right earnest can be the key factors in both the communication and development process since they can be the instruments for getting facts to the people upon which decisions can be based.[50]

6. Understanding Local Social-cultural Issues

Before launching any programme of health education, the health educator must assess the local problems and possess the knowledge about the beliefs, conceptions and misconceptions, which the people have formed about diseases, their causation and cure. This is possible provided the multi-disciplinary studies of rural communities are encouraged. Such studies would throw light about the cultural background of the people. He can arrange his programmes accordingly and this will save him from antagonism and hospitality.

7. Create Good Relations with Mass Media

There is less coordination between health education and the means of mass media communication, which need strengthening on positive lines. It needs to be recognized that most of our health education programmes and activities are so ritualistic in nature that they rarely correspond to the realities of the situation. In most situations the health educator's knowledge of the cultural content of health education programme is often so deficient that they find it hard to deliver the health education messages in a culturally acceptable manner. It needs to be stressed that the cultural aspect of health education programme is of the greatest importance in the Indian situation. Anthropological and sociological studies in the area of health education are so few in our country that health educators find it extremely hard to understand the many changing aspects of the communities they deal with. There is, thus, an urgent need to study the social and cultural context of health and disease, and to design health services in such a way as will gain the acceptance and support of the people involved. The social scientists can help the health educator in the following ways:

(1) to understand the role of socio-cultural factors in health, including people's beliefs about etiology, diagnosis and therapy of prevalent diseases;
(2) to understand the food culture including people's belief regarding consumption or rejection of various foods on socio-cultural consideration;
(3) to understand people's attitudes towards acceptance or rejection of health education programmes; and
(4) to help them plan and develop culturally relevant health education programmes.

South-East Regional Office of WHO has also expressed its dissatisfaction over the lack of importance to health education in its report "Health Situation in the South-East Asian Region, 1994-97."

Despite these achievements, health education and promotion practices are faced with major constraints—the low priority accorded to health education at the policy level, high illiteracy levels, inadequate resources, poor social status of women, and limited capacity for health promotion research are but only a few examples. To overcome such constraints, new thinking and innovative approaches are required. As we move into the 21st century, the challenges for health promotion go beyond the wider articulation of the concept of health promotion, to building infrastructure and achieving adequate levels of resources, both technical and financial, in order to respond effectively to the increasing demands for health promotion in the Region. "Settings for Health" represent the organisational base of the infrastructure required for health promotion.

Partnership, which effectively respond to the health needs of specific population groups, such as workers, women and school children, need to be more vigorously pursued. Healthy public policies need to be developed to ensure supportive environments for individual and community health action, and to protect people from lifestyle-related problems such as those due to tobacco and alcohol. Documentation and dissemination of health promotion outcomes are also critical to the legitimization of the cause of health promotion in the Region.

New health challenges mean that new and diverse networks need to be created to achieve intersectoral collaboration. Such networks should provide mutual assistance within and among countries, and facilitate the exchange of information about which strategies have proved effective. All countries need to develop the appropriate political, legal, educational, social and economic environments required to support health promotion. In this venture of health education, mass-media if properly used can help solve the problem."

Health promoters and educators need to be convinced that the mass-media can operate in the public interest and should play a critical role in social afflicts, including health issues. The health concerns of readers, listeners and viewers are very much the concerns of the print and broadcast journalists. The basis of the relationship between the health and media sectors should therefore be one of partnership, not one of user-helper.

Health and media are not naturally inclined to work in unison. Historically, medical scientists trained in the methodical and meticulous search for knowledge have been somewhat skeptical of any effort at popularizing their work. Some doctors even view the media with suspicion and ambivalence. Media people, on the other hand, need to have their Source material in language understandable to the layman; they have motive to dwell on technical details, and often loose patience with lengthy scientific papers.

Yet media and health in a close partnership have much to contribute to the public's welfare. Without the involvement of the media, the health sector cannot hope to inform the public on health issues or to help stimulate a community's involvement, which is critical to the success of any health effort. Without the technical input of the health sector, the media cannot fulfil their obligations to serve the interest of the public and these public interests certainly include health.

The complexity of the media, with their obsession for meeting dead lines and their own technical constraints, is little appreciated or understood by health professionals. Those in health who work in partnership with the media need to acquire a rudimentary knowledge of how media works—not in order to become media specialists but to be more empathetic in their dealings with the journalists and broadcasters. This in turn will call over a good hard look at the core curriculum of the training of health promoters and educators.

Whether the health professionals can play their rightful role in battling successfully against lifestyle-related illness—including AIDS and whether health education and promotion practitioners will enter the 21st century adequately prepared of the communication challenges, will depend on the actions that health authorities take now.[51]

In the new millennium, we need to harness all the resources especially the mass media in a planned manner. This would require active collaboration between media and health specialists. Jack Ling[52] in his article, "Health, and the Media" has rightly stressed that the health sector should focus on making technical subjects digestible and understandable to the layman. In particular, the health professionals should identify existing, credible channels of communication, including traditional ones, in order to reach the public. The media offers the public health community more than just access to air-time and newspaper space; they are also a source of communications expertise that is needed to ensure the success of large-scale health promotion campaigns and transmit technical information about health to a mass audience.

What is more useful is the follow-up of media-transmitted message that can be effected by village health workers. For instance, primary health care workers can be an effective channel of communication by delivering in person the same messages that have been delivered to a target audience in print or over the radio, thus increasing the overall impact of the educational drive.

A dialogue has to be initiated between decision-makers in media and in public health. The object of that dialogue should be to heighten awareness among the media personnel about the important responsibility they hold for the health and well-being of their people, and equally to alert health professionals to their own responsibility for ensuring that their health initiatives reach all people. Without this whole-hearted backing form the media in conveying health messages to the greatest number of people, we risk having only Health for Some and not Health for All.

However, the success of health education would depend in the long-run upon the shoulders of the providers of health care to the people. They should be motivated to do this job as a part of their medical duties. S.S. Sooch in his Article, "Revamping Health Care" in the *Daily Tribune*, (26 January 2000) rightly remarks that there is a general feeling that most of the health care providers in the government-run hospitals are indifferent, apathetic and insensitive and a few even out-rightly arrogant in their behaviour. A sense of compassion and human touch is simply missing. A series of crash courses should be arranged to expose the entire staff to the art of public relations.

Experience over the past few decades has indicated a number of barriers to effective communication, which include the vast population and the large size of the country; the diversity of languages, religions, customs and beliefs; low literacy levels; low income levels; and limitation of mass media. While developing and revising IEC strategies we should take these constraints into consideration and keep also in view the following principles of effective communications:

(i) To communicate in the language of the people, if possible, in the dialects of the people;
(ii) To provide specific information about the service facilities to be rendered to the people;
(iii) To make the messages simple, clear and meaningful to the audiences;
(iv) To conduct two-way communications;
(v) To make the communication a combination of telling, showing and doing, wherever possible (i.e. Use audio-visual aids, charts, films, etc.);
(vi) To lay stress on group approach and interpersonal communication in the rural community; and
(vii) To follow up the communication, as every communication needs a feed-back.

Health Education is vital to provide health to all in 21st century. This is the cheapest and most effective tool of health care. The success of Primary Heath Care in 21st century depends upon the identification of community needs through community needs assessment surveys and later on providing health education to the community so that they can solve their problems themselves.[53]

Notes and References

1. John J. Hanlon, Principles of Public Health Administration, SI. Louis, 1960, p. 402.
2. WHO: Technical Report Series, No. S-9, p. 4.
3. S.L. Goel, Health Care Policies and Programmes, Deep & Deep Publications, New Delhi, Vol. 2, p. 6.
4. WHO: Technical Report Series, No. 156, p. 3.
5. WHO: Etienne Berthet, A new role for teacher, *World Health*, May 1979, p. 23.
6. WHO, Esmat Mansour, "Towards a World without Polio", January-February 1995, p. 27.
7. Adopted from: Behavioural Sciences, Medicine and Health Education by Leo Baric in (Ed.) Behavioural Science and Diseases: The Health Education Council, London, 1972.
8. McCormick, James: The Doctor-Father Figure or Plumber, Croom Helm, London, 1977.
9. A report prepared for the 1965 Annual Meeting of the Association of Schools of Public Health, Health Education Monographs, No. 21, 1966.
10. WHO: Hiroshi Nakajima, The State of the World's Health", *World Health*, March-April 1995, p. 3.
11. World Health Organisation (1988), Education for Health—A Manual on Health Education in Primary Health Care, Geneva.
12. Baric Leo (1972), Behavioural Sciences in Health and Disease (Ed.), The Health Education Council, London.
13. Wood, T.D. and C.L. Brownell (1925): Source Book in Health at Physical Education, Macmillan Company, New York.
14. K.S. Sanjive, Planning India's Health, Orient Longman, New Delhi, 1971, p. 94.
15. S.L. Goel, Health Care Policies and Programmes, Deep &. Deep Publication, New Delhi, Vol. 2, pp. 7-8.
16. World Health Organisation (1954), WHO: Technical Series Report, No. 89, Expert Committee on Health Education of the Public, Geneva.
17. A.B. Hiramani, Health Education—An Indian perspective, Delhi, B.R. Publishing Corporation, 1996, pp. 47-48.
18. H.S. Dhillon and Dennis D. Tolsma, 1991 Meeting Global Health Challenges—A position paper on health education, XIV World Conference on Health Education, Helsinki, Fenland, June 16-21, 1991.
19. WHO, 1963, New Approaches to Health Education in Primary Health Care, Technical Report Series, 690, WHO, Geneva.
20. V.D. Sarangapani, Health Education: Concept and Scope, in K. Mahadevan (Ed.). Health Education for Quality of Life, Delhi, B.R. Publishing Corporation, 2002.
21. *Ibid.*
22. Economic Commission for Asia and the Far East, Communication in family planning, Bangkok (Asia Population Studies Series, No. 3).
23. K. Mahadevan (Ed.). Health Education for quality of life, Delhi, B.R. Publishing Corporation, 2002.
24. WHO: Pablo R. Imperio, Primary Health Care, *World Health*, 1986, p. 9.
25. WHO: Education for Health: A manual on Health Education in Primary Health Call, Geneva, 1988, p. 22.

26. *Ibid.*, p. 23.
27. WHO: S.L Goel, Health Care Policies and Programmes, Deep &. Deep, New Delhi, Vol. 2, p. 8-9.
28. WHO: F.J.W. Miller, The Target, *World Health*, August-September 1975, p. 15.
29. WHO: S.L Goel, Health Care Policies and Programmes, Deep &. Deep, New Delhi, Vol. 2, pp. 9-10.
30. WHO: September-October 1995, p. 4.
31. WHO: Dr. Halfdan Mahler. Health For All—Everyone's Concern, *World Health*, April-May 1983, pp. 2-4.
32. WHO: S.L Goel, Health Care Policies and Programmes, Deep &. Deep, New Delhi, Vol. 2, p. 10.
33. McCormick. James, The Doctor-Father Figure or Plumber, Croon Helm, London, 1977.
34. WHO: Abdulmoneim Aly, Health Education through Religion, *World Health*, July 1989, p. 27.
35. WHO, *World Health*, Feb-March 1979, p. 24.
36. WHO: June 1988 (Booklet inside), Education for Health, pp. 8-12.
37. UNICEF. UNICEF New, Communication: A Tool for Development, Issue 84/ 1975/12, p. 18.
38. WHO, *World Health*, Nov. 1975, p. 14.
39. *World Health*, Jan-Feb. 1989, p. 9.
40. *World Health*, May 1979, p. 25.
41. WHO: S.L Goel, Health Care Policies and Programmes, Deep & Deep, New Delhi, Vol. 2, pp. 12-15.
42. K. Kaliy, Appraisal Communication in Health Education: Perspective on methods in K. Madhawln, *op. cit.*, pp. 312-13.
43. Bosnian proverb.
44. WHO: Technical Report Series, 1954.
45. Borbr, Health in Independent India, p. 217.
46. WHO, *World Health*, April 1977, p. 20.
47. Based on personal discussion and interview.
48. WHO, SEARO: SEA/RC 23, p. 88.
49. UNICEF, Health and Basic Services, Keys to Development, *op. cit.*, p. 46.
50. For further details refer to author's article, Role of Communication in Family Planning: Setting up of Mother's Club in PEN, Family Planning Association of India, Haryana Branch, May 1977.
51. Jack, C.S. Ling, The Media its Role, in *World Health*, January-Feb. 1989, p. 25.
52. *Ibid.*, March 1980, p. 18.
53. S.L. Goel, Health Care Policies and Programmes, Deep & Deep Publications, New Delhi, Vol. 2, pp. 23-29.

3

CHAPTER

Preventive Health

Informed opinion and active cooperation on the part of the public are of the utmost importance in the improvement of the health of the people. "Enshrined in the WHO Constitution of 1948, this statement is today just as valid as ever. Under the Seventh General Programme of Work for the period 1984-89, WHO is called upon to foster activities aimed at encouraging people to want to be healthy and to know how to stay healthy. Public Information and health education are two sides of the same coins in WHO's newly formed Division of Public Information and Education of Health (IEH). The task of IEH will be to advocate WHO's policies, to lend support to all technical activities involving WHO and its Member-States, and to encourage positive action at the community level. All this will require the participation of the media as well as high degree of interpersonal communication."

—Jack Ling, Director, JEH

Health Education is as essential to health promotion as Research and Development in industry. Without health education, no progress in science and technology can promote an effective health care system. Health Education is the pivot around which the whole of the health system must revolve. Let us explain with example. Dr. Mohamed Abdelmoumene in his Article, "Health First" in *World Health,* November 1988 observed (emphasis added).

The second half of the twentieth century has witnessed profound changes in the character of medicine-change impelled by the giant strides that have been made by science and technology. Not only have there been stitch fundamental discoveries as the unraveling of the structure of DNA; there have also been breakthroughs in diagnostic techniques thanks to new immunological process or clinical imagery, and in industrial techniques employed in the manufacture of biological and pharmaceutical products.

CHART 3.1

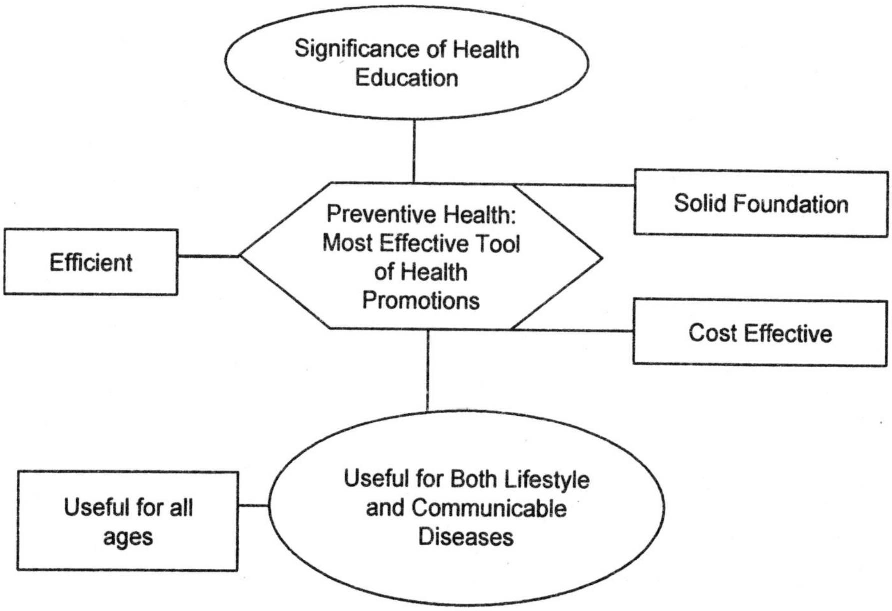

At the same time, without minimizing the importance of scientific progress, we have to recognize that, as far as public health in the past few decades is concerned, medical interventions (apart from vaccinations) have not been the chief contributors to the improvements in health registered in the industrialized countries. Where fault lies? The problem has been that the developments in science and technology must accompany with corresponding health education to individual, community, patients, etc. The dramatic decrease in heart disease recorded in certain developed countries has been due essentially to a change in dietary habits and lifestyles created through constant health education. Similarly, some counties have shown a marked drop in frequency of lung cancer because of a reduction in smoking due to educating the smokers about the ill-effects of smoking. On the other hand, unfortunately, the threat posed by other abuses, such as drug taking and alcoholism continues unabated.

These considerations underlie efforts all over the world to strengthen activities aimed at curbing harmful habits and encouraging healthier lifestyles through well laid out health education system. These steps must be taken in collaboration with the powerful media networks, with educators and schools, with professional and local organisations, and with trade unions.

"Most of the world's major health problems and premature deaths are preventable through changes in human behaviour, and at low cost," WHO's Director-General, Dr. Hiroshi Nakajima, declared recently. Viewed in its social and cultural dimension, health is seen to be not a gift that comes automatically, nor a consumer product that can be bought, but the result of the conscious education aimed at each human being, each family, each community. . . .

What must be done today is to educate everyone with the will to be healthy. This involves educating peoples the true meaning of health in the lives of individuals and nations, and encouraging everyone to find in their environment the motivation and the means to sustain their wish to be healthy.[1]

To want to be in good health, to give this capital importance in life, to be able to tell oneself resolutely "health comes first"—these are ideas that can be acquired and developed. They are of inestimable value, because they make impossible a dialogue between individuals and the institutions, which must serve them, a dialogue through which both can make progress."[2]

ADVANTAGES OF HEALTH EDUCATION

We mention here the following points to prove the important role of health education in health delivery system:

(1) Health Education develops a permanent base to support the delivery of health services.

(2) Health Education kindles interest among people about their health.

(3) Health Education, being preventive in nature is cost effective.

(4) Health education promotes Community Participation in the health programmes of the Community.

(5) Health Education can reduce dependence on health system, as 75% diseases are preventive.

(6) Health Education creates a chain effect as it passes on from individual to family to society.

(7) Health Education removes many mis-conceptions entangled into the minds of people.

(8) Health Education can promote partnership among health professionals and health receivers.

(9) Health Education can promote individuals to take timely action to avoid complexities.

(10) Health Education can check the rush for secondary and tertiary health care system.

(11) Health Education being a two-way process can help in providing knowledge to health professionals.

(12) Health Education can help professionals in creating right attitudes among people about their health.

(1) Health System Develops a Permanent Base to Support the Delivery of Health Services

People in the developing countries lack health education and that is why they approach doctors, hospitals, health centres when they feel any physical or mental problem. They take medicine and forget later on about their health. The result is the appearance of that very health problem or side effects, Why? The answer is that the people do not possess the knowledge of health without which their health base-remains shaky. If we want, permanent base for our health system health education would help in equipping the people with the essential knowledge. This knowledge would be quite useful for keeping their health in perfect order.

I. Health education with its roots in health, education and community development, has always approached health with two fundamental philosophies: (i) "start where the people are," and (ii) "involve the people." As health education grew in sophistication with its ties to learning theory and behavioural science, these tenets were translated into (a) the principle or relevance, and (b) the principle of participation.[3]

II. Health education initiates and supports the self-study, documentation and setting of priorities by the community in the planning process. It then enables the adaptation and evaluation of appropriate technology during the implementation of health programmes. Finally, it reinforces an increasing self-reliance and community development process that also leads to improved inter-sectoral coordination.

This process calls for three types of health education in support of the Primary Health Care (PHC) process:

(a) The first is communication designed to awaken, arouse or predispose the latent will of people to participation in controlling their own health.
(b) The second is any combination of training, technical assistance and community organisation that will enable action.
(c) The third is communication and feedback designed to reinforce successful change and to maintain the process of increasing self-reliance and healthy lifestyle development.

(2) Health Education Kindles Interest among People about their Health

A Lay Health Resource

It is imperative that this alliance between people and health providers should be democratic and not manipulative. If they are given the right and responsibility to participate and are appropriately supported, people have the wisdom, the ability and the will-to-deal with their own development. The challenge to policy-makers and health workers is to get the best out of the "lay health resource" that people represent. Ordinary men and women are the most abundant, most effective and most economical tool for meeting health needs. For example, it has been estimated that well over half of all health care is self-care or care provided by the family.[4]

Achieving community participation is neither cheap nor easy. It requires a long-term investment in health education in training and reorientation. Sometimes social and cultural values or beliefs interfere. Sometimes bureaucracy and excessive centralization make it hard for the community to see what is expected of it. But these difficulties are surmountable, and the results are worth the effort and the time. People are the true measure of the success of policies and programmes. At the same time, people are the determinants of success. Experience teaches us that, whether in the most sophisticated cities or in the most remote villages, when people act with determination and understanding in pursuit of goals they deem essential, they achieve success.

Previously insoluble problems are solved and resources are mobilized. Miracles happen! We must learn to harness the energy, wisdom and will of the people we serve.

The great challenge we face is to establish and sustain systematic and routine practical measures, which will bring about a democratic alliance between people and their health services. The growing world-wide trend towards greater democracy and democratic values seems likely to bring this goal nearer.[5]

(3) Health Education being Preventive is Cost Effective

Once the people understand about their health, their would be less need of hospitals and medicine. Lowell S. Levis in his Article, "Listen to the Community" feels that—

When the community is fully involved in all aspects of health development, new ideas and practices are widely and rapidly diffused through health education. Social networks are activated. People with similar values and experience trust and accept advice from each other more readily than they do from "authority figures", whose motives and social credentials may differ from those of the population they serve. Perhaps in the final analysis, reaching the hard to each on their own terms may be the most valuable contribution of community participation. Modern public health practice is increasingly appreciating the practical as well as the ethical benefits of community partnerships. The challenge now is to try innovative ways of strengthening these partnerships. Listen to the community: they can help us to help them. There is no mystery about community participation in health. The health care of ordinary people, for example, is mostly provided by self-care, or through family and friends, or through religious and voluntary groups.

Only a small proportion of health care (perhaps as little as 10-15%) is provided by health professionals. Communities therefore have considerable responsibility for promoting good health through their investments in education, economic growth, social resources like recreation, and environmental protection. No professional service system could effectively or economically replace this "natural" social resource for health.

Professional planning and services should now be brought into clearer alignment with the community's priorities and preferences. This is not easily accomplished. It involves many stresses and strains on health professionals who, in the past, have not taken into account the community's resources, priorities and views on how to proceed.[6]

This requires continuous health education of the community. Let us illustrate with an example given by Dr. Christian Aurenche: The mission hospital in Tokombere, a rural and mountainous area in Northern Cameroon, had a qualified and dedicated staff. But in spite of an ever-increasing number of patients seen, greater use of medicines, progress in the quality of health care and higher health expenditure, the health status of the population had not been improving.

In 1976 Dr. Christian Aurenche started to work in Tokombere. He launched a new approach. Instead of the traditional situation where the hospital is the centre of the health care system, he made the village the centre and the villager the first health actor, while the health professionals offered technical support for the villagers. To achieve this, the attitudes and ways of work of the health workers had to change. Instead of spending their time in only looking after the sick, the health workers became actively involved with the community in studying and solving its own health problems. Village health committees took shape. Mobile health staff provided practical information on health and what could be done to improve it.

The training of health workers had to change. Instead of receiving lectures on how to work with communities, they had to go to the villages and learn. They also had to learn to accept that initiatives taken by the community had to be taken seriously and supported.

Nikojai P. Nupalkov feels that prevention is always better. To quote: Prevention health actions are always, in the long-run, the most effective; the earlier you start treatment the better are the results. For more than a decade, WHO has been trying to develop an integrated approach to the prevention of different non-communicable diseases through early detection and treatment. It makes sense to screen a population, not for one particular disease but for all those that mostly affect people in the second half of their lives, using an integrated system of diagnosis and treatment. The CINDI-Countrywide Integrated Non-communicable Disease Intervention Programme, the Inter-Health Programme and the MONICA Programme are closely related to each other. The WHO MONICA project (Monitoring of trends and determinants in Cardiovascular disease) is a ten-year study which began in the mid-1980s; the drive against lifestyles that are potentially harmful to health; and CINDI is rather more oriented towards the needs and problems of the developed countries, since it started in countries of Europe and the Americas which had more developed systems of public health services.

But the principle is one and the same—protecting the health of certain groups in the population, not only by detecting the diseases at an early stage but also by monitoring these groups in order to formulate the best approaches to prophylactic and treatment measures, while at the same time neutralizing the effect of the causative factors responsible for these relatively common diseases[7]

(4) Health Education Promotes Community Participation in the Health Programme of die Community

People when motivated through health education, are encouraged to participate in their own health improvement. Poor health in young people does not derive from illness but from lack of hope, which results in a turning inward and isolation. These problems can be improved by continuous health education. Health Education would empower the community. A Declaration on Health Development in the South-East Asia Region in the 21st century by South-East Asia Regional Office of World Health Organisation, New Delhi resolved:

The active role of communities in the development process is essential. The negative image of patients and communities passively receiving health care judged appropriate by others, having no voice in assessing their heath needs, planning for services, and providing and evaluating services is bleak indeed. Fundamental to the development process is the involvement of the people who are most affected. At least two strong factors are at work here. One is the importance of respect for the people, human dignity and trustful sharing. The other is that often the critical determinants of health or illness are in the hands of the community, both in understanding the nature of the problems and participating in finding solutions to those problems. To ignore these two major contributions to be made by the community is to miss the essential resource for health and development.

Examples of community participation include village development committees, mothers' clubs, village drug cooperatives, village funds for nutrition, community-based health insurance schemes and health care schemes. The community-based approach is also being developed to address emerging problems such as health for the elderly and home care for persons with chronic degenerative diseases. These innovations are being shared among the Member-States in the Region.

The involvement of health-related sectors is facilitated when the community is mobilized. To mention some examples, the Basic Minimum Needs approach of Thailand involves four major sectors (health, local government, education and agriculture). In Indonesia, the Family Welfare Movement's cadres are volunteers who play important roles in health, women and family development. The involvement of district administrators in Bhutan has been instrumental in the promotion of anti-smoking environment and in the development of a model village approach, which seeks to improve the village environment, including water supply, sanitation, housing and roads. The mandating of rural development committees in India, with men and women elected by the rural community

(Panchayati Raj) through a constitutional amendment, is expected to lead to enhanced community participation in development, including health.[8]

Immunization against childhood diseases starts at birth or as soon after that as possible, and the schedule is completed by the age of 18 months. There has been a gradual increase in the number of children immunized as well as the numbers receiving the third doses of OPT (diphtheria, pertussis and tetanus) and poliomyelitis vaccines. Nutrition and growth supervision of the children is carried out monthly. Children are weighed, immunized and given appropriate nutrition intervention where the child's growth is not proceeding satisfactorily.

Health education of the mother is an important part of these visits. Attendance at these pre-school clinics is fairly regular during the first 24 months, and tends to drop after the first immunizations are completed. As most of the services are preventive, the importance of people's participation is vital to the life of the programme. Over the last five years, the number of mothers and children who come to MCH facilities has been increasing steadily. This has been the result partly of providing rural health facilities within easier reach, but the FWES' increasing contact with the community and their role in motivating the mothers to use the facilities have also been vital factors.

Promoting better health for mothers and children, and through them better health for the whole family, is the vital nucleus of action towards better health for all. Let us hope that increasing cover age in antenatal care, delivery under supervision, family laughing and immunization will lead the country to the desired goal of a drastic reduction in infant deaths and sickness.[9]

Let us explains with experiment done in Manila:

Health care delivery in the City of Manila has undergone a process of evolution since its inception. In the beginning, it was geared towards looking for sick people among the population; unwilling though they might be, they were then compelled to receive the health and medical services that the government felt they should receive. Early health administrators, following this paternalistic line, felt duty-bound to deliver the health care that was programmed along this concept of donor-recipient relationship. In later years, the emphasis shifted to educating people to go to health centres and hospitals set-up by the government. Ever larger sums of money were called for to meet the endless demands for more health services. However, despite the expansion of the health programme and the greater complexity of health services, and despite the increasing number of health centres and free clinics provided by both the government and private sectors, there has been only a slight reduction in mortality and morbidity—rates over the years. Communicable diseases continue to be prevalent in the community. High-cost, curative, hospital-based medical care received priority and few resources were earmarked for preventive health care.[10]

We believe that understanding, patience and dedication can overcome these barriers. We believe that people's apathy and indifference result from their inability in the past to recognize their own potentials as partners in community development and progress. When they see that the government has welcomed them as full-fledged partners in community affairs, our people in the depressed areas can be aroused to act positively. We are optimistic that Manilans will respond sincerely to the chance of a life-long working partnership between the government and the community to enable them to attain a better quality of life.[11]

(5) Health Education can Reduce Dependence on Health System as 75 per cent Diseases are Preventive

Most of the communicable diseases and lifestyle diseases can be prevented through appropriate health education to the community. Health Education should be practical and reinforced with examples and case studies; such health education when conducted scientifically can reduce the cost on these preventable diseases.

In the space of a few decades, there have been remarkable reductions in morbidity and mortality due to infectious and parasitic diseases in most developing countries in all regions of the world. However, other threats to health in the form of the so-called "Western degenerative" or "lifestyle" diseases are emerging at rates that far outstrip what would be expected from the fact that people are living longer.

In many developing nations, already beset with economic, social and other health problems, the rates of heart disease, diabetes and hypertension are as high as or even higher than in major developed nations. These chronic diseases impose a destructive drain on communities through their association with sickness and premature death.

Primary preventive activities will focus on behavioural and structural changes related to smoking, healthy nutrition, and levels of physical activity in the community. Secondary prevention targets include improved case detection, expanded health education services, and an upgrading of follow-up and rehabilitation facilities.[12]

Health Education about smoking, drinking, drug abuse, etc. can help in controlling large number of diseases. Suzanne Cherney rightly feels:

The prevention of AIDS hinges on educational messages and policy decisions, which, many people, feel, condone or even encourage questionable behaviour. Global Programme on AIDS curriculum package, for example, may not be utilized so long as teachers and parents believe that school AIDS education increases sexual activity among adolescents. (A GPA review of existing studies shows that if anything, it does the opposite).

GPA thus invests a great deal of time in explaining why prevention methods such as school AIDS education are effective and not harmful. GPA also advocates compassionate care and support of those living with HIV and AIDS, and urges close collaboration with the communities most affected. It argues for the empowerment of women, millions of whom are unable to negotiate safe sex or leave a relationship that puts them at risk. GPA advocates against too-against coercive measures such as mandatory

HIV testing which not only flout human rights but threaten to make the epidemic worse, by driving people away from prevention and care programmes.[13]

Changing Behaviour through Health Education

Some disease control interventions are based solely upon changing human behaviour through educational or promotional techniques—for instance, campaigns against smoking or for breast-feeding. Virtually all kinds of health intervention involve educational components as part of the disease control package, but the extent of educational effort required ranges from providing simple information (when and where a clinic will be held) to efforts at increasing understanding (the importance of immunization), and even to attempts to change lifestyles (diet, sex)[14]

Health Education may take into account the data generated by epidemiology, which would make health education relevant and specific. Each one of us is born, grows lip, perhaps marries and has children, and dies as a single individual. Our health is personal matter, and we do our best—each as an individual—to prevent our own ill-health.

But the health status of a village, a district, a city or the whole planet is a collective thing. It can only be assessed by bringing together all possible information about every individual in order to determine what patterns there may be in the distribution of disease—or indeed of good health in a given community.

This is the role of epidemiology—the study and the application of all those "facts of life" that bear on our well-being. In collating those facts and establishing that patterns that put lives at risk, or that cause certain diseases and encourage their spread, research which may seem remote and arcane is helping medical science to put together a global jigsaw of health.[15]

(6) Health Education Creates a Chain Effect as it Passes on from Individual to Family to Society

Health Educations aimed at people particularly opinion leaders, rural and urban elite, NCOs, etc. has its chain effect as it passes on quickly provided it is structured in a simple and a practical way. The manages in health education need be framed in such a way that these can be comprehended easily. This experiment has been a great success in South Korea through Mother's Club.

Creation of Women's Club as in Democratic Republic of Korea (DRK) Women can be effectively approached only by women workers. The experiment of mother's club has been sufficiently rewarding and useful in the People's Democratic Republic of Korea as agencies of socio-economic development. The process of social and economic development is a process of human development for people is the target as well as essential variable in development. Communication being a two-way process, provides for participation at whatever stage of enlightenment the individuals composing a society find themselves. Mother clubs if established in India in right earnest can be the key factors in both the communication and development process since they can be the instruments for getting facts to the people upon which decisions can be based.[16]

Some of the principles of successful community Health Organisation for health education are:

(a) deal with Health problems which the community recognizes as its problems;
(b) provide for community self-determination;
(c) engage the community in an active way in the solution of the Health problems;
(d) move at a pace that is comfortable for the community;
(e) encourage health promotion in the community through solving of health problems; and
(f) encourage community self-understanding and integration of health services.[17]

(7) Health Education Removes many Misconceptions Rooted into the Minds of People

There are many misconceptions rooted in the minds of people which need to be removed by constant health education otherwise these can cause damages silently.

> "Unprecedented challenges face the youth of today", said Dr. Hiroshi Nakajima, Director-General of WHO, in a message to the World Assembly of youth last December. And he added that young people may be given opportunities "to demonstrate their creativity, energy and commitment to solving their own problems and helping to build a healthy future for the entire community in which they live."

For many years the health of young people has been neglected because these were considered to be relatively free from diseases and less vulnerable than young children or older people. However, they are highly vulnerable to social conditions, which have changed, so markedly in contemporary times and their health is threatened in many ways by new lifestyles. They have to face such hazards as unwanted or too early pregnancies, sexually transmitted diseases and AIDS, tobacco, alcohol and drug use, and accidents and injuries stemming in part from risk-taking behaviours. At the same time, the enormous competitive pressures for economic and educational opportunities may be leading them to more psychological disorders and even to suicidal behaviour.

But, just as hazards are unprecedented, so is the willingness of young people to give their time and energy to improving the surrounding world, and in many instances the health of their families and communities. Such commitment to social development and to promoting the health of other people is a value that deserves to be capitalized upon more than any other. It improves the well-being of young people by enhancing their self-esteem and the rewards that come from a sense of accomplishment, it offers a constructive rather than a destructive channel for their energy, and it provides an opportunity to experience healthy and responsible interactions among generations. Young people are willing and able to take greater responsibility of their health and their lives, but whether they do so is heavily dependent on the behaviour of others. How well we listen, how well we respond to their needs, how much we trust them, how much we facilitate their action; that is the challenge to society and that is the urgent choice which those who are past youth must make. The purpose must be to focus the attention of the world on how we can help youth to choose health, and in so doing give health to all.[18]

Information and education on health are of the utmost importance for all groups, communication with young people, that is, the provision of information and the readiness to discuss that information with young people, will provide the biggest health dividends. If young people make healthy choices at that point of their lives, they are likely to remain healthy in adulthood and old age. It is rare to lose a good health habit, as one grows older.

By the same token, it is very difficult to undo the damage of bad health habits learnt and practiced when one is young. By and large, young people are well motivated and much more idealistic about matters such as health than their elders. All they ask is the knowledge and the means to pursue a healthy lifestyle. Our challenge is to get them to ask the questions, and then to respond in a way that prompts them to ask more and more questions. . ..[19]

Having access to the computer, for example, leaves young people in complete control of the learning situation, and that is an essential factor in the process of achieving autonomy. If we want to help them to become responsible for their behaviour, we must state this intention clearly from the outset. Our methods need to convey a sense of deep respect for the life experiences of individuals, and to encourage them to find out for themselves how best they can improve their own health. Let it be emphasized that this aspect is not just something that has emerged from technological progress, but is simply a matter of having respect for other human beings.[20]

(8) Education can Promote Partnership among Health Professionals and Health Receivers

Development is a multi-dimensional phenomenon, which cannot be achieved unless the community itself is involved. Resources for health available with any government are limited especially in the developing countries like India. Communities, according to their capacity, need to mobilize human, financial and material resources to supplement the resources provided by the national government and other extra-community sources in order to effectively carry out health improvement efforts. Substantial, financial and human resources can be mobilized from the community, some which may otherwise remain unused, such as the enthusiasm and energy of youth and women for community action. Thus, the community participation is most widely seen, as a way to mobilize resources for that would otherwise not be available. A local health centre promoting to meet the diverse needs of the people may be faced with expenditure it could not meet if the entire effort had to be financed out of the public purse. So, in order to cut costs, the intended beneficiaries themselves contribute to the extension of community activities.

Community participation involves members of communities in planning, implementing and monitoring of activities with the help of health professionals. Thus, community is wholly involved in the programme rather than being asked to either contribute or to take advantage of the services offered under it. Community participation is the process in which individual families assume responsibility in their own programme. They come to know their own situation better and are motivated to solve their common problems. This enables them to become agents of their own health development instead of passive beneficiaries of health development aid. They, therefore, need to realize that they are not obliged to accept conventional solutions that are not suitable. They have to acquire the capacity to appraise a situation, weigh the various possibilities and estimate what their own contribution can be. All this would be possible if health professionals provide them continuously health education.

Purposes

Based upon our earlier observations, let us mention the important health improvements that can be served by encouraging people's participation in Health Education—

(i) Creating will and determination among the members of the community for improvement in their present and future health status;

(ii) Identification and development of the local resources, thereby generating self-reliance among the community;

(iii) Achieving integrated area co-ordination among various agencies interested in community health;

(iv) Mobilizing the available manpower for productive and useful health activities;

(v) Keeping the members of the community constantly informed about the health developments in the area;

(vi) Arranging functional literacy programmes which can help them in understanding new technology in the area of health;

(vii) Organizing various clubs of youth, women to serve as centres of discussion and development;

(viii) Providing an open forum for the community to discuss its problems and find indigenous solutions, which may be efficient and economical;

(ix) To develop local leaders who can further educate and mobilize the people in the area;

(x) Encouraging the people to adopt modern changes, which can accelerate their health development;

(xi) Arranging extra-curricular activities to generate social awareness through well designed publicity; and

(xii) Encouraging the people to develop themselves rather than depend upon the Government for all health activities and thus become self-reliance, which is the key to development.

Though people's participation is a pre-condition for success of health programmes and there must be an inbuilt mechanism to involve people in their conceptualization, planning, implementation, monitoring and management of resources (funds). This may increase the efficacy and acceptance of the health programme on one hand and reduce the operational and administrative costs on the other.

Meaningful participation is concerned with achieving power, i.e., the power to influence the decision that affects one's health. So power is the key variable to influence decision-making and lack of it not only causes but also perpetuated the ill being of the poor. Thus, participation, power and well-being are inter-linked. Indian experience has been altogether different as policies and programmes meant for health development of poor have rendered only intoxicating impact and have genuinely not been concerned with sharing power.

The people's participation in health development process has been elusive. This has been caused by two factors:

(1) Lack of honesty the part of NGOs and government or traders of development; and/or

(2) People's apathy owing to many reasons who more often than not, are either deviated or resisted to join the moves seeking their participation.[21]

Akbar Moafefi in his article, "The Corner-Stone", observes that Health education based on man's active involvement in his community is the most effective and economic way of building up family health and understanding.[22] Man, from the beginning, delegated two functions to the professionals and the state-defence of the land and restoration to health. It did not take long for him to realize "war was too important an affair to be left to generals" (Clemenceau). The defence of land thus became everybody's job, and professional soldiers taught everyone how to defend his land. It is time that the professional healer also taught people how to take care of their own health; how to use available resources, how to collaborate and participate in health improvement, how and when to seek professional services, how to avoid diseases which are easily avoidable. It is the job of the health and to work towards it.

This is the most positive, the most enduring and the economical approach to health. It is based on the integrity of man and confidence in his capacity to solve problems. The family whose members are in constant communication with each other and the community are the best channels for this type of action, for the problem-solving approach. Actions initiated by the people themselves have the greatest probability of enduring.[23]

(9) Health Education can take a Timely Action to Avoid Complexities

People do not understand as to what to do when they are faced with serious health problems like cancer, AIDS, etc. They are caught up at a point when very little can be done for them. Health Education would have helped them to know about the health problem quite early through many symptoms. A timely help could have saved his life as it has been rightly said that a stitch in time, saves the time.

(10) Health Education can Check the Rush for Secondary and Tertiary Health Care System

At present patients move in hospitals like flies causing problems for themselves as well as the hospital authorities. The rush is because people lack health education and with little disturbance in their physical or mental system, they seek relief in hospitals, which is not available. Why? The reason is that they reach the hospitals when they have become too late. Because of lack of health education, they never follow the rules and principles regarding exercise, food, body cleanliness, mental exercises for relaxation, etc. resulting into serious ailments. It is therefore, essential, that the people should undergo health education and read literature on health, which can keep them fit. In this way, there would be less rush at secondary and tertiary level. This would enable the doctors to provide quality health care.

(11) Health Education being a Two-way Process can Help In Providing Knowledge about People to Health Professionals

Need of Empowering the People Especially the Disadvantaged Sections of the Society Participation has a goal and objective, which the community commonly shares. This common sharing makes the members of the community come together to take collective action to achieve the common goal. The goal sets the parameters and defines, in different situations, who the participants are? The roles different participants perform depend upon their capacity and capability skills, technical knowledge, formal position, education, control over funds, connection with those in power, etc.

The hierarchy makes the powerful participants active and others passive. This affects participation of those who make decisions for others. The poorer groups, who are generally the most affected of the development process, are the least endowed and least powerful. The poor are automatically excluded from the participation process. Decision-making is the first step in the development process. Therefore, a key objective of participation is to find out ways to include the hitherto neglected groups, who are directly affected by the negative impacts of development in the decision-making process.

Participation is a process of giving weightage to the poorer groups in the development process so that they may have say and control over decisions, which affect their lives; participation is a process of empowering the poorest. The indicator of genuine participation is the extents the poorer groups have power over decision-making and over resource management. 73rd Constitutional Amendment Act has taken a bold step in providing reservations to the weaker sections of the society. As a result, majority representation has been provided to them to undo the socio-economic handicaps thrust on them, in the traditionally exploitative society. These weaker sections of the society have also been given an opportunity to get elected to the posts of Adhyakshas and Upadhyakshas, if this provision was not made in the Act, the disadvantaged groups would have been reduced to mere numbers, having no great say in the decision-making process. Due to their illiteracy, ignorance and social backwardness, they could not have mustered enough courage to stand up to the cause of their communities. Thus, for the first time the local governments have been transformed into a system of people's governance of themselves. They can also mobilize the prospective beneficiaries to participate in the process of planning as well as execution. They can, therefore, effectively initiate a process of bottoms-up approach to development.

There should not be mere participation but empowerment should be entrusted to poor people. Arvind K. Sharma rightly mentioned:

> "This reappraisal attributed poverty not just to a violently iniquitous distribution of wealth and resources but equally to an oppressive system of governance in which power was unequally distributed. This, it was asserted, prevented the majority from participating in the political process; and, therefore, this majority has no opportunity to influence the decisions, which affect them. The silent majority remains an object of development, not its agent."[24]

(12) Need of Attitudinal Changes among Personnel both Political and Administrative Responsible for Delivery of Health Services

A reorientation of the attitudes of the doctors towards the citizens has become very much necessary for both the prevention of the citizen's complaints and their prompt redress. Doctors should pay great attention to the opinions of the people. Reorientation of the attitudes of the Doctors towards the citizens is a very difficult task. It will require thinking on several fronts such as in service training, recruitment from a wider social base, special assignments in rural areas and the like. The doctors of today should not only possess traditional service virtues like efficiency, integrity and loyalty but should also shake-off all the feelings of exclusiveness and superiority. There should be a desire to establish contacts with the citizens to understand their problems. Unless the change in the attitudes of doctors as a whole is brought about, all other measures to deal with the citizen's grievances will be of limited use.

In order to restore the faith of the people in the fairness and capacity of the doctors, the Prime Minister had inaugurated a Conference of the Chief Secretaries in November 1996 on "an agenda for an effective and responsive administration." The objective of the conference was to make public service more efficient, clean, accountable and citizen-friendly by evolving a concrete action plan. The adoption and implementation of the proposed action plan would require strong political will and commitment from the Central and State Governments.[25]

The select committee, of British Parliament, clearly demarcated parliamentary activities of a Member, which needed to be insulated from influence of outside bodies or corruption. The Committee short-listed seven ideals of Public Life as follows:

Selflessness

Holders of public office should take decisions solely in terms of the public interest. They should not do so in order to gain financial or other material benefits for themselves, their family or their friends.

Integrity

Holders of public office should not place themselves under any financial or other obligation to outside individuals or organisation that might influence them in the performance of their official duties.

Objectivity

In carrying out public business, including making public appointments, awarding contracts or recommending individuals for rewards and benefits, holders of public office should make choices on merit.

Accountability

Holders of public office are accountable for their decisions and actions to the public and must submit themselves to whatever scrutiny is appropriate to their office.

Openness

Holders of public office should be as open as possible about all the decisions and actions that they take. They should give reasons for their decisions and restrict information only when the wider public interest clearly demands.

Honesty

Holders of public office have a duty to declare any private interests relating to their public duties and to take steps to resolve any conflicts arising in a way that protects the public interest.

Leadership

Holders of public office should promote and support these principles by leadership and example.

The attitudes of change agents need be:

(1) Willingness to consult and involve poor, backward and illiterate people.
(2) Acceptance of the fact that illiterate people are not unintelligent.
(3) Readiness to understand people's view points, their problems and need.
(4) Ability to bear with hardships to work with limited facilities and resources.
(5) Readiness to go beyond the fixed programme activities and objectives to take up water, food, education, etc., and proper orientation to extend the role from that of medical and health aspects to concern in social-structural and cultural dimensions of development.
(6) Ability to share knowledge and skills with all other workers of the project team, village health workers, community volunteers and community in general demystification of the 'professional' and the 'technical'.
(7) Genuine sincerity and commitment to the development of the rural, poor and backward sections of the society thus setting a model.

It is of utmost national importance that the doctors are honest and upright in the discharge of their public duties. It is at this time that the civil servants should serve the nation honestly by giving a sense of continuity. If they fail, the future of the nation may be dark.[26]

Fostering Trust

It is the fallacy of modernity that we believe we communicate better through machines. Human beings communicate through bonds of mutual confidence. It is the prime task of the health communicator to facilitate a state of communal trust.

Unfortunately, the staff of the public health services belongs to the educated elite. Therefore, typical bourgeois values permeate the hierarchy from the top to the level of the field-worker. Reality is seen through the reports of the latter, who knows that his superiors only welcome "facts" which are consistent with their social values and views. Large amounts of pseudo-information are concentrated around the false fact that poverty and ill-health are caused by ignorance. This allows the establishment to launch masses of educational programmes, the purpose and result of which only distract attention from the need for a structural change in society and a redistribution of wealth. In the process, the livelihood of the health education establishment is sustained.

Health and nutrition messages processed by the system have been devised and meted out according to the measure stick of the middle-class bureaucrat behind a desk. With their frequent characterizations of rural or village people's actions as mistakes, habits as bad and attitudes as wrong, they reflect a feudalistic lack of trust in the ability of common people to cope with their lives. There is little doubt that the pattern of working life in an organisational bureaucracy of which health services are a part tends to retard emerging moves towards change.[27]

(13) Health Education can Help Health Professional in Creating Right Attitudes among People about their Health

Advising People

The health professionals may advise the people to act in a way, which may be beneficial to them and to the health institutions concerned. Public relations through its various channels need to inject the desired changes to generate health development, dynamism and modernization. Thus, the advice to be effective should be preceded by extensive planning of the public relations strategies to be followed.

The right to participate in the affairs of the health is meaningless unless the citizens are well informed on all sides of the issues, in respect of which they are called upon to express their views. One-sided information, disinformation, misinformation and non-information—all equally create an uninformed citizenry, which makes democracy a farce when medium of information is monopolized. This is particularly so in a country like ours were about 48 per cent of the population is illiterate and hardly 6.5 per cent of the population has access to the print media, which is not subject to precensorship.[28]

Personnel Communication

The art of developing common understanding about health issue of people is vital to bring about change of attitudes and behaviour among them. Sociologists have classified the diffusion process, which leads to a widespread acceptance of the programme into five stages:

1. Awareness (the individual's first introduction to a new idea or practices);
2. Interest (the stage at which he actually seeks further information and background data);
3. Evaluation (the stage of assessment on theoretical grounds);
4. Trial (a limited phase of experiment), and finally
5. Acceptance or adoption.

Thus, the impersonal methods are relatively simpler and even less time consuming. The radio, TV, newspapers, posters, and pamphlets can also help in improving public relations. Experience with personal and impersonal methods of public relations has revealed that if both the methods are used simultaneously, one can obtain better results than simply using one of the other methods. Alastair Metheson, Deputy Director of UNICEF's division, remarks on the basis of his research that "to get people to act in ways that conform to new values almost always requires that mass communications be reinforced by personal influence."[29]

(14) Health Education Supports Planning and Action

Health education initiates and supports self-study, documentation and setting of priorities by community in planning process. It then enables adaptation and evaluation of appropriate technology during implementation of health programmes. Finally, it reinforces an increasing self-reliance and community development process that also leads to improved intersectoral coordination.

This process calls for three types of health education in support of the Primary Health Care (PHC) process. The first is communication designed to awaken, arouse or predispose the latent will of people to participate in controlling their own health. The second is any combination of training, technical assistance and community organisation that will enable action. The third is communication and feedback designed to reinforce successful change and to maintain the process of increasing self-reliance and health lifestyle development.[30]

CONCLUSION

We may conclude with the following points to make health education a reality:

1. The movement starts with the people.
2. Do the felt needs truly reflect major issues?
3. What are the priorities? A dialogue is engaged with professionals.
4. Central support comes into play. Plans are formalized.
5. Implementation starts. Other sectors are involved. Resources are coordinated.
6. Action develops. But is the technology appropriate?
7. How effective are the activities? What are the changes occurring?
8. As progress is monitored, new needs emerge. The community is ready for the next stage.
9. The cycle for increased involvement and self-reliance develops at another level.
10. The community takes action to develop new resources.

11. Are programmes developing in the right direction? Central and local activities are evaluated.[31]
12. Greater involvement of all sectors helps fill gaps. Self-reliance becomes a reality. And the cycle continues.

Notes and References

1. WHO, Lawrence W. Green, New Policies in Education for Health, *World Health*, April-May 1983, p. 13.
2. WHO, Dr. Mohamed Abdelmoumene, Health Trust, *World Health*, November 1988, p. 3.
3. WHO, Lawrence W. Green, New Policies in Education for Health, *World Health*, April-May 1983, p. 13.
4. WHO: *World Health*, April-May, 1983, p. 16.
5. Hiroshi Nakajina, A Grand Alliance, Editorial, *World Health*, May June 1992, p. 3
6. Lowell S. Levis, Listen to the Community, *World Health*, May-June 1992, pp. 10-11.
7. WHO: Nikolai P. Napalkov, "Live Better-Live Longer", *World Health*, March-April 1995, p. 13.
8. SEARO: Declaration on Health Development in the South-East Asia Region in the 21st Century, New Delhi, 1997, pp. 22-23.
9. WHO: N.N. Mashalaba, Contract with the Community, *World Health*, February-March 1979, p. 31.
10. WHO: Evangeline G. Suva, Experiment in Manila, *World Health*, July 1983, p. 5.
11. *Ibid.*, p. 7.
12. WHO: Lifestyle Hazards, *World Health*, June 1989, pp. 18-19.
13. WHO: Suzanne Cherney, "AIDs: A glance back, a look forward", *World Health*, March-April 1995, p. 19.
14. WHO: Richard H. Morrow, New Weapons, *World Health*, June 1989, p. 10.
15. WHO: The facts of life, *World Health*, June 1989, p. 16.
16. For further details refer to author's article, "Role of Communication in Family Planning: Setting up of Mother's Club in PEN", Family Planning Association of India, Haryana Branch, May 1977.
17. Dr. S.L.Goel and S.S. Dhaliwal, Urban Development and Management, New Delhi, Deep & Deep, 2002, p. 272.
18. WHO: Herbert Friedman, Youth of Today, *World Health*, March 1989, p. 3.
19. Ann Kern, Get them to Ask questions, in *World Health*, March 1989, p. 5.
20. Robert Perreault and Maire, Claire Lauren Dear, Tele Health, *World Health*, March 1989, p. 7.
21. Dr. S.L. Goel and S.S. Dhaliwal, Urban Development and Management, New Delhi, Deep & Deep, 2002, pp. 273-77.
22. WHO: Akbar Moarefi, The Comer-Stone, *World Health*, August-September 1975, p. 30.
23. WHO: Akbar Moarefi, The Corner-Stone, *World Health*, August-September 1975, p. 33.
24. Sharma, Arvind K., 'Peoples Empowerment', IIPA, July-September 1996, p. 236.
25. Ray, C.N., 'Citizen's Charter in India: An Overview', IIPA, Oct.-Dec. 1998, p. 804.
26. Dr. S.L. Goel, Urban Development and Management, 2002, pp. 284-86.

27. WHO: Andreas Fuglesang, 'Folk-wisdom and pseudo-information', *World Health,* Jan.-Feb. 1989, p. 7.
28. Dr. S.L. Goel, Urban Development and Management, 2002, p. 280.
29. UNICEF, UNICEF News, 'Communication: A Tool for Development Issue', 84/ 1975/2, p. 18.
30. WHO: A panorama of planning and action, *World Health,* April-May 1983, pp. 16-17.
31. *Ibid.,* pp. 16-17.

4

CHAPTER

Health Management Information System (HMIS)

> "Knowledge is power an when you assemble knowledge in the right place in a timely fashion, it is also profit. The combination of human and computer-based capital resources which results in the collection, storage, retrieval, communication and use of data for the purpose efficient management of operations."
>
> —*MIS*

First let us understand the meaning of the term Management Information System.

The significance of information can be seen from the Nepoleonic Phrase-an army marches on its stomach and the administration marches on information. Information is the life blood of an organisation. Information is the data transmitted before or after processing. Management is the planning, implementation and control of the use of a set of resources to achieve objectives. A system is a set of sub-systems having independence so as to form a complex unity. Management Information System is thus a system in which required data are collected, analysed and transmitted to help the managers at various levels in the process of planning, implementation and evaluation. According to R.R. Duersch: "It is a system which provides management with the information it requires to monitor progress, measure performance, detect trends, evaluate alternatives, make decisions and to take corrective action."[1]

Information is the planner's raw material, forming the basis for the diagnosis, structuring his objectives and permitting him to evaluate the programme efficiency and effectiveness. Information is the tool of the management realm being the essential link between means and ends. It can be studied, analysed, organized, stored for future reference, summarised

CHART 4.1

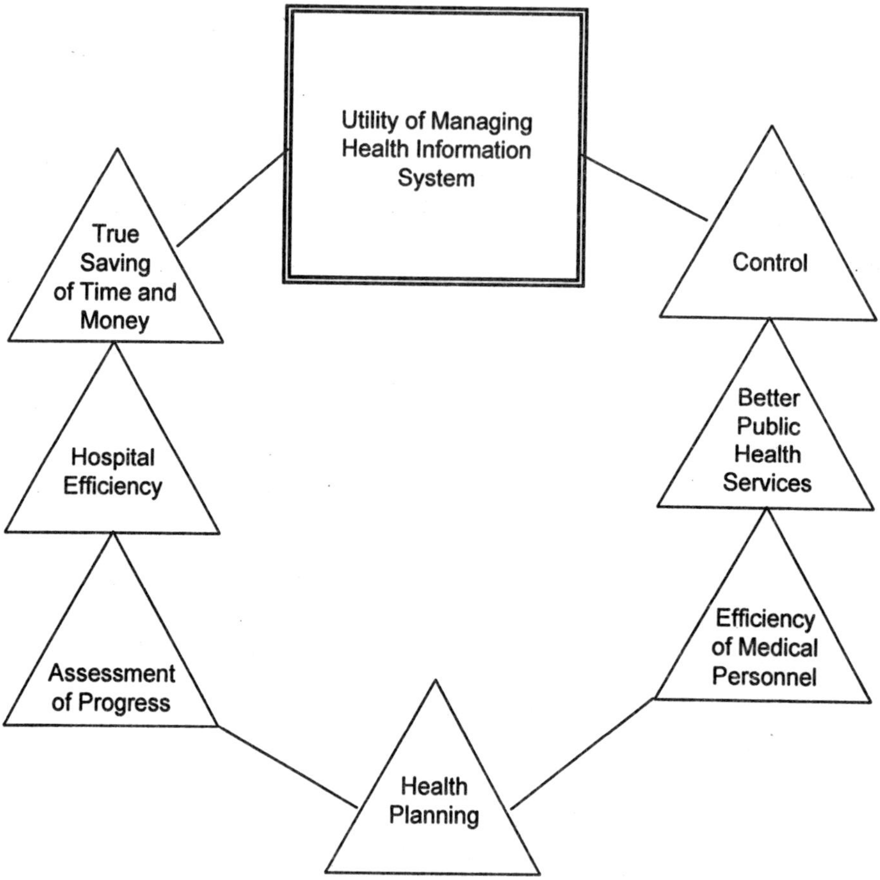

and/or displayed. Information is substantially different from mere data in that data is raw information while information is the aggregate of facts or data organized into knowledge or intelligence. One of the roles of management must be to sift out the information found within the data, and even before to ensure that the data collected will in fact furnish information needed.[2] Peter Drucker has rightly said that the manager has a specific tool: information? It has been rightly mentioned that Information is now recognized as a valuable resource and has been termed as one of the 8 m —men, materials, machine, money, methods, markets, moments and messages—a term used for information." Information is a relative term. To quote Harper Marion: "'Information may involve anything from the most minute and finite to the Universal. Processing information today calls not only for distinguishing the forest from the trees, but distinguishing leaves and chlorophyll—while still not losing sight of forest."[3] The degree to which a planner can be successful in terms of the provision of services will depend upon the degree to which he is able to obtain information about them, which is valid and reliable. The term system has been defined as a coherent, integrated whole, being a combination of number of entities or elements. Similarly, in the information area, there are a number of elements which have to be considered in an integrated manner, as components of one system, so that they are viewed in totality as means of providing administrator with required information in the appropriate form and at an appropriate time.

The latest advances in information technologies have allowed for the development of applications that have had tremendous repercussions in the healthcare field. Along with access, means must be provided to ensure that information is trustworthy and relevant. Certification of information quality can remain voluntary, preserving citizens' rights and promoting diversity. Collaboration among all Internet stakeholders is crucial to reducing conflicts of interest and for cost-effective distribution of quality health and medical information.[4]

Meaning

> "A management Information System is a combination of planned procedures, processes suitably designed forms, an appropriate organisation structure and managers who are capable of utilising the facts which are produced in a suitable form."

According to G. Murdich, "MIS is a system that collects, stores, processes data and provides information to managers for planning, controlling and decision-making."[5]

Prof. Murdich has rightly said that MIS would ensure in:

(a) Providing to manager's information on the impact of men, money, materials, equipment and facilities on the various systems and the business as a whole.
(b) Maintaining Central Data banks and model banks for integrated planning, control and decision-making.
(c) Sensing, through designated communication channels, the effectiveness of systems operations.
(d) Providing timely feedback to managers on performance of all systems by means of summary, key elements and exception reports.
(e) Scanning the environment by formal intelligence operations to keep managers informed of environmental changes impinging the various systems of the business.[6]

A Management Information System (MIS) has been defined as "the combination of human and computer-based capital resources which result in the collection, storage, retrieval, communication and use of data for the purpose of efficient management of operations.

During September-December 1962, the Advanced Systems Development Division of IBM conducted a survey to determine the scope and goals of an Advanced Management Information System. The major information problems were found to fall into seven categories:

1. Complexities in the information flow cause major communication problems and inhibit responsiveness and growth.
2. *Duplication of effort*: Identical reports are generated, data files are created and maintained at several locations.
3. *Variations in field Processing*: At the present time, field locations vary the processing of similar information and vary information flows.
4. *Inaccessibility of data*: Useful and necessary data are available, but often in a form or location that makes them uneconomical and unfeasible to retrieve.
5. *Time lapse*: Data are simply not being moved fast enough. Time lags are caused by mail, multiple audit points and varying closing periods. In many cases the data are no longer of value when they are made available.
6. *Inaccurate sources data*: The sheer volume of data makes it humanly impossible to consistently accurate and efficient.
7. *Limited information support*: The relation between the creation of information and servicing of all those who could benefit from it is poor.[7]

A health management information system is a process whereby health data (input) are recorded, stored, retrieved and processed for decision-making (output). Decision-making broadly includes managerial aspects such as the planning, organizing and control of health care facilities at the national, state and sub-state levels and clinical aspects which can be sub-divided into: (i) providing optimal patient care, (ii) training of medical personnel to generate appropriate human resources, and (iii) facilitate research and development activities in various fields of medicine.[8]

HIMS is an essential management tool for effective functioning of the health system. During the Eighth Plan the Central Bureau of Health system for sending district level information on morbidity reported by the government primary health care institutions through National Informatics district computer network. Though some states responded initially the system was never fully operationalised in any state. The HMIS system did not take root due to the several inherent deficiencies. The major problems faced in the implementation of HMIS were:

(a) HMIS proforma requires continuous maintenance of detailed Sub-centre Registers, numbering 13, along with the Reporting formats. This involves substantial recurring expenditure for printing of forms and registers. The States/UTs expressed inability to meet the recurring expenditure for printing of forms and registers.

(b) Lack of hardware, software and trained personnel at the district and lower levels and the NIC facilities were inadequate to meet computing requirements of HMIS.

(c) Separate programme-wise Information System—required by some users.

(d) No legal provisions for collecting data from non-government sector.

(e) No compulsion of State/UT level to implement the system.

As a result there is no system through which reliable data on morbidity in different districts/states could be collected and analyzed and used for decentralized district-based planning. So far there has not been any effort to use the currently available IT tools to build up a comprehensive HMIS and use it to improve efficiency and functional status of the health system.[9]

Standards—The growth of informatics technology and the corresponding growth of its applications in the health field are both so rapid that they often occur before norms and standards are set-up and agreed to. Standards for health data, for software and hardware, and for the procedures involved, all require to be set-up so that the multitude of application areas may relate to each other. This is essential for sharing and exchanging data and for making economies in the use of hardware and software. A number of international organisations are working in this all important domain of standards, and a great deal of investigation and hard bargaining is still to come.

The use of informatics in the health sector also influences the way in which health care is to be provided. It therefore has an effect on the norms and standards for the "evaluation of the medical actions taken." The article by Professor Jean-Raoul Scherrer and Dr. Francois Borst, of the Centre for Medical Informatics at the University Hospital of Geneva, Switzerland, argues that the uses of health informatics call for the standards of "medical management" to be developed or revised.

In a number of policy statements, Dr. Hiroshi Nakajima, Director-General of WHO, has emphasized the importance of informatics to health and has underlined health as one of the principal pillars of the technology. WHO is engaged on a number of collaborative activities with member-states that are either directly concerned with informatics or include an informatics element. The WHO secretarial itself is a heavy user of informatics support, and is actively establishing an electronic mail service with networks to its collaborating institutions.

Though we have bound a number of informatics solutions to old challenges, many other challenges still remain. Making computing support available in local languages, providing tele-links to remote and outer-city areas, establishing codes of ethics that govern the access to and uses of medical data and computerised systems, and drawing up appropriate legislation—these are but examples of what remains to be done.

The advent of computing, and particularly the informatics explosion of recent years which has put the new technology within reach of millions of users in developed and developing countries alike, has been compared to the coming of electricity. We are still discovering new uses for it, and it is indispensable. This is already the case for the business and financial sector, and it is only a matter of time—a very short time—before it will be true too for health informatics.[10]

Thus Tenth Five Year Plan (2002-07) focused on:

Building up a fully functional, accurate Health management Information System (HMIS) utilizing communication link will send data on births, deaths, diseases, requests for drugs, diagnosis and equipment and status of ongoing programmes through service channels within existing infrastructure and manpower and funding; it will also facilitate decentralized district-based planning, implementation and monitoring.

Building up an effective system of disease surveillance and response at the district, state and national level as a part of existing health services.

The Union Ministry of Statistics and Programme Implementation (MOSPI) during the year 2001 constituted the National Statistical Commission (NSC) under the Chairman of Dr. C. Rangarajan.

The Commission observed that a computerised Health Information system at all treatment facilities is an essential prerequisite for establishing an effective Health management Information System. The HMIS has a good potential to provide a comprehensive database on working of health programme at the decentralised level up to the district. The HMIS if properly implemented would reduce delays in the information flow, provide qualitative information in a standardised form, avoid duplication and facilitate quick retrieval of information by all agencies concerned. Some of the key recommendations of the Commission are:

(a) A comprehensive assessment of the Health Management Information System (HMIS) should be made by a small Committee quickly and HMIS be reintroduced in the country in a phased manner with necessary modifications. The combined HMIS format should be separated into programme-wise modules. While revising the program modules, care should be taken to meet the data requirements of both the Central and State Governments. Flexibility should be given to the States and UTs to include additional items to meet their State specific data requirements.

(b) Steps should be taken to rationalise and minimise the number of records and registers maintained by the peripheral health workers such as ANMs and public health inspectors to reduce their burden and to improve the quality of data. The minimum data set on which data from the grass-root levels should be regularly collected along with their periodicity should be clearly identified.

(c) A suitable mechanism to collect the data at the grass roots level and its upward transmission to the district, State and the National level should be evolved and for that methods of data collection, transmission, and processing must be modernised. As NIC facilities are inadequate to meet the requirements of HMIS, adequate funds need to be provided for necessary hardware, software and connectivity and training of personnel.

(d) The Central Bureau of Health Intelligence (CBHI), which is at present a part of Directorate General of Health Services (DGHS) should be separated and upgraded to a full-fledged Directorate of Health Statistics (DHS) directly under the Department of Health. An officer from the Indian Statistical Service at the Additional Secretary level should head this Directorate and act as the Statistical Adviser to the Ministry. Also required posts of supporting officers should be created. The DHS should be the nodal agency in matters of health statistics and should advise the Department in all matters related to the collection of Health Statistics; coordinate with the National Statistical Office the Central and State Governments as well as international agencies in matters related to health statistics.

(e) The CBHI upgraded as DHS should be strengthened with adequate Electronic Data Processing (EDP) personnel and existing personnel should be trained in EDP operations, to enable the processing, tabulation and presentation of the large volume of data on health. Adequate funds out of the national health programmes should be earmarked for development and maintenance of information system as well as for verification of field level performance data through independent agencies.

(f) In order to facilitate effective implementation of the HMIS in the States and UTs, the State Department of Health and Family Welfare in every State should have a Statistical Division headed by a senior level statistical officer. In the districts, a health statistics cell should be set-up in the Office of Chief Medical Officer (CMO) to implement HMIS and to take care of all health and family welfare statistical activities of the district.

Following important recommendations emerged:

(i) Computers at NIC district centre are hardly available for entry of HMIS and other health data. It is, therefore, necessary that the requisite hardware with accessories and the latest operating softwares are provided to the District Chief Medical Officer and Directorate of Health Services at State/UT HQrs. with common software.

(ii) The trained personnel may be available at district and state level for operation maintenance of computer hardware and softwares. Each programme should have a component of training in "General awareness to computer, data entry, programming, etc." at district and state level. The requisite fund may be kept at the disposal of District Chief Medical Officer and Directorate of Health Services/State Bureau of Health Intelligence at State/UT HQrs. Distt. Programme Manager to ensure data entry in Distt. CMHO office computer.

(iii) It was strongly felt that 15% of the total cost of hardware may be earmarked for annual maintenance and a fixed amount in every district may be provided towards purchase of computer consumables and other stationery items. There should be a nodal agency at the national level and also at the level for all the programmes responsible for drawing funds from different programmes and make available the registers and formats.

(iv) HMIS format to be revised to independent programme-wise modular formats keeping in view that the modular formats may be uniform over States/UTs and contain gender information and also information by specific age groups wherever applicable.

(v) NIC to Centrally Develop Data entry software with flexibility for add on information.

A Management Information System (MIS) has been defined as "the combination of human and computer-based capital resources which result in the collection, storage, retrieval, communication and use of data for the purpose of efficient management of operations.[11]

During September-December 1962, the Advanced Systems Development Division of IBM conducted a survey to determine the scope and goals of an Advanced Management Information System. The major information problems were found to fall into seven categories:

1. Complexities in the information flow cause major communication problems inhibit responsiveness and growth.
2. *Duplication of effort*: Identical reports are generated, data files are created maintained at several locations.
3. *Variations in field processing*: At the present time, field locations vary the processing similar information and vary information flows.
4. *Inaccessibility of Data*: Useful and necessary data are available, but often in a form, location that makes them uneconomical and unfeasible to retrieve.
5. *Time lapse*: Data are simply not being moved fast enough. Time lags are caused by mail, multiple audit points and varying closing periods. In many cases the data no longer of value when they are made available.

6. *Inaccurate sources data*: The sheer volume of data makes it humanly impossible to be consistently accurate and efficient.
7. *Limited information support*: The relation between the creation of information and servicing of all those who could benefit from it is poor.[12]

MIS has become necessary for organisations to meet the following emerging developments:

(a) Increased complexity of organisations.
(b) Development of technological revolution.
(c) Emphasis on research and development.
(d) Diversification of functions and activities.
(e) Information explosion.
(f) Complex management issues.
(g) Development of computer, Internet, E-commerce and E-Governance. The combined result of all these developments is the need of designing the management Information systems:

> "The purpose of an MIS is to raise managing from the level of piecemeal spotty information, intuitive guesswork and isolated problem-solving to the level of systems insights, systems information, sophisticated data processing and systems problem-solving. Managers have always had 'sources' of information; the MIS provides a system of information. It is thus a powerful method for aiding managers in solving problems and making decisions."[13]

APPLICATIONS OF HEALTH INFORMATION USE IN HOSPITALS[14]

1. Essential for Health and Hospital Planning and Development

One trend all modern hospitals have in common is that the amount of processed information generated per patient is constantly increasing. One survey in a Japanese hospital has shown that the number of clinical tests given to their patients has doubled every seven years for the past 30 years. Similarly, the variety of drugs that are used at hospitals is constantly increasing. Much of this is due to the great advances that have been made by modern medical science and, fortunately, this is reflected in better hospital care. But the reverse side of this coin is that hospital personnel must now cope with an enormous amount of information per patient—a phenomenon often referred to as the information explosion.

Naturally, the information that directly concerns the patient's care is of paramount importance. But it also serves other useful purposes essential to health care.

First, when such information is properly compiled and aggregated, it provides basic data for efficient hospital administration. How each patient is treated can yield important statistical data, while the number of patients handled, categorized by sex, age, and diagnosis, provides basic information required by administrators to plan for the future of the hospital. Similarly, compiled data about clinical testing are vital for the efficient management of the hospital laboratory, and information as to the type and number of prescriptions issued allows the hospital to estimate the drugs the hospital will need for the year.

Second, health information provided by the hospital is needed by civic health administrators at the district level. Such data, accumulated from all the district's hospitals, are essential in formulating health planning for the district, by matching with population statistics, other demographic data and the health resources of the district. The more limited these health resources are, the more accurate will be the data necessary to conserve them. This medical information then progresses upwards—to the level of national health planning. Thus each root of this informational evolution starts with the physicians' first encounter with the patients.

Third, this medical information, containing not only data about the patient's illness but also the success or failure of therapy, is a valuable source of clinical training for medical students, nurses and allied health care personnel who are privy to such information. It is not an exaggeration to say that a large part of clinical training involves the proper use and the accessibility of this medical data.

The fourth and last point is that medical information is a source of new medicine and therapies. The development of new therapeutic drugs is built upon the careful observations of experienced physicians, and the comparison and analyses of the effects of previously administered drugs, gleaned from the patient's data. This in turn leads to continued medical progress in, say, uncovering a new entity of a disease or a new method of diagnosis.

So, these medical data gleaned from patients from the bedrock of medical science and improved health care, and most of such information is generated in hospitals.

In spite of the importance this medical information has for health care, it is still processed manually in a majority of hospitals the world over. This inefficient method results in delays in reaching crucial treatment decisions, for instance when test results fail to get back to the physicians in time, or in delayed action by administrations when a prompt response is needed. In the fast-paced, populous world of today, it is no longer possible to compile accurate statistics manually from such routine data as grading the patients by sex, age and diagnosis. Simply counting such entries can overwhelm the staff of a small hospital. What of the hospital information systems of the future? They will be even more sophisticated and versatile since constant advances are being made in information handling technologies. Even small hospitals will be able to afford them, and they are destined to become a convenience as common as the telephone.[15]

2. Health Information for Epidemiology

Epidemiology is the health discipline that deals with the "distribution and determinants of disease frequency" in human populations. It should be quite obvious from this definition that epidemiology is essentially a quantitative science that deals basically with the need to collect, process, analyse, evaluate and disseminate statistical information about disease occurring in communalities.

It is a fact that no other health discipline handles such huge volumes of data. Large cohort studies often involve monitoring thousands of individuals over a long follow-up period to determine disease incidence. Probably the largest such study ever conducted was the Salk vaccine field trial of 1954 for the prevention of poliomyelitis, which involved the participation of nearly a million school children.

Epidemiology has traditionally been closely associated with health statistics and, in turn, with the use of computers because of the need of handle data. Computer programmes for data-processing and statistical analyses have been in use or mainframe computers for more than 20 years. Many of these statistical programmes could not also run on microcomputers, making it possible to perform "number-crunching" activities of epidemiological data on desk-top machines.

The principal sources of epidemiological data include health surveys, institutional records containing demographic and medical data. The information collected on forms has to be subsequently checked, coded and processed, and experience has shown that errors commonly occur at this point.[16]

3. Making Health Professionals Experts in HMIS

Health professionals are increasingly interested in the use of computers and especially micro-computers, for health statistics and epidemiology, not least because the price of today's microcomputer hardware now makes these machines affordable to them and, in some cases, to students. Microcomputers can now be found on the office desks of doctors and in the research laboratories of health scientists. These individuals have been asking about microcomputer-based statistical software that they could use with their desk-top machines to carry out data handling and management functions.[17]

4. Expert System in Medicine

Medicine is a discipline that requires both judgement and action. Information science can help in several aspects:

- it can help the physician in collecting complete and relevant data;
- it can support the physician by providing access to the rapidly increasing sets of medical knowledge through different kinds of data bases; and

- it can facilitate the management of medical records which may be used for clinical follow-up of patients, clinical research, evaluation of medical action and education.

In all these aspects, information science gives indirect help to medical decision. But there are many other practical uses designed to help the physician directly in what he considers as his personal privilege: the decision process itself.[18]

5. Co-ordination World Health Organisation involving all members in information sharing

The new science of informatics—the science of the collection, evaluation, organisation and dissemination of information by computers—has innumerable applications in the field of public health. Here are just three examples of the use WHO making of computer technology to share information with its 192 member-countries. An example of informatics support to WHO's International coordination activities in the field of water and sanitation is the Country External Support Information System (CESI). The system is a sector management information tool which is maintained by WHO and used by governments and external support agencies. Its purpose is to improve the planning (including resources allocation) and management of water and sanitation projects.

CESI is a computerized database of drinking water supply and sanitation projects in developing countries which have received or are seeking external support. The system was developed to run on microcomputers by WHO's Division of Environmental Health (EHE) in collaboration with the Division of Information Systems Support (ISS) at the Organisations headquarters in Geneva. The EHE Programme in WHO collects information about continuing and completed projects from external support agencies (bilateral and multilateral funding institutions, US agencies, and non-governmental organisations). Extra data on projects under preparation come both from the agencies and from the governments of developing countries.

In essence CESI offers the opportunity for all those operating in the sector to share information regularly, so that aid can be directed where it is most needed and inefficient overlap can be avoided. It should soon be feasible for CESI to exchange information electronically with other systems. Meanwhile, data from agencies with manual record systems or non-compatible computers are received in printed form, for manual entry by WHO. CESI output is also sent regularly to participating agencies in printed form or on computer diskettes.[19]

The computerized EPI Programme Information System (CEIS) was developed in 1984 to enable a microcomputer to monitor, evaluate and report the activities of WHO's Expanded Programme on Immunization (EPI). Programme managers both in WHO and its member-states need information for planning, evaluation and disease control. The CEIS contain six core indicators, immunization coverage, disease incidence, coverage surveys, training courses, funding and demographic data.

In developing countries, blindness is a major health problem whose control depends on the application of simple measures by frontline health workers, because specialist medical care is not always readily available. To help primary health workers in managing common and potentially blinding eye disorders, WHO's Collaborating Centre for Prevention of Blindness and Trachoma at Brown University, providence, Rhode Island, USA, has developed a prototype system to run on a hand-held computer, which incorporates a set of WHO guidelines for primary eye care, including diagnosis and treatment. With the aid of the expert knowledge that can readily be extracted from this system, the health worker manages patients with eye problems by one of three actions: definitive treatment with no referral necessary; initial treatment with referral to a secondary care centre; or referral with no treatment.

The prototype of the hand-held computer version of this system has been field-tested with primary health workers in Egypt and Tunisia, where the prevalence of serious eye diseases such as trachoma is relatively high.[20]

6. Equipping Employees with Hospital Information to provide Decent Health Care

A health information professional must understand why information is important before using a computer to process it and communication technology to transmit it. All hospital personnel directly involved in looking after patients are obliged to process a large amount of information, so as to provide good care. Physicians. for instance. must obtain each patient's demographic data and a history of the illness, note the signs and symptoms manifested. and compile a past treatment history and associated information in order to arrive at a diagnosis for treatment. Nurses. in turn, need much of this information to formulate a proper care plan. After which they must note the patient's daily progress. Laboratory technicians require details as well. to conduct tests that the doctor has ordered. the results of which are sent back to physicians. Pharmacists too need certain data. to supply the necessary medication. All these examples show that a large part of the daily work of doctors, nurses. laboratory technicians, and pharmacists consists of information handling, perhaps up to 40 per cent of their hospital working day.[21]

7. Time Savers

Fortunately, new technologies are now emerging which help to process this information far more accurately and efficiently. To the computer are now added allied machines that can undertake, for instance, imaging in the audio-visual field and rapid data transmission. Gradually, all these time-savers have been brought into hospitals to solve the problems created by the information explosion. Such technologies have been melded into a uniform system which is designed to meet hospital needs and is generally called a hospital information system.

The basic concept of such a system is to create a cumulative file of each patient's data, which can be quickly updated on a continuing basis. This type of data file in computer terminology is called a database. Once each patient's database is created and regularly updated. Data handling at the hospital improves tremendously, enabling a section requiring specific information on a patient to obtain it rapidly from the database. The information is delivered by a printout from a computer terminal in a standardized form. Or the physician may type an order into the computer data-base, which the computer then transmits to the laboratory as an instruction to perform clinical tests for a certain patient, the laboratory also receiving pertinent data that is stored in the patient's database. Similarly, when a physician uses his or her computer terminal to write a prescription into the patient's database, the computer transmits the prescription immediately to the pharmacy, while the prescription information is kept and accumulated in the database, which provides this information to the administrator in the form of hospital supply statistics. It Statistics become far easier to compile, and the data can be easily copied on to a diskette for transmission to the district level, where similar medical data from all the district hospitals can be compiled by another computer into a statistical analysis of any district-wide health matter.[22]

8. Operating Efficiencies of Organisations

A health care system is a complex network of integrated, though largely autonomous, public and private sector components. These includes individuals, institutions such as hospitals, community health agencies, occupational health departments, public health departments, clinics and doctors offices, laboratories, medical, nursing and other health professional schools, accrediting and licensing bodies, local and central government bodies and vendors of goods and services.

Health care is gradually recognizing at it needs someone to establish and implement a long range information systems plan which is consistent with the organisation's objectives and direction. That person has to determine the investment to be made in information technology and provide a rigorous and disciplined framework for evaluating information benefits *versus* information costs; anticipate and understand the consequences of new information technology; and plan and coordinate all information resources within the organ—Important not just computers. Even more important, such a person must explain the impact of information technology to staff at all levels of the organisation.

A multitude of forces—for instance, aging population which is living longer, and a doubling of medical knowledge Every five years thus forcing health care disciplines into more and ore specialisation which fractionalize are and complicates communications are generating increasing demands for more reliable and timely information, and more effective systems to coiled, process and distribute data. Health care services need information systems which enhance the operating efficiencies of their organisations and help to determine the efficacy of their procedures. In turn this calls for individuals who truly understand the information needs of the many people dedicated to the delivery of care, the promotion of health, the prevention of disease and the postponement of disability.[23]

SETTING UP A TASK FORCE

A Task Force on HMIS was constituted by the Ministry of Health and Family Welfare during March, 2000 under the chairmanship of DGHS with the TOR's to:

(a) Suggest a format of reporting from Districts and States that could capture health information required for purposes of planning, monitoring and review.

(b) Suggest the manpower structure at District, State and national levels for a commonly agreed system of data collection, data entry and data analysis.

(c) Agree on the formats of data collection at various levels and its analysis.

(d) Reconfigure the system of statistics and data gathering at the national level to provide for a more effective and efficient internal organisation that meets the requirements of States.

(e) Develop illustrative structures of coordination among various health data interventions including IDSP at district and State levels.

(f) Weed out unwanted data collection systems and replace them with a consolidated and comprehensive data system; which can thus satisfied; the need.[24]

ESSENTIALS GOOD HEALTH INFORMATION SYSTEM

1. Accuracy and Timeliness

The information collected must be accurate and must be available in time, otherwise its use would be limited.

2. Quantitative Adequacy

Information collected should be adequate to suit the needs of the organisation. The collection of more information than required would cost more and thus increase unnecessary expenditure. Therefore, we must collect only as much information as is needed by the various levels in an organisation.

3. Designing of Tools According to the Needs

A good information system should not be a prestigious show-piece. It should be according to the needs of the organisation.

4. Cyclical Flow

The information must flow constantly, otherwise its use would be limited.

5. Economic Value

The economic value of information is measured by the gain achieved from using such information. One expert even remarked that "at least 50 percent of the cost of running our economy is information cost. Herbert A. Simon says: "Information should be gathered upto the point where the incremental cost of additional information is equal to the incremental profit that be earned by having it.[25]

6. Recipient's Point of View

Information conveyed to a receiver should infuse the desired knowledge in him. The value of information must be measured by the receiver in terms of its uses to him.

7. Managerial View

Management Accounting Information has to meet these requirements:[26]

(a) It must be informative in the sense of decreasing the amount of uncertainty.

(b) It must demand action. The collected information is worthwhile, if and only if, it indicates action relevant for the achievement of certain goal.

(c) It must motivate an appropriate action. Unsatisfactory results must be prevented by its use.

OPERATIONALIZING OF MIS

MIS has the following elements:

- Inputs (data)
- Analysis and Processing
- Storage and retrieval
- Output
- Flow

Both the input and the output are directly related to information requirements of organisation. The information includes both the inflow of the input as well as the outflow of the information. The information processing, analyse and storage can be manual, mechanical and electronic. Let us now discuss the steps for Design and Installation of MIS. The following steps are necessary for installing MIS:

1. Analysis and determination of system's requirements
2. Design of MIS
3. Procurement of necessary material
4. Installation
5. Operation and follow-up

We must keep in mind that all these five steps are interrelated. The system in improved through the interaction of these steps,

1. Analysis of System's Requirements

It analyse, in depth, the systems requirements. Such an analysis will require answers to questions like:

- What are the objectives of the organisation?
- What are the activities to be carried out?
- What type of evaluation is required to assess the impact of its activities?
- Who will collect the data?
- How will the data be collected?
- Where, how and by whom will the data be processed?
- How accurate and reliable should such data be?
- What will be the frequency and timeliness of the report?
- Who will use the information generated and how will it be used?

2. Design of Information System

The next step is the actual design of an information system covering all its five elements already mentioned, in such a manner that it fulfils with minimum cost and in the required form, the information requirements of the administrator. The following points may be kept in mind:

(a) The data generated at various levels should correspond to that actually needed for management at that level.
(b) The necessary links between the various sub-systems of the management information system should be provided.
(c) An appropriate method for the processing and analysis of basic data should be designed. The workers may be trained to understand the meaning and the value of the data, so that they can play an active role rather than being mere passive transmitters of data.

3. Procurement of Necessary Material

The third step is the production of necessary material and. the provision of required facilities so that the system could be put into operation, e.g., for a manually operated system the formats have to be produced.

4. Installation

The information system should set-up, keeping in mind and retaining as far as possible existing procedures and system. It may replace the other components which require change.

5. Operation and Follow-up

The output of the system is examined against the objectives for which the system was designed. It should be the endeavour to continuously improve upon the system taking into account the changed situation.

MAJOR THRUST AREAS SUGGESTED/RECOMMENDED DURING XI FIVE YEAR PLAN

1. While prioritizing Efficient Health Information System (HIS), to begin the States/UTs should strengthen the existing State/UT health statistics unit in their respective health and FW directorates with identified nodal officers, trained personnel and computer so as to effectively coordinate for validated health data base and capacity building in State/UT and closely link with CBHI. Subsequently States/UTs to make efforts for establishing a dedicated State/UT Health Statistics Division, equipped with adequate infrastructure. This Division be responsible for efficient HIS, validated health database of the State/UT. monitoring and evaluation as well as capacity building, while keeping close linkages with CBHI and various reporting unit within the State/UT.
2. At district level, Chief Medical and Health Officer is responsible for all health statistical activities under whom the existing Distt. Health Statistics cell be strengthened by the States/UTs and efforts be initiated to equip this cell with a dedicated trained officer as its incharge and a Group C staff oriented in computer operation and atleast one computer with accessories. This Distt. Health Information Unit can then coordinate for efficient health information system in the district, including on the spot supervision and related capacity building of PHCs and other Health units in the district.
3. At PHC/CHC/Dlapensary level, the States/UTs should make efforts to orient and reorient the medical officers and health supervisors towards health data management through continued supportive supervision and wherever necessary through in service training program organized by State/UT, CBHI and other Institutions. A close coordination with all the existing government/non-government health institutions in respective jurisdiction will ensure maximum coverage of health and medical data with requisite quality and timeliness.
4. Since ANMs at grass root levels are heavily loaded due to their

multitasking operations it is necessary to reduce their workload by providing two MPW(F) in each sub-centre as per IPHS requirements. They should be given the responsibility of maintaining registers for all health and family welfare related database. The acute shortfall of MPWs (64211 out of sanctioned strength of 81561) has been a cause of concern not only to provide basic health services but also to document the quantifiable services as a pivot for health management information system. Similarly there is an urgent need on part of all the States/UTs to fill in all the post of MPW (male) at both, Sub-Centre and PHC levels, that will be responsible for collection of health related information.

5. There is a acute shortage of CHCs too. To maintain the norm of having one CHC per 1,00,000 population, the present requirement is at least 7415 CHCs, against only 3043 CHCs. Moreover, in the 3,043 CHCs that we do have. only 440 have a pediatrician, only 704 have a physician, only 780 have a gynecologist and 781 a surgeon. So not only is the infrastructure inadequate, we don't even have the staff to use the existing infrastructure. Such a large shortfall in medical and paramedical personnel has got an important bearing on the low priority of the documentation of the information, which should on priority basis be attended by all concerned state/UT and central level health authorities.
6. Central and State/UT Governments may bring an act for compulsory registration of all private/non-government medical institutions and practitioners with the State/UT Government and mandatory for them to furnish medical health reports to appropriate Government Health Facility in their vicinity.
7. For Monitoring of Information and Evaluation System (MIES) an integrated format on different health indicators is being developed under RCH/NRHM with an aim to ensure uniformity in the health information collection system avoiding the multiplicity of formats, weeding out redundant information and thus leading to qualitative dissemination with varying periodicity
8. In order to maintain data quality which is required to be used as inputs for any decision-making, the exercise of validation at different levels hardly needs any emphasis. Since NRHM had already initiated the concept of establishing Programme Management Units at state and sub-state levels, their involvement in the validation process should be ensured. In addition, possibilities may also be explored to associate and identify a nodal officer in the district health offices so as to assume the ownership of data being transmitted from the district to the state.

9. What is most important is to remove any underlying apathy to collect the health information and document them with greater speed and accuracy. This can be achieved by putting the right people at the right place having a data sense and data use. The States have got a greater visible role to play to ensure this important aspect of HMIS. To improve the quality of data, the grassroots level functionaries need to understand the importance and use of data generated at their level so that the recording and reporting of data by them could be improved. Also, the monitoring system at all levels need to be strengthened and emphasis should be on monitoring of all programmes/ components, strengthening feedback mechanism and utilization of data at all levels for monitoring and planning purposes. States/UTs may ensue all measures to fully utilize the in service training programs of CBHI on Health Statistics and Medical Coding (ICD-10) as well as Medical Record Management, being organized for various categories of medical/non-medical staff involved in handling medical/health data, for which purpose CBHI communicates its annual training calendar well in advance to all States/UTs. For this purpose, every State/UT should prepare district-wise inventory of such training needs, people trained and remaining to be trained and utilize this inventory for promptly recommending the names of untrained personnel to various CBHI in-service training courses. The GIS mapping is an essential tool now-a-days. NIC has already developed GIS maps up to the village level. The facility should be availed by all the State/UT authorities for GIS mapping on various health indicators.
10. The Birth and Death Registration System in the country is still way behind and there is an urgent need to improve the system. The Civil Registration System must be improved and strengthened. For this purpose the ASHA, recruited under NRHM can also be utilized for recording and reporting the birth and death cases to the appropriate authority with a suitable honorarium.
11. The capacity building of the Health manpower starting from grass root level is extremely essential and allocation of funds for providing the training must be earmarked in this plan period. The training on the electronic data management system should also be provided in association with D/o IT and NIC.
12. ICD-10 coding system be implemented throughout the country for comparison at both, national and international levels and the use of ICO-10 be concurrently monitored by hospital administration for timely corrective measures at various levels, including meeting the ICO-10 trained manpower needs.
13. As already decided by the MOHFW/GOI, it will be desirable to

strengthen IDSP as a national health information system with appropriate computer connectivity rather than pursuing the HMIS which was conceived about two decades back and could not succeed for various reasons. In the present context, this Union M/o Health and FW is committed to ensure the efficient implementation of IDSP which is one of the major projects undertaken with World Bank loan. Apart from the work on surveillance, also attempt to collect information on financial, logistics, manpower and implementation aspects in the health sector.

14. Like CBHI has developed a central website for health information, the States/UTs may also initiate efforts to develop similar websites along with district specific health information, while utilizing the available expertise of 15, States/UTs may initiate steps towards computerizing the Hospital Information System in a phased manner to begin with state/regional level hospitals. This will facilitate efficient hospital database on morbidity and mortality based on ICD-1O, essential for District/ State/National Statistics on morbidity and mortality. likewise at the grass root level, on a pilot basis the .use of Hand Held Electronic Device can be explored in association with the Ministry of Information Technology.
15. A National Institute of Health Information System, as already recommended by NCMH may be considered, for which purpose, CBHI be properly upgraded with necessary supports from public health, statistics and national health programmes to play the role effectively. This institute will also be responsible for Human Resource Development and research studies. NIMS, ICMR may be involved in taking up evolution studies and operation research periodically. The recommendation of National Statistical Commission to upgrade the CBHI as a full-fledged Directorate of Health Statistics as a nodal agency to provide sufficient inputs on health statistics should be seriously pursued. The M and E division of the Department of Family Welfare which is responsible for collecting and collating all Family Welfare information including RCH should be merged in the proposed National Institute of Health Information System. Keeping in view the recommendations of NRHM, the synergy between the Health and Family Welfare Information System need to be made and this Institute should be responsible for Monitoring and Evaluation of all health related programme including RCH.[27]

Advantages

The following advantages can accrue from a good information system:

(a) Timely availability of information develops a high degree of confidence between top executives and the members of the management.
(b) The management need not resort to frequent meetings to sort out various issues.
(c) The executive time can be saved and devoted to critical issues.
(d) It helps in reviewing actual performance and enables taking corrective action.
(e) It helps in reviewing strength and weakness of an organisation, knowledge of which it is most essential in formulating future plans and strategies.

Confederation of Indian Industries, in their background paper, "Rethinking Government" rightly suggested that the recent information and technological revolution is helping the Governments to:

- Stimulate economic competitiveness.
- Streamline and integrate citizen services providing convenient "one stop" access to services and information.
- Enhance the quality and effectiveness of traditional government services (e.g. social services, public safety, courts).
- Deal more successfully with fiscal constraints.

The importance of informatics to development has been recognised and expressed in many different fashions. The overall message, however, is that informatics technology is an all embracing technology and one which will affect strategic and operational issues. It is not a sector of development but has become a key tool and strategy to development. No country can afford not to join the information revolution, nor can it avoid its all-pervasive impact. As to the question of whether developing countries should embrace informatics, having recourse to the most advanced technology is not a luxury for the poorest countries. They are the ones that most need to own such technology, since they can then shape its development and ensure its social relevance and cultural coherence.

Top executives today, have to manage the ever increasing rate of change and large scale and complex organisations. In the managerial world of increasing complexity both in magnitude and direction, information becomes the key to management effectiveness. Therefore, we must give priority in designing and installing MIS to suit the requirements of specific organisations. The success of MIS would depend upon "First, The quality of leadership that corporate executives provide. Next, the planning and control tools that management has built into the computer system programme. Third, the role operating management plays. Finally, calibre of the computer and systems staff."

It is difficult to direct or manage successfully an information system department. Quality information systems are expensive to produce and, in many cases, even more difficult to maintain. Systems generally take a considerable amount of time to develop, test and implement. They require a high level of professionalism and expertise from the technical staff, who are often only all too aware of their importance to the organisation and are therefore sometimes perceived as being difficult. Traditionally, not enough effort has been expended on the professional management of the information system function, and it is now necessary to rectify this mistake. This requires training for information system executives in the discipline of management.

In addition, there is frequently no service culture among information's system staff. Their focus on technical excellence has outweighed their concern for business issues in general and specifically for their users. Although this has been tolerated for many years, it is now perceived as being a mistake which needs urgent rectification.

There are many other challenges, which top management and information systems managers or directors have to face, in order to operate an efficient and an effective information system service. Many of these have been mentioned in this Chapter. These challenges have always been well handled, for many different reasons, and frequently mistakes have been made. As well as listing some of these mistakes, we suggest some possible courses of action which may be taken to alleviate some of the problems.

It is hoped that by having thought about these traps, organisations will be more alert to the problems and perhaps they will make sufficient resources available in terms of funds, people and time so that better information systems decisions, and thus ultimately better administrative decisions, are made.

Information, possibly the most valuable asset of a global society, seems to have a life of its own. Once limited to oral transmission, then by papyrus, movable type, and now the Internet, information is bound up with human progress. Yet we are vulnerable to its misuse. Like a virus, it can quickly multiply out of control, it is difficult if not impossible to eliminate, and it can only be managed with varying degrees of success. Though information has become essential for the maintenance of health, it can take dangerous forms that must be addressed if they are not to cause harm.

To realize the potential of the Internet as a source of valuable healthcare information for the general public, patients, and practitioners, it is imperative to establish a validation system and standards of quality. International cooperation is needed for the establishment of standards, such as those governing the publication of medical literature.[28]

MIS should be designed to ensure smooth and proper flow of information into the desired channels. The information must be made available to the management at the required time and in right quantity and quality. It is also to be borne in mind that supplying unnecessary or unwanted information is also a sign of inefficiency of the system. Information Services should be recast according to the priorities of the administrative system and should be aimed strictly at problem-solving.

Besides, there is always a communication gap between the statisticians (so-called information specialists) and the management people. There is a need of understanding between these two wings, otherwise, information generated would serve no practical purpose.

The reason for the failure to fully utilize management information system can be laid on management's own doorstep. These reasons include the following:

1. Management is conceptually unprepared for the revolution in information technology.
2. Management does not plan adequately. The planning is mostly parochial rather than corporate-wide in scope.
3. There is not enough fresh thinking and too much reliance on canned approaches.
4. The wrong people are selected to plan and install the system. The wrong people include specialists who fail to appreciate the business or management who fails to become sufficiently involved.
5. There is an overemphasis on hardware and an under emphasis on the design of comprehensive system.[29]

A useful MIS must have a reasonable cost compared to its worth. The economics of information system requires constant balance between the value of the information carried in the system and the cost of designing and operating it. An MIS cannot act or think for management, and can only shape thoughts and assist in the evaluation of situations.

It is difficult to direct or manage successfully an information system department. Quality information systems are expensive to produce and, in many cases, even more difficult to maintain. Systems generally take a considerable amount of time to develop, test and implement. They require a high level of professionalism and expertise from the technical staff, who are often only all too aware of their importance to the organisation and are therefore sometimes perceived as being difficult. Traditionally, not enough effort has been expended on the professional management of the information system function, and it is now necessary to rectify this mistake. This requires training for information system executives in the discipline of management.

CONCLUSION

The importance of informatics to development has been recognised and expressed in many different fashions. The overall message, however, is that informatics technology is an all-embracing technology and one which will affect strategic and operational issues. It is not a sector of development but has become a key tool and strategy to development. No country can afford not to join the information revolution, nor can it avoid its all-pervasive impact. As to the question of whether developing countries should embrace informatics, having recourse to the most advanced technology is not a luxury for the poorest countries. They are the ones that most need to own such technology, since they can then shape its development and ensure its social relevance and cultural coherence.

People dealing with health are those who ought to be most at ease with informatics and telematics, if only because their development owes a great deal to the biological model which has inspired cyberneticians, systems specialists and computer information scientists. In addition, we can think of organic life as a process of absorption, processing and transmission of information. Life stops when the body can no longer receive or emit information. Today the proper and efficient use of relevant information has become indispensable for the survival of human societies as well.

The main issues which strategies and policies in informatics and telematics for health have to face are those of finance, management, training and research. What ought to be emphasized is that the need for these new technologies is, at times, inversely proportional to the level of development of a country. Informatics may well become one of the basic ingredients of any health policy, and even turn out to be a very efficient instrument for primary health care strategies.

One does not have to undertake sophisticated cost analyses to assess what can be gained by investing in informatics support to such areas as the management of drinkable water or the control of epidemics. No country, as poor as it may be, can afford not to make a minimal effort to use informatics and telematics to effectively improve the health of its population, especially at a time when human resources have become the main key to development.[30]

Notes and References

1. Raymond, J. Coleman and M.J. Rilley (ed.) Management Dimensions, Holden-Day WC 500, Samseone Street San Francisco, California, p. 15.
2. James J.O. Brien, P.E.: "Management and Information System", Van Nostrann, New York, 1970, pp. 2-3
3. Harper Marion: "A New Profession to Aid Management", Charles Collidge Parlin Memorial Lecture, p. 13.
4. Consumer Informatics, Health Informatics Series, p. 80.
5. Robert G. Murdkick, "MIS for MBO", *Journal of Systems Management*, March, 1977.
6. *Ibid*.
7. IBM Corporation Office Products Division, "Preliminary System Design for Project OMNT", New York, The IBM Corporation, pp. 10-11.
8. Report and Recommendations of Sub-Group, on Health Informatics for the XIth Five Year Plan (Convenor, Dr. Prof. Arvind Pandey, Director, NIMS).
9. *Ibid*.
10. Salah Mandil, "Health Informatics", *World Health*, Aug. 1989, p. 5.

11. W.C. Churchil, *et. al.*, "Proposed Research on MIS", Management Science Research Report, No. 54, p. 2.1.
12. IBM Corporation Office Product Divisions, "Preliminary System Design for Project OMNI", pp. 10-11.
13. R.G. Murdich, Information Systems for Management, Prentice Hall, 1985, p. 14.
14. *Ibid.*
15. Shigekoto Kaihara, "Information Explosion", *World Health*, Aug. 1989, pp. 6-7.
16. *Ibid.*, p. 9.
17. *Ibid.*, p. 11.
18. Roger Salamon, "Expert Systems in Medicine", *World Health*, Aug. 1989, p. 12.
19. *Ibid.*, p. 17.
20. Shigekoto Kaihara, "Information Explosion", *World Health*, Aug. 1989, p. 11.
21. Shigekoto Kaihara, Information Explosion", *World Health*, Aug./Sept. 1989, p. 6.
22. *Ibid.*, p. 7.
23. Denis Protti, "A Need for Information Professionals" in *World Health*, August, 1989, p. 26
24. Planning Commission Working Group on Health Informatics Including Telemedicine for XIth Five Year Plan (2007-12) Report, August 2006, p. 1.
25. Herbert A. Simon: Theories of Decision-Making in Economics and Behavioural Science, *The American Economic Review*, 49, June 1959.
26. John Debold, ADP, "The still sleeping Gaint", *Harvard Business Review*, Sept. 1964, p. 61.
27. Proceedings of the Meetings of WG-HMIS held on 5th July and 1st August, 2006.
28. Consumer Informatics, Health Informatics Series, pp. 80-81.
29. John T. Garrity, Getting the most out of your Computer, New York, Mckinsey, 1964, p. 13.
30. Mahdi Elmandjra, "Informatics and Telematics: the Future", *World Health*, Aug. 1989, p. 28.

APPENDIX 4.1

Health Performance Network

The National Knowledge Commission (NKC) is convinced that extensive use of IT in health care will promote the delivery of efficient health care in the country. However as the use of IT in the management of health care and medical knowledge will increase, the health care establishments will develop and use their own health IT systems. It has been the experience of western countries that these individually developed systems are often not interoperable with other establishments, which makes the health care system inefficient and expensive. NKC believes that India has a unique opportunity to learn from the world experience and adopt only the proven best practices in the field.

In this context NKC constituted a working group, under the chairmanship of Dr. N.K. Ganguly, Chairman Indian Council for Medical Research (ICMR) study of the use of IT in future health care. The working group studied the future need, conducted several meetings and deliberations and held consultations with various national and international experts. NKC believes that the use of IT in health care needs a national direction for its proper implementation and makes the following recommendations for developing a Health Information Network.

1. Initiate Development of Indian Health Information Network

India needs to develop a web-based network, concocting all health care establishments, in both private and public sector. When fully functional, all health care transactions will be recorded electronically and this data will be available in the health data vault to authorized users when they need it and where they need it.

The proposed Knowledge Network with gigabit capabilities may provide the backbone and network infrastructure on which the Health Information Network may ride. The network will be a hub and spoke model. All health care establishments in a district will connect to a central data repository at the district level. All the district nodal data repositories will connect with a state level data bank, which in turn will connect with a central data bank.

There should be active involvement of private and public health entities to effectively address the creation of this network, portals, electronic health records, health data vault, security, privacy and other related issues in future, which will encourage the participation of the following:

- Citizens
- Health care providers and payers
- Education, research institutions and investigators
- Government departments and institutions
- Public health agencies and NGOs

- Pharmaceutical industry and medical device makers
- Telemedicine institutions
- Software and hardware developers

The ready availability of information will accrue enormous benefits to public health planning, medical education, cost control, medical research, drug development, prevention of fraud, disaster management and improved patient care.

2. Establish National Standards for Clinical Terminology and Health Informatics

For a web-based interoperable national grid it is imperative to have common clinical nomenclature, or else disparate programmes developed by the industry will not be interoperable. The clinical standards will establish a common lexicon to be used in electronic transactions. This will enable all geographically scattered entities to communicate in one common language and facilitate data transmission and collection. It is important to develop common nomenclature standards for the traditional medical systems, as large number of people depend on these systems for their medical needs. Besides the common clinical language, adoption of a common national standard in health informatics will facilitate the messaging, collation and analysis of data.

3. Create a Common Electronic Health Record (EHR)

An electronic health record (EHR) is the record of a persons from birth to death where all heath care encounters are recorded. Health transactions are presently recorded in a paper format, like a hospital patient chart, prescriptions, laboratory tests, etc. The technology to capture and store this information electronically already exists and has been developed by many private and public organizations in India. For uniform data capture, storage and subsequent use, it is recommended to create a common national EHR based on common clinical and IT standards. The record should be able to capture data generated by the traditional medicine health providers. To promote the early adoption of the health IT, this EHR may he given free of cost or at subsidized rates to all users. The other IT tools and applications can be developed by the private industry and should be compatible with The National HR.

4. Frame Policies to Promote use of IT in Health Care

The use of IT in health care needs an impetus from the government otherwise the development and penetration will be slow and arbitrary. These policies should be formed, not to hamper, but promote the health IT business in the country and generate employment in this sector. The central government should declare a time period after which all transactions in health care in the country will be in electronic format. Sufficient time should be given for the health establishments to adopt electronic transaction. NKC feels 7-10 years is an adequate time for all parties to evolve electronic transactions after which all health establishment should be able to comply.

5. Create Appropriate Policy Framework to Protect Health/Data of Citizens

The integrity of data at the primary data collection site will determine the usefulness of this enterprise to ensure that only correct patient and other health data is collected, it is of utmost importance to gain. The confidence of the citizens that their health data will not be misused by the health providers, insurance companies, employers and the government. Both technological and legal framework is important to achieve this. While encryption, anonymity and other IT security measures should be in place; it is also important to have rules in place. It is important to maintain confidentiality and security of the personal health data and to govern the access and use of data.

6. Medical Informatics to be Part of Medical and Paramedical Curriculum

Medical education needs to make full advantage of the power of ICT. A well-structured health informatics curriculum needs to be made an integral part of medical education are all levels. Basic ICT facilities, such as good quality access to Internet and e-Journals, need to be made compulsory for all medical colleges in the country. For capacity building, IGI fools should be effectively deployed to train the large number of health workers. Short and medium-term courses need to be developed and made available on the net to address training needs of all health workers in the field. It should be made affordable, accessible and easily available for small players. There is a need to evolve common formats for data reporting to facilitate IT enablement of medical manpower at all levels. Education-related portals should also be set-up for training of medical manpower.

7. Create an Institutional Framework for Implementation

An autonomous body with the Ministry of Health should be responsible for planning and implementing the project in a time bound manner. This body should be autonomous and a non-profit organization with representation from private, public and voluntary sectors. All stakeholders should be represented in this body and it should have the resources to promote and implement the plan. It should also have the authority to ensure the smooth functioning of the Indian Health Information Network. The objectives for this institutional body will be:

- To formulate an implementation plan.
- To coordinate the participation of all stake-holders.
- To create linkages with e-governance medical education network.
- To ensure financial viability of the project.

- To set-up a comprehensive and interactive national health portals.
- To suggest common national standards.
- To protect confidentially and security of data.
- To facilitate the ownership, access and flow of data.
- To maintain and upgrade the system in future.

The next step in the development of Indian Health Information Network is to formalize the institutional body with appropriate professional people with domain expertise, adequate budget, time tables, and measurable milestone to implement these recommendations. The body may consider conducting pilot programmes before scaling at the national level.

Source: National Knowledge Commission, 2006-07, Government of India.

5

CHAPTER

Telemedicine

With the area of 32,87,268 sq.km, population of 1.1 billion, urban-rural divide, inaccessible hilly regions, islands and many tribal areas, India is an ideal setting for telemedicine assisted health care delivery. Growing number of medical, paramedical colleges and schools with lack of adequate infrastructure, learning materials and teachers needs is a matter of grave concern. E-health technology has the potential to create a national level GRID which can form the backbone to be shared by healthcare providers, trainers and beneficiaries. A strong fiber backbone and indigenous satellite communication technology in place with large mass of human potential trained in IT and local presence of telepathy industry, E-health application and implementation should not be a problem technically. Further a number of pilot projects over last five years with successful outcome stand to its testimony. A ground work on telemedicine in the country has already been laid with the efforts of ISRO and Information Technology Department partnering with many State Governments and specialty Institute/hospitals. Policy standardization and infrastructural issues have already been researched. However, a country level plan is long due to steer the Telepathyship by the Captain (M/o Health and Family Welfare/ Government of India) with its crew (technology and healthcare providers/ educators) and passengers (citizen) in right direction (policy, implementation, application, security, social and legal issues) to reach at the destination (Quality Healthcare and Wellness).[1]

Health Telematics is defined as a composite term for health-related activities services and systems carried out over a distance by means of information and communications technologies for the purpose of global health promotion, disease control and health care, as well as education, management and research for health.[2]

Telemedicine, the practice of transferring medical data using interactive audio, visual, and data communication systems, is quickly

CHART 5.1

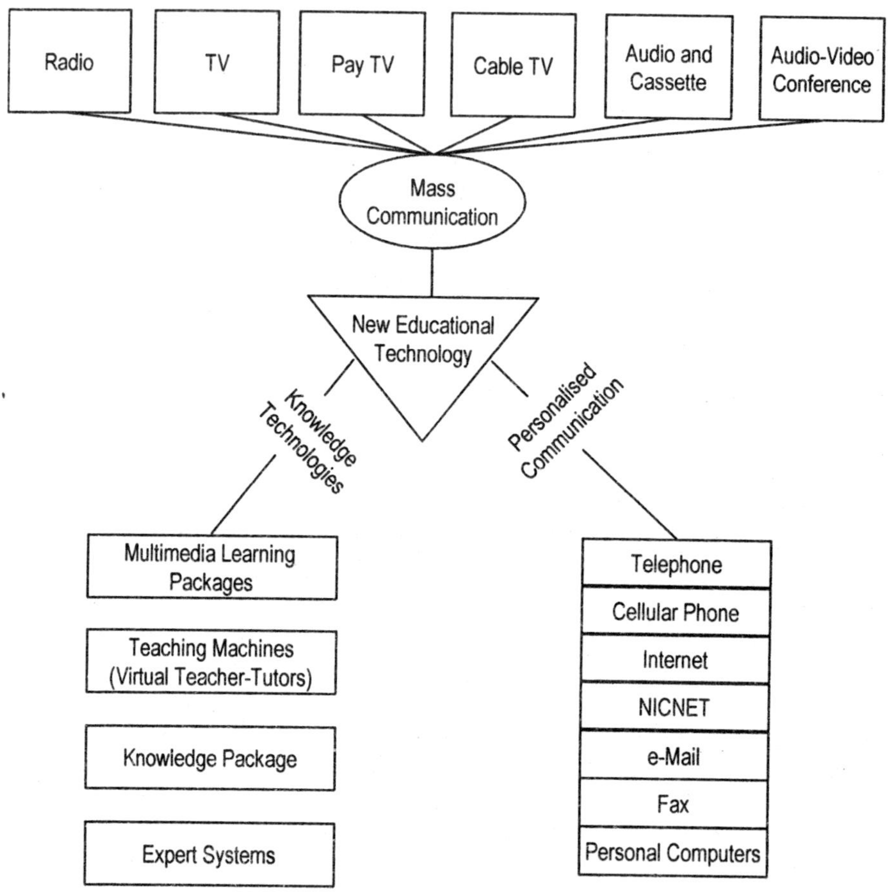

becoming indispensable in modern medicine, healthcare delivery, and education.

Telemedicine has been defined as the use of telecommunications to provide medical information, services, and care to people located at any place.

At the University of Kansas telemedicine Program, telemedicine technology has been used for several years for oncology, mental health care to patients in rural jails, hospice care, and most recently, to augment school health services by allowing school nurses to consult with physicians.

Cyber medicine, defined as "the science of applying Internet and global networking technologies to medicine and public health" adds a new dimension to telemedicine. The global coverage of networks extends the scope of information available to patients. In this evolution, physician-physician and patient-physician communications are enhanced by patient-patient relationships (e.g., through e-mail exchanges or formalized discussion groups). Curative and palliative care are complemented by predictive and preventive medicine in which the active patients, not only the health care providers, are at the center of the health network. For example, health assessment tools can directly provide the individual with a personalized analysis of his or her lifestyle habits and risk profiles for common diseases, as well as orientations for changing behaviour (e.g., stress management, body weight reduction, smoking cessation, etc.).

Self-medication and self-care become part of a global healthcare process in which the gatekeeper role of the general practitioner (primary care) is bypassed by the creation of direct links between patients and specialists (secondary care) from one side, and patients and non-physicians (e.g., nurses, community pharmacists, patients' groups) from the other side. It also paves the way for a new business, the e-health business, for which providers are looking for future clients in the promising market of citizen-oriented health products (e.g., dietetic and pharmaceutical products, fitness programs, behavioural programs, etc.).

Although a variety of telecommunication media can be employed for telemedicine systems, in general these systems link clinicians and patients together synchronously or asynchronously. Systems that provide a synthconous or "serial" link allow one clinician to interact with one patient at a time. This often necessitates a predetermined appointment for the interaction to occur so that both parties are available. Although this approach lessens patients' travel burden, it is still labor-intensive. In general, "serial" systems are video-based, either with direct video links or streaming video through the Internet.

Telemedicine systems that operate asynchronously or "in parallel" allow one clinician to monitor multiple patients simultaneously. These systems are partially or fully automated and usually have a computer system interacting with the patients. Using predetermined algorithms, these automated systems supplant the routine monitoring of patients and notify appropriate personnel when problems are detected. Although the degree of personal clinician inter-action varies with these systems, by necessity it is limited compared to face-to-face interactions. Personnel costs are decreased with these systems, and patient monitoring, albeit automated, can be increased. These systems often employ store-and-forward technology.[3]

Telemedicine in its true sense is the transmission of medical information in the form of audio, video, text and images of patients from one location to another, using telecommunication channels. The main communication is between two or more clinics, hospitals, institutions and health centres, within a country or outside, for consultation, advice and opinion. Telemedicine also means transfer of expertise from one point to another and it is the fastest means of communication for consultation for improvement and efficiency in diagnosis and treatment. In addition, high quality medical services of specialists and super-specialists can be readily available using telecommunication and computer technology.

The Telemedicine system can improve rural health care especially primary and secondary care of patients attending community and district hospitals. The technology can improve professional interaction between rural health professionals and their colleagues with urban medical specialists. We must understand that the quality of interaction between distant physicians becomes significantly improved when they communicate via telemedicine networks because it conveys more than just their voices through telephone conversation and discussion. The Store and Forward architecture in Telemedicine system allows consultants and specialists to share images, sound clips and graphical data of the patients, not confined to verbal discussion. The interactive and synchronous video conferencing allows physicians and distant specialists to interact with each other along with their patients and not just voices on telephone. We must realize that in Telemedicine technology the whole nature of interaction between the physicians along with the information (patient's record) conveyed to them is greatly enhanced. In fact, this is a face-to-face discussion or advice and opinion between the patients and their physicians located at different and distant places.[4]

Dr. Prakron Vuthipongse, permanent Secretary, Ministry of Public Health, Thailand, in Inter-country Workshop on Tele-Medicine for Health Development in 21st century from 30th March-3 April, 1998 at Bangkok said that as a decision-maker he was aware of the advancement in today's technology, especially in its applications which will help to bring letter quality of health care to people in remote and rural areas in a cost-effective manner. He also said that the initiation of Tele-Medicine in the Ministry of Public Health has emerged from the fact that, in remote and rural areas, there has been mal-distribution of medical specialties, resulting in poor health care services. He expected the workshop to come up with fruitful recommendations on regional and national plans of action as well as on inter-country cooperation.[5]

However, this very conference cautioned about the use of Telemedicine: Health Telematics raises certain ethical issues, such as the acceptability of transmitting personal information across cultural boundaries; young doctors getting professionally affected, and the confidentiality of the relationship between the patient and the treating doctor. Full cooperation of the medical and paramedical staff involved, as well as patients is essential. Even in the most advanced form, Health Telematics might not provide a blanket solution for each situation. There would be cases where human intervention is needed. It also raises concern on widening the gap between the poor and the privileged.[6]

Thus, in the new millennium the use of tele-medicine offers a potential source of latest knowledge, however, we must use it with great caution and thought.

Dr. R.A. Mashelkar, Director General, Council of Scientific and Industrial Research, delivered the convocation address at the 30th Convocation of Indian Institute of Technology, New Delhi. He said,

"Knowledge without innovation is of no value. It is through the process of innovation that knowledge is converted into wealth and social good. Innovative nations lead the world today. When one looks at India, one feels that centuries of subjugation have perhaps undermined our capacity for innovation and creativity, which has got to be revived. We cannot allow the 'I' in India to stand for imitation and inhibition, it must stand for innovation. This requires an all pervasive attitudinal change towards life and work—a shift from a culture of drift to a culture of dynamism, from a culture of idle prattle to a culture of thought and work, from difference to confidence, from despair to hope. Revival of creativity and the innovative spirit needs to be made into a national movement today, in the same spirit and on the same scale as marked our freedom struggle.[7]

Dr. R. Chidambaram, Chairman, Atomic Energy Commission and Secretary to the Government of India, Department of Atomic Energy, delivered the Convocation Address at the Third Annual Convocation of Shivaji University, Kolhapur, he said, "For a nation to grow and advance rapidly, it has to strive for excellence in all its spheres of activity.[8]

Dr. Shivayogi P. Hiremath, Vice-Chancellor, Kuvempu University, Shimoga (Karnataka) delivered the Convocation Address at the Graduation Day—1999 of JJM Medical College, Davanagere. He said, Doctors on the net is a common caption in most of the Western Countries. Why are so many people turning online for medical information? Experts suggest that there is something inherent in the quick turnover medical office visits that it leaves patients wanting more and more connection, more personal interest, more explanation and more help."

A doctor has to be a constant student and should always work hard to keep abreast of the field by regularly attending the Continuing Medical Education (CME) programmes.[9]

ADVANTAGES OF TELE-MEDICINE

1. Accessibility

Providing healthcare services via telemedicine offers many advantages. It can make specialty care more accessible to underserved rural and urban populations at a low cost with high quality. Video consultations from a rural clinic to a specialist can alleviate prohibitive travel and associated costs for patients. Videoconferencing also opens up new possibilities for continuing education or training for isolated or rural health practitioners, who may not be able to leave a rural practice to take part professional meetings or educational opportunities. Continuing Medical Education is essential as the technology is changing fast.

2. Useful for low income and unserved childrens

A TCP Press Release, September 13, 2007 observes, "Telemedicine is a powerful tool that helps overcome major obstacles low-income and underserved children and families face in obtaining the health care they need", said Wendy Lazarus, Founder and Company-President of The Children's Partnership. "For children living in medically undeserved areas—both rural and parts of urban areas—telemedicine can address health care provider shortages, transportation costs, and lost time from work and school, by using technology to bring the care to where the children are."

3. Useful in Emergencies and Disasters

It is not too much of a stretch of the imagination to realize that telemedicine will soon be just another way to see a health professional, just as seeing friends and family while talking to them on the phone is becoming commonplace. Farther down the road, it has been theorized that we each could have a 'personal Diagnosis System' as part of our home entertainment centers. This system would monitor our daily health status and automatically notify a health professional if we become ill.

4. Outreach to remote areas

Telemedicine in clinical practice is a new concept to India while it has been in practice in the developed world for quite sometime where it is also culturally accepted. We have a situation where a patient irrespective of the distance he/she is located, can get almost instant specialist/ superspecialist advice for his/her ailment which facility hitherto was available only to those living in metropolitan cities. In the absence of availability of proper guidance from a specialist, we have lost many precious lives. The importance of Telemedicine will be appreciated only when its benefits trickle down to our remote rural and semi-urban areas where 80 percent of our population lives. It is doubtful whether there is any other single development, which will allow social justice in our Health Care programme, if the technology is implemented properly. The technology helps us make full use of the specialist/superspecialist services available for bringing solace to millions of people living in semi-urban and rural areas.[10]

5. Consultative Services to Individual patients

The FDA (The Food and Drug Administration, USA) an authority which regulates the medical field as well, define Telemedicine as "The delivery and provision of health care and consultative services to individual patients and the transmission of information related to care, over distance, using telecommunication technologies and incorporating:

1. Direct clinical, preventive, diagnostic and therapeutic services and treatment,
2. Consultative and following-up services,
3. Remote monitoring of patients.
4. Rehabilitative services, or
5. Patient education.[11]

6. Helps in continuous medical Education through Distance education.

While considering the educational paradigm shift, the Report of the Task Force of International Council on Distance Education (1996) identifies four major factors as drivers of educational change:

1. The Explosion of Information.
2. Emergence of Information Technology.
3. The Changing Nature of Work.
4. Changing Student Population.

All the developed countries are now moving from the industrial to the post-industrial or information societies. Some of the changes in fields such as computer applications are so fast that the packages become out-dated within 2 to 3 years and new technologies/applications offer more economical, generalized and integrative solutions to current issues. In fact, the speed of changes is making any long-term visualization very difficult. Our vision of the 21st century, therefore, cannot go far beyond and, therefore, we may restrict ourselves to the first quarter of the 21st century that networking with broad band communication with integrated multimedia can afford.[12]

7. Patient Empowerment and Professional Education

To enter into a win-win mode of cooperation with proactive patients. Healthcare professionals should be prepared for in-depth revision of their education and training programme and accept deep change!; in their attitude with patients. Appropriation communication and Internet technique is a technical prerequisite for all physicians who need to collaborate with other professionals and patients through health information networks. Physicians' background on the principle of evidence-based medicine is another prerequisite to be able to respond to the checklists and to the structured questions that might arise from their patients. Knowledge on the general aspects of prediction (e.g.. genetic counselling), prevention and environmental disease relationships should complement highly specialized knowledge on disease prevention and treatment strategies.

Physicians should be ready to direct patients to sources of high-quality Health-related Web sites including bibliographic databases, evidence-based Knowledge sources such as the Cochrane Library or dedicated interest groups. Physicians also should share their favorite sources of information with other Professionals and patients, Providing information on the Internet is no longer

8. Potentialities of the Holistic View of Media

With the integration of a variety of communication media into the education system, distance education has come to play a major role in universalizing medical education. The technological environment of distance education has changed more significantly with the introduction of live, interactive media. These media are markedly different from other distance education media, in the sense that they are directed towards group interaction rather than individual interaction. With the explosion of technology, distance education is increasingly being defined not by the technology used for delivery but by the nature of interaction involved in the educational process (Garry E. Miller, 1994).

Teleconferencing, because of its interactive nature is also referred to as "virtual conference." Virtual conference creates an analogue of communication forms that typically occur in a face-to-face conference, including paper presentation, discussion, moderation, questioning and answering, etc.[13]

IGNOU has been using Interactive ETV for its students and counselors. Many experiments have been conducted to experiment the utility of these technologies like CEC-ISRO-UGC-IGNOU Teleconference (December 1524, 1994), NOS, DECU-ISRO Talk back Experiment, (December, 1996), etc. Based upon these experiments D.R. Goel and D. Sarang made the following observations which need analysis. To quote them:

(i) The technical, instructional, economic feasibility, legal viability and social acceptability was established and it proved the operational possibilities of an interactive Distance Education system.

(ii) Potency of teleconferencing as an instructional tool in direct classroom, enrichment education and professional training was realized through the experiments.

(iii) In most cases technical coordination among the technologists and pedagogists was very successful.

(iv) Except in few cases of improper use of media-materials due to technology unfamiliarity on part of the academicians and learners, occasional technological shortcomings and personnel management, the experiments were successful in preparing for the operational level.[14]

However, it may be added that its large scale use needs caution, advance preparation and financial resources availability, pooling of resources, understanding the environment of the country, and the needs of the learners.

9. Training in latest medical technology

Conventional classroom training is considered to be too slow and inefficient to keep pace with change. Moreover, administrative hurdles, which include setting up infrastructure and finding tutors, have stymied the growth further. Traditional distance education modes like postal coaching have also failed, as these are non-interactive.

Special packages can be developed for different specializations and given to special category.

Limitation

There are many limitations to use telemedicine:

(a) Medical personnel who have neither high qualifications nor experience can cheat the public to make money.
(b) Facilities of telecommunication are the essential feature of telemedicine. It is non-existent in many areas of developed countries and more so in developing countries.
(c) Funding for telemedicine is limited. Funds are being allocated mostly for direct hospital services.
(d) Efforts are being made but still not very effective by pooling the resources from health, education, government and business to make use of the facilities. It means pooling of resources.
(e) All the medical personnel are not competent in handling health care through telemedicine.
(f) There have been many frauds in telemedicine. There is a need of law and policy for medicine.

RECOMMENDATIONS OF ELEVENTH FIVE YEAR PLAN

Information Technology is now one of the major components of the technological infrastructure for health management. All sub-sectors dealing with the generation, transmission and utilization of demographic and epidemiological data such as bio-informatics, bio-statistics, HMIS and the decision support systems (DSS) are finding increasing use in health planning and management. The nationwide network of NICNET provides rapid reporting mechanism for health information; MEDLARS Biomedical Informatics Programmes provides ready access to medical databases to post-graduates and research workers as well as practicing physicians. Planning Commission has provided additional central assistance to the UHSs in Karnataka, Andhra Pradesh, Tamil Naidu, Punjab and Maharashtra for strengthening of libraries and networking them through IT. This effort has to be augmented and all medical colleges need to be brought into the network.

Indian Space Research Organisation (ISRO)

ISRO has been actively engaged in applying space technology for healthcare and education through specific initiatives which include *inter-alia*:

(a) Providing telemedicine technology and connectivity between remote/rural hospitals and super-specialty hospital for tele-consultation, treatment and training of doctors and para-medics.

(b) Providing technology and connectivity for continuing medical education between medical colleges and post-medical institutions/hospitals.
(c) Providing technology and connectivity for mobile tele-medicine units for rural health camps in the areas of opthalmology and community health.

A number of initiatives in tele-medicine have been made in the private sector, SGPIMS, Apollo Hospitals, Asia Heart Foundation, Escorts and others are presently engaged in extending consultations through tele-medicine and are conducting regular tele-education, tele-consultation and tele follow-up sessions with patients.

Need for strengthening telemedicine/e-health initiatives in India

Despite the massive public health infrastructure, healthcare in rural areas remains a critical challenge. The magnitude of healthcare services required in the context of the existing shortage of medical officers and trained para-medics clearly demonstrate the need for strengthening tele-medicine and other e-health initiatives over the next Plan. The National Rural Health Mission provides an opportunity for taking tele-medicine to the healthcare facilities at the primary, secondary and tertiary levels of care. Computerization of health related data would be an essential first step.

With the establishment of about 300 Telemedicine nodes by Government/Private/Trust agencies of which 175 nodes by ISRO all over the country and the experiences gained by each of the implementation agencies have brought to bear some of the important issues that needs to be addressed for future implementation strategies for the development of telemedicine and e-health for augmenting the present healthcare delivery system in the country.

Major thrust areas for 11th Five Year Plan

- Establishment of e-Health department in M/o H&FW in states D/o H&FW with support of state IT Department.
- Computerisation of health care delivery system and health records at state, institutions, district and taluk/block level for the flow of information over the network.
- Computerisation of three tier healthcare system: CHC/PHC and SC.
- To acquire and implement IT equipments like servers and client systems, multicast video conferencing facilities, data storage and archival facilities in all the specialty hospitals, medical institutions and other centres of excellence who will be providing teaching and training facility.
- To identify agencies within the medical institutions/speciality hospitals/research institutions to develop content for medical education/CME/training modules.

- To acquire and implement terrestrial/wireless/satcom technologies required for various connectivities from taluk/block to district to the state capital.
- To plan for one dedicated medium weight class Communication satellite (HEALTHSAT) for satcom-based connectivity which will have the capability to meet the broadband connectivity requirements for various applications of the National Grid.
- The cost of HEALTHSAT with launch, operations and maintenance of the satellite is around Rs. 400 crores. Apart form this, the various connectivity charges by other technologies have to be incorporated. The present cost of a standard telemedicine node including computer hardware/software and video conferencing system is around Rs. 4.0 lakhs at the district hospital level. Whereas at the CHC/PHC level the cost will be around Rs. 1 to 1.5 lakhs. Hence number of nodes which will come up during the 11th Five Year Plan upto the block level may have to be worked out.
- All tele-medicine network should evolve around a National tele-medicine grid. Ultimately, every individual would need to have a unique ID.
- Formal specific training programmes in tele-health for all levels (grass-root to policy-maker depending on requirements) and facilitate a support system to provide current information to doctors in the management of patients through new data bases, software packages, etc.
- Medical Council of India to include Information Technology in healthcare in the curriculum of all medical and para-medical degree courses. Information Technology to be also included in all IT and MBA courses.
- Introduce at least one mobile van in each district.
- Trauma care, ambulance on National Highways to be provided with technology for transmitting audio-video images using EDGE, GPRS, MMS, etc. Pilot studies using tele-medicine and ambulances would be required.
- Setting up of a Tele-health Corporation of India. Given the highly specialized and technical natural of tele-medicine, a Tele-medicine Board of India needs to be established under the aegis of the Ministry, which will include a set of technical experts with representatives from major healthcare organisations and NGOs working for tele-medicine. The basic objective of this Board would be to oversee the growth of tele-medicine, develop R&D tools, provide software, manage the National tele-medicine grid and interact with international organisations.
- E prescriptions at all levels by the end of XII Plan but to cover atleast PHCs and above during the XI Plan. This will necessitate availability of computers and net facility at all healthcare facility.

- Minimum standards of treatment to be documented and made available on the Ministry of Health website. Details should be available regarding new drugs, banned drugs, new identifications, list of essential drugs, adverse effects, standard treatment protocol, drugs of choice, etc. Skill, knowledge and care should be the corner stone of what we strive for.
- Magnitude of care may vary at different levels but the standard of care to remain the same. This will be possible once the standard treatment protocols are available and will help in identifying the kind and nature of drugs to be placed at each level and the financial requirements for making available these drugs at different health facilities.
- Synergy amongst all existing initiatives and programmes between different Departments/Ministries in the area of health.
- TCI network being created under Department of IT.
- North-Eastern Council initiatives with support from ISRO.
- E-governance initiatives like common service centres under Department of IT.
- Integration of existing infrastructure like CBHI, IDSP, NICD, etc. in the Ministry of Health and F.W. to have proper synergy between them and avoid duplicity in data collection, compilation and transmission.
- Proposed Tele-medicine project by Delhi Government.
- Any other State initiative/Central project which will cater to health needs and requirements.[15]

10. Role of Telemedicine in Disasters

The United Nations telecommunications agency recently deployed 50 satellite terminals, which are capable of providing telemedicine services, in remote areas of southern Peru as part of its efforts to restore vital emergency communication links to the region in the wake of last month's deadly earthquake. The 50 "plug and play" terminals, which are portable devices the size of a small suitcase, allow users to make calls to telephones, access the internet and provide other voice, data and video services, such as telemedicine.

The Geneva-based International Telecommunication Union (ITU) said in a statement that the terminals are being deployed to areas where telecommunications were served because of the damage caused by the quake. Rescue operations in Peru have been hampered by the often mountainous terrain. "We take very seriously the role of telecommunications in mitigating disasters", said Sami Al Basheer Al Morshid, Director of ITUs Telecommunication Development Bureau.

"Whenever a country is affected by a disaster, we quickly mobilize and dispatch transportable telecommunications resources that can be used for general communications by government authorities and to provide e-services such as telemedicine that are crucial for saving human lives", he

Chart 5.2

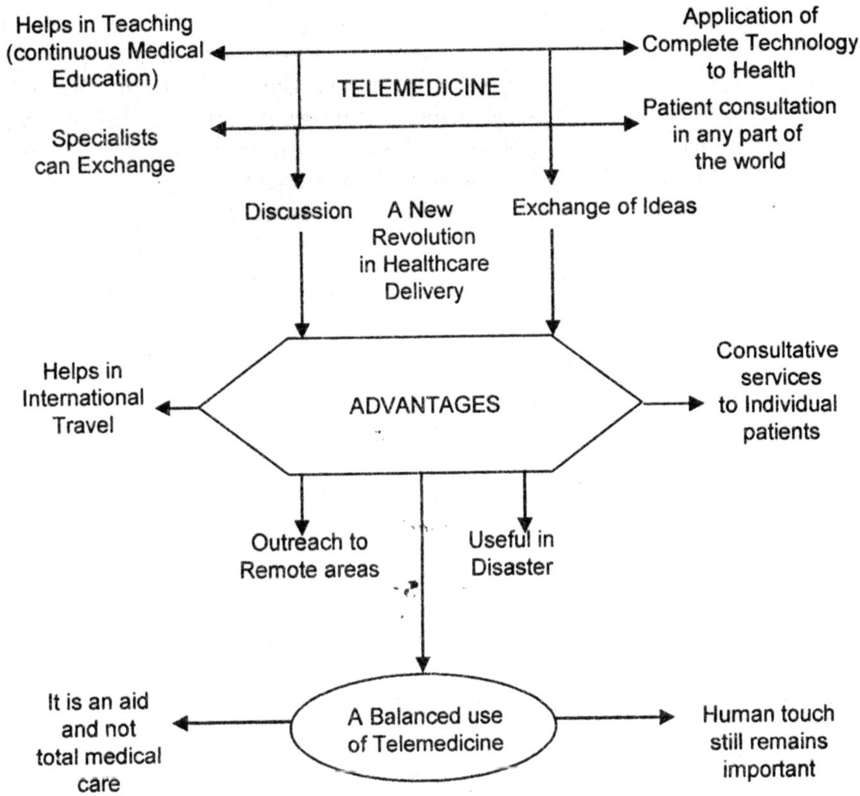

added, voicing hope that the contribution would help Peru cope with the recent massive earthquake. So far, the ITU has allocated more than $ 500,000 to cover the costs of deploying the terminals and paying for their use, but officials said this figure may rise.

Cosmas Zavazava, head of the Emergency Telecommunications Division of the ITU, told the UN News Service that the agency is planning to launch in December a framework for cooperation in emergencies that will include a fund to pay for the deployment and use of equipment. The 15th August quake, which measured 7.9 on the Richter scale and struck 161 kilometers south of the capital, Lima, has resulted in the death of over 500 people and injured more than 1000 others, according to the UN office for the Coordination of Humanitarian Affairs (OCHA). In addition, preliminary assessments indicate that over 37,000 houses and four hospitals were destroyed, while 16 hospitals were damaged.

Source: United Nations Press Release, September 7, 2000).

11. Role of Telemedicine in Travel especially International Travel

We often see people in the airport preparing for foreign travel who seem far removed from the robust young people featured in travel ads. They are in wheelchairs, supported by oxygen, and many require considerable physical assistance. Yet they are traveling long distances and may be entering a truly alien landscape of medical response, relative to the one that has cared for them thus far. These intrepid travelers are not rare. This chapter does not address the issues of the medical traveler coming to the United States seeking health care. That broad topic is related but is not the subject of this section. The medical evacuation and medical assistance programs available for repatriation will be given only short coverage. The focus of this chapter is the emerging resources of electronic information and telecommunications to support the traveler with regard to health needs. Electronic information and telecommunications applied to health care define telemedicine. No matter where you are, you should be in an electronic continuum with familiar, competent, and interactive health care. In this brief chapter, the scope of medical issues in travel will be considered along with the comparative anatomy of health services in the United States and abroad. Most important, the excellent resources in telecommunications and electronic information will be reviewed along with those services that the public demands and the steadily improving technology may bring to bear in the near future. Ideally, our medical care should be as portable as our medical conditions.[16]

CONCLUSION

With the integration of a variety of communication media into the health and medical system, telemedicine has come to play a major role in improving the health and medical care system. The environment of health and medical system has changed more significantly with the introduction of hire and interactive media, i.e. Telemedicine. Teleconferencing because of its interactive, nature is also referred to as virtual conference. The Telemedicine if properly planned and implement can change the health and medical system in India.

It's not too much of a stretch of the imagination to realize that telemedicine will soon be just another way to see a health professional, just as seeing friends and family while talking to them on the phone is becoming commonplace. Farther down the road, it has been theorized that we each could have a "Personal Diagnosis System" as part of our home entertainment centers. This system would monitor our daily health status and automatically notify a health professional if we become ill.

NOTES AND REFERENCES

1. GOI, Planning Commission, Reports and Recommendations of Sub-Group II on Telemedicine for the XIth Five Year Plan.
2. WHO: SEARO, Health Telematics, Report of a WHO Inter-country Workshop on Tele-medicine for Health Development in the 21st Century, Bangkok, Thailand, 30th March-3rd April, 1987, p. 4.

3. Patrice Degoulet, Marius Fieschi, Marie Christine Jaulent, Springer, 2004 and Joel Menard, Patient Empowerment Cybermedicince and Citizen Education, Consumer Informatics, Health Informatics Series, pp. 129, 132.
4. B.D. Gupta, Introducing Telemedicine, Deep & Deep Publication, 2005, pp. 1-2, 52.
5. WHO: SEARO, Health Telematics, Report of a WHO Inter-country Workshop on Tele-medicine for Health Development in the 21st Century, Bangkok, Thailand, 30th March-3rd April, 1987, p. 2.
6. *Ibid.*, p. 5.
7. AIU, *University News*, Sept. 20, 1999.
8. AIU, *University News*, April 21, 1997.
9. AIU, *University News*, Aug. 19, 1999.
10. S.K. Sharma, Forward, Introductory Telemedicine, B.D. Gupta, New Delhi, Deep & Deep, 2004.
11. B.D. Gupta, *op. cit.*, p. 7.
12. UGC: Contribution of Education in National Development—Ninth Five Year Plan and Future Perspective, New Delhi, 1996, pp. 47-48.
13. M.D. Ushadevi, Virtual Conferencing Hearing through Mediated Technologies, *University News*, Sept. 29, 1997, AIU, New Delhi, p. 6.
14. D.R. Goel and D. Sarangi, "Interactive Distance Education: A Summative View of Indian Teleconferences", in *University News*, 35(42), Oct. 20, 1997, p. 11.
15. Planning Commission, Working Group on Health Information including Telemedicine (WG-HTM) for XIth Five Year Plan, 2007-12.
16. Health Informatics Series.

6

CHAPTER

Medical Tourism

Tourism has been in existence from times immemorial. There were many objectives of tourism. Different people preferred tourism for different reasons. Some traveled for sight seeing, some for business, some to attend government meetings, some for adventures, etc. Very few used to travel for natural tourism, i.e. people go to Switzerland for good climate for health, some used to come to Himachal Pradesh to get cured from Tuberculosis. There are many places in the world where there are mineral springs where bathing can cure many skin and other diseases. My recent visit to Budapast (Capital of Hungary) made me learn that there are more than 200 places where mineral bath can cure a number of diseases. Medical Tourism, i.e. patients going to different countries for treatment is fast becoming a world-wide industry involving huge money. The medical treatment in USA being costly, people from that country are seeking treatment at a quarter or one-tenths of the cost at home. From Canada, people come for treatment as the waiting time is very great. People are coming from poor countries where treatment is not available.

Pope John Paul II, states that: "The world is becoming a global village in which people from different countries are made to feel like the next door neighbours. In facilitating more authentic social relationships between individuals, tourism can help overcome many real prejudices and foster new bonds of fraternity. In this sense tourism has become a real force for peace.

Medical Tourism can be defined as cost effective private medical care for patients needing specialized hospital care services because either those services are very costly in their own country or are not available in their country.

Medical Tourism is perceived to be one of the fastest growing segments in marketing "Destination Incredible India" and is poised to be the next big success story after software. The key competitive advantages of

CHART 6.1

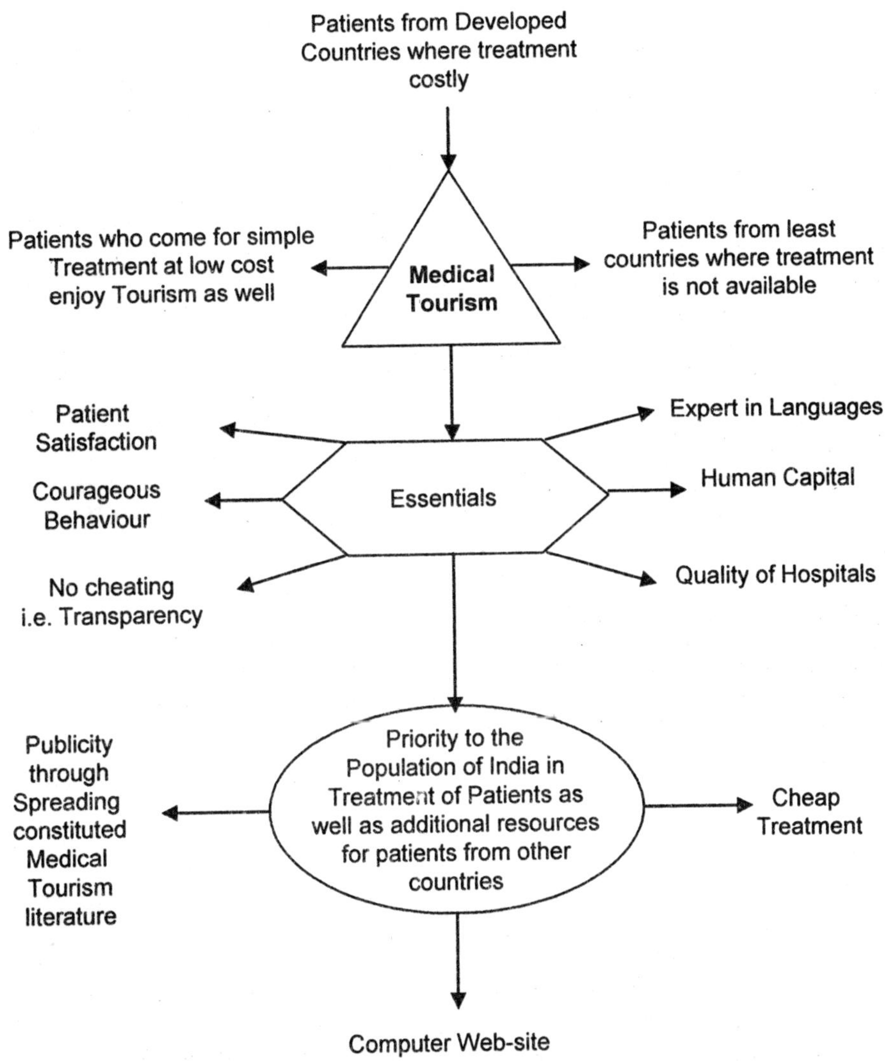

India in medical tourism stem from its low cost advantage, strong reputation in the advanced healthcare segment such as cardiovascular surgery, organ transplants, eye surgery and the like of tourist destination available in the country. Health tourism or the feelings of wellness is a new emerging concept. Spas, stress relief, centres for rejuvenation are different services growing in demand. Many people come to India for the rejuvenation and overhauling the human machinery through Indian system of medicine. However, India has to compete with Singapore, Thailand, Malaysia which have highly developed hospitals and well developed tourists spots. Every state of Indian Union is developing first class hospital services to cater to the needs of foreign tourists.

Promotion of health tourism will require a judicious blend of both quality health services and developing tourism industry. This will entail quality services, sound infrastructure, qualified personnel, health providers, cost effective management, etc. in the realm of tourism, the building blocks will be marketing, communication, hotel services, etc.

The Ministry of Health and Family Welfare in close coordination with the Ministry of Tourism is evolving strategies to give a strategic push to open the Indian Healthcare Sector to foreign tourists. The policies adopted by other countries for accreditation of their hospitals are also being examined to gain from their experiences in taking this forward in India.

Some measures for rationalizing the flow of tourists have already been taken. It has been decided that there should be a fast track clearance for the medical patients at the airport. Earlier foreigners coming to India for medical treatment were being granted tourist visa by Indian Mission abroad as tourists' visa is non-convertible, non-extendable and valid only for a period of six months, reports of difficulties being faced has been received. It was, therefore, felt necessary to facilitate foreign nationals who wish to utilize specialized health care facilities to come to India for medical treatment. The matter was considered by the Ministry of Home Affairs and it was decided to introduce a new visa category called "Medical Visa (MED-Visa) and Medical Attendant Visa (MED)-Visa)." A medical category visa may be issued with the following conditions:

(a) The Indian Missions/Posts abroad may scrutizine the medical documents very carefully and satisfy themselves about the bonafide purpose for which medical treatment visa is being requested;

(b) Mission may satisfy that the applicant has sought preliminary medical advice from his country of residence and he has been advised to go for specialized treatment. In case the foreign national desires to go for treatment under Indian System of Medicines, his case could also be considered; and

(c) This type of visa should be granted for seeking medical attendance only in reputed/recognized specailised hospitals/ treatment centres in the country. Although not exhaustive, following illustrative list of ailments would be primary consideration: serious ailments like neuro-surgery; ophthalmic disorders; heart-related problems; renal disorders; organ transplantation; congenital disorders; genetheraphy; plastic surgery; joint replacement, etc. The basic idea would be that the mission may satisfy about the need for foreign national to come to India for medical treatment/health enhancement.[1]

REASONS FOR DEVELOPMENT OF MEDICAL TOURISM

1. Cheap treatment.
2. Priority treatment not wasting time.
3. Enjoy the beautiful and historical places of the country where patient has gone for treatment.
4. Competency of treatment in a particular country.
5. Beautiful location like Dental treatments in Kerala, an Indian state with good scenic spots.
6. Traditional system of the country may be more popular and can treat the patients in a more effective manner.
7. Easy travel and tele-communication has provided the facilities to travel in any country of the world.

India is considered the leading country promoting medical tourism and now it is moving into a new area of medi-city that is developing all types of health and medical facilities at one place purely for treating nationals from other countries. The main purpose is to provide low cost and high quality treatment to earn for the development of the country. All care is being taken to develop these medi-cities in most of the states of Indian Union with meticulous details so that the medical and health services may be second to none. In addition, medical outsourcing where sub-contractors provide services to the over-burdened medical care systems in western countries.

India's National Health Policy declares that treatment of foreign patients is legally an "export" and deemed "eligible for all fiscal incentives extended to export earnings." Government and private sector studies in India estimate that medical tourism could bring between $ 1 billion and $ 2 billion US into the country by 2012. The reports estimate that medical tourism to India is growing by 30 per cent a year.

The largest of the estimated half-dozen medical corporations in India serving medical tourists is Apollo Hospital Enterprises, which treated an estimated 60,000 patients between 2001 and spring 2004. Fortis is coming in a big way backed by a reputed group of Ranbaxy Ltd. They are setting up chain of hospitals. It is Appollo that is aggressively moving into medical outsourcing.

With the growth of medical-related travel and aggressive marketing, Bangkok became a centre for medical tourism. On my personal visit three times, I found that the people are highly dedicated and provide mechanical services from the core of their heart. Soft spoken lady doctors take care of the patients with utmost care and affection. Bangkok's International Medical Centre offers services in 26 languages, recognizes, cultural and religious dietary restrictions and has a special wing for Japanese patients. The medical tour companies that serve Thailand often put emphasis on the vacation aspects, offering post-recovery resort stays.

The newest and fastest-growing area of medical tourism is a visit to the dentist, where costs are often not covered by basic insurance and by only some extended insurance policies. India, Thailand and Hungary attract patients who want to combine a filling, extraction or root canal with a vacation.

PROBLEMS

Experts have identified a number of problems with medical tourism:

1. Patients have to pay cash from their pockets as it would take time for insurance claims to be processed.
2. Consultations about post-operative care has to be done through telephone or computer which may not be the problem.
3. It is not clear whether the laws like consumer protection Acts or other laws to take care of negligence apply to foreigners or not. In addition, such actions are going to take very long time. They are in a need of going Consumer Protection Act to take care of the complaints of foreign patients to build confidence in them.
4. There are growing accusations that profitable, private-sector medical tourism is drawing medical resources and personnel away from the local population.
5. There is lack of proper standardization and accreditation system of hospitals in India.
6. India must devote more facilities to Indian system of medicine which can attract more medical tourists as this is unique for India.
7. Organ Transplantation is becoming high racket. People from affluent countries can come to developing countries for this purpose. This can create danger for people in India as doctors can sell the organs to foreign tourists at a high cost causing malpractices and dangers to life to Indian poor people.
   The first successful kidney transplant was done in 1954 and the earliest liver and heart transplant operations took place in 1967. Kidney transplantation has been established as a regular procedure, with sizeable cost-benefit advantages over continuous dialysis. But both heart and liver transplant programmes, while increasing enormously in numbers, still await confirmation of their risk-benefit importance by careful studies. Other invert or live tissues are also being transplanted such as corneas, bones, eardrums, bone-marrow, lungs, the pancreas and skin. Every year 14,700 kidney transplants take place, while the total number of liver and heart transplants exceeds 3,000 each and is expanding rapidly. Short-term survival rats are satisfactory for kidneys, heart and liver transplantation, but long-term results, both from the clinical and psychological standpoints, are still lacking; all the same, a five-

year survival rate of 60 percent is well within reach both for liver and heart transplants.

In addition to the difficult technical, legal and scientific problems related to transplantation, many questions arise about the ethical relevance of the procedures involved, and these have been answered only in a partial and uncertain way. Although there is a growing consensus that organ transplantation is not only morally permissible but even desirable, important reservations have been voiced about the ethics of some vital factors related to the procedure, such as the definition of death, the circumstances of organ retrieval, and the appropriateness of investing very large sums in order to treat very few, when such expenditure could possibly be used more profitably for the benefit of larger groups of individuals.[2]

8. There is a danger of transportation of diseases through foreign nationals which can become a big problem like Congress Grass from USA.
9. Foreigners in the guise of patients can lay hand on the secrets of the country.

ESSENTIAL INFRASTRUCTURE FOR MEDICAL TOURISM

I. Human Capital

Doctors in developing countries like India are more motivated by money than developing expertise. Human capital in the form of super-specialist doctors, general doctors, nursing and other para medical staff must work with sincerity, dedication, ethical values so that patients coming from advanced countries can get good treatment and going back after treatment talk highly of the hospital and its staff which can encourage other patients to choose India as its destination. The success or failure of tourism depends to a great extent upon the quantity and quality of human elements. There is a need of intensive training for all the staff where foreign tourists are expected to be treated in the art and science of communication as well as how to exhibit their competence.

Dr. Anoop Misra in an issue as "AIMMS: Ailing Institute" in *The Tribune*, Oct. 7, 2007 rightly feels "The overall academic level as well as service was deteriorating, we could not give the treatment prescribed in medical literature. No new equipment was in sight. Machines were neither working nor properly serviced.

Suggestions

1. Medical Education must be geared to promote quality education to get highly talent doctors and other paramedical staff.
2. Doctors must be trained in the art and science of communication to promote assurance and faith.

3. Medical Personnel must be trained to work as a team and not quarrel among themselves.
4. There is a need of training in the art and science of dealing with foreign peoples.

2. Environment of the Hospital

The environment of the hospital must be soothing. It should be located in natural surroundings where patients feel comfortable. It should be neat and clean, there should be playcards to locate the particular facility. In addition, the reception staff must be courteously and is able to guide the patient properly. Lavatory facilities, drinking water, sitting facilities should be made available. Environment has a great role on the health of the patient. The following may be done to beautify the hospital environment:

(i) Plants in pots may be kept at various locations. These may be changed according to the season. The weeds should also be regularly removed through contract arrangements.

(ii) Proper spraying, may also be done to ensure infection free atmosphere. Some sprays with fragrance may also be used. Spread of rodents, flies, mosquitoes should be checked.

(iii) Proper play cards may be displayed for the guidance of visitors.

(iv) Dustbins and waste paper baskets may be provided to avoid littering and proper disposal of waste materials.

(v) Preparation of Tea/Coffee or any other article may be banned in the individual rooms. Tea/Coffee, etc. can be had only in the canteen. Canteen should be equipped with proper exhaust fans to avoid pungent smells.

(vi) Good ideas may be written on the board specially provided for the purpose at the entrance of the building to infuse good thoughts.

If there is space surrounding the hospital it should be well maintained. There should be regular removing of the congress grass and weeds and planting of flowering plants depending upon the season.

3. Facilities in the ward

Foreign nationals who have efficient hospital system in their country but is costly and that is why, they are coming to India. However, the facilities in our wards both government and private are lacking in many respects. Since foreign tourists are coming from countries with well facilitated wards, would find it difficult to adjust in the wards in India. In India, all facilities are either of poor quality or non-functional. These irritants would create bad image among foreign nationals coming for medical treatment.

Suggestions

1. Rooms of wards must be furnished with good beds, linen, sofas, chairs, etc.
2. Food may be served as per the taste of the patients.
3. Behaviours of medical staff to patients must be polite.
4. Services should be prompt with smiling faces.
5. Cleanliness must be maintained.

4. Financial Charges

In foreign countries, charges for all the facilities are well defined and they stick to it as they are sincere in their approach. In India we see a lot of bungling in hospital charges. They charge for facilities which even they did not provide. The financial charges should be extremely fair otherwise the hospital would get bad reputation. We should economise on every facility so that foreigners are treated at a lower cost plus profits to the hospital and thus raising revenue for India.

5. Excellence in Service

A certain degree of informed zeal and identification with tasks entrusted to a functionary with a view to ensure higher levels of performance are the hallmark of excellence in medical and health personnel. The excellence would attract foreign tourists. In the words of Pt. Jawaharlal Nehru:

> "No administrator I, suppose, or anyone else for the matter of that, can really do first class work without a sense of function, without some measures of a crusading spirit: "I am doing this, I have to achieve this, as a part of a great movement in a big cause". That gives a sense of function, not the sense of the individual, narrow approach of doing a job in an office for a salary or wage, something connected with your life's outlook or anything, perhaps being interested, as people inevitably are, on one's personal preferment in that particular work."[3]

Suggestions

1. Services must be provided promptly and timely.
2. Medicine must be of excellent quality.
3. Paramedical staff must speak with the patient to avoid monotony.
4. Only competent people be engaged.

6. Effective Communication

Ideal relation involves a state of communication, in which the doctor and the patient can converse with mutual confidence. It demands doctor's interest, consideration, empathy, friendly objectivity, understanding and the patient's full faith and co-operation. If a doctor clumsily alarms his patient while explaining the treatment or the patient gets frightened, it is a failure in communication. Of the two participants fail to understand each other, either due to language difficulty, lack of vocabulary, wrong use of technical terms, etc. The doctor may fail to understand the idiom, dialect, phraseology or use of words. The patient will either take such a doctor as stupid, in-attentive or uninterested or a snob. Often the patient does not understand what the doctor wants to know and in turn the doctor gets impatient and starts shouting in a loud voice. The problem arises specially when the doctor uses medical terms or Jargoan which he fully believes to be correct. But a doctor who shouts, ridicules or shows indifference would forfeit patient's respect. The doctor has to keep him cool and has to extract the information as to what the patient really means.

7. Improving patient satisfaction

Hospitals should try to establish cordial, equitable and, therefore, mutually profitable relations between the hospitals and their beneficiaries. The patients mostly complain of discourteous behaviour of hospital staff especially at the lower level . . . This irritates the patients and their relatives. The test of the efficiency of a hospital is the satisfaction of the beneficiaries. The sympathetic and courteous behaviour of hospital staff would have a soothing and lasting effect on the patients and their relatives. It is suggested that all hospital personnel must inspire confidence and put the nervous patients and their relatives at ease.

The hospital today is more than the combination of medical and therapeutic treatment by specialists, greater and refined medical and surgical knowledge and ever better and more effective facilities and equipment. It includes these factors as the core of its efficient operation but an additional dimension—one which is too often ignored or at least minimised—is the human and social element in the structure of the organisation.[4]

The ideal of service must be encouraged among the personnel responsible for health care. It is the responsibility of the hospital authorities to set the pattern for the philosophy of patient care. It was rightly mentioned by Gardner that,

> "No society can reach heights of greatness unless in all fields critical to its growth and creativity there is an ample supply of dedicated men and women."[5]

Most of the patients complained of a great distance between the doctors and the patients. This gap between the doctors and the patients must be bridged through personal attention given by the doctors to the patients. According to K.G. Agarwal, "Hospital effectiveness which can be measured in terms of patient satisfaction does not depend on the improvement of hospital service aspect along but on the medical care aspect as well. Hospital effectiveness has a positive association with the hospital social system. The hospital social system is almost the measure of its organisational health . . . some element of democracy must be introduced in the hospitals. This might take care of the alienation of hospital staff that we see all around these."[6] K.K. Kaul, Professor and Head, Smt. Patel Paediatric Centre, Government Medical College, Jabalpur (M.P.), has rightly said,

> To restore their reputation, hospitals need to develop a strong system of public relations and intimate involvement with the community they serve.[7]

The participation of people in the formulation and administration of local and national plans and programmes that affect their well-being is particularly important at a time when developing countries like India are rapidly widening the scope of public services and adopting technological advances for improving their administration. Both developments could make public administration increasingly complex and more difficult for the mass of citizens to understand. Imaginative measures are needed to promote and sustain the interest of citizens in the hospital administration to give them a sense of participation in the decisions that immediately affect them and to enable them to contribute to better administration. Citizen participation in hospital administration is also an important safeguard against the abuse of administrative authority. It is a method for tapping human and material resources for development that might otherwise remain inert.

8. Dealing with foreign patients in a dignified way

The best treatment and medical services must be provided to the foreign patients as he is under emotional strain and surcharged with suspense and anxiety about the consequences of the disease or calamity that has come up suddenly. Such an approach would alleviate a large part of sufferings borne out of the fear and suspicion of the unknown.

9. Supporting Services

In addition to quality care for the patients, there is a need of providing other supporting facilities if we are to ertcourage foreign nationals for medical care.

(a) Directory containing the names of medical institutions, their specialization, charges, accreditation, etc. should be provided to the foreign nationals so that the foreign patient can make up his mind about the place and particular hospital. The names, description of the Institute and other things mentioned in the directory must be verified by the government so that we can release the directory with complete responsibility. If anything goes wrong with the foreign patient, besides the hospital, government would be equally responsible and would have to cut a sorry figure before the international market.

(b) Nodal Person with telephone numbers to facilitate correspondence—The foreign national coming to India may feel insecure in his mind. As soon as he intimates his interest in getting treatment in India in a particular hospital, he should be informed the name of modal officer with telephone numbers so that he can fix all the details with him. The purpose is that no time is lost in useless activities as this would incur extra cost unnecessary charges to a foreign national. He should come and get treated and leave the hospital as early as possible to economise.

(c) Hospital conveyance to pick up the patient—As already intimated, hospital conveyance can pick up the patient from the Airport or Railway station as already fixed. This would save him from botheration and he can proceed straight to the hospital room and his treatment can be started, thus we have to take meticulous care for foreign patients as firstly he is in a foreign land and secondly, he is not in good health.

(d) Deputing for the care foreign nationals persons who can understand the language and feelings—Foreign national coming for treatment is alone and must feel frustrated. In order to keep him comfortable, such persons should be deputed who understand him and can develop good rapport within. The effort must be to provide home environment.

Medical Tourism is a budding area, there is a need to promote this by this very corporation with some trained people in the art and science of tourism development.

10. Hospitals must pay heed to hygiene

Phuspa Girimaji in an article "Hospitals must pay heed to hygiene" in *The Tribune,* dated 14th Oct., 2007 observes that Imagine conducting eye surgeries in operation theaters that are not fumigated. Worse, using instruments, cotton pads and linen which are not even sterilized. The very thought makes one shudder at the consequences. But that was how surgeries were conducted at Dr. Mohan Lal Memorial Gandhi Eye Hospital in Aligarh. Given the conditions in which the operations were done, it was a miracle that out of 52 patients, only 14 lost their sight.

Said the National Consumer Disputes Redressal Commission in its order, "The inquiry reports leave no doubt that there was deficiency in service on the part of the hospital and the staff is not maintaining the autoclave equipment and other materials which were used before and after the operation." Condemning the hospital for its recklessness in treating patients in unhygienic conditions, the apex court regretted that despite several orders of the Supreme Court highlighting the need for maintaining the highest standards of hygiene, health service providers continued to provide poor service, thereby putting the life and limbs of the patients at risk."

Observed the commission: "We hope that the Indian Medical Council as well as the Health Departments would take appropriate steps in improving the standards and maintenance of cleanliness and hygiene in public and private hospitals so that damage may not be caused either to the life or limb of any patient.

11. Marketing

Medical Tourism plays an important role in economic development of the nation. This would generate employment particularly in medical sector but other sectors like transport, hotel, etc. would also be benefited. Therefore, first and foremost requirement to promote medical tourism is to do attractive marketing. Marketing is the first step to make foreign nationals aware of the potentialities of medical and health care in India with complete details. The persons associated with marketing must be dynamic who can convince the foreign nationals about the efficient medical care available in India. Since, India wants to introduce medical tourism on large scale, it is advisable to make use of our embassies abroad. We should not feel pessimistic as marketing to attract foreign nationals take time. For this purpose, some success stories must be used to illustrate the point.

12. Safety

Medical Tourists must be ensured about their safety. For this, law and order administration must be given orientation in the art and science of taking care of the safety of foreign nationals. This becomes all the more important for female as there have been many incidents earlier of rape, molestation, cheating, etc.

13. Courteous Behaviour

All the foreign nationals coming for medical tourism must be dealt with courtesy, humility and affection. Indians must develop good rapport with them so that they feel at home and develop a sweet memory of the country. Good behaviour costs nothing but pays in the long-run

14. Reasonable charges for medical services

We should not be greedy to fleece or cheat the foreign nationals by asking them to pay high charges. This can make more money in short-terms but in the long run, foreign nationals would stop coming and all our resources would become idle. Therefore, we should be satisfied with the golden eggs of the hen and not kill the hen itself.

15. Quality Medical Care

Foreign nationals coming for medical tourism should be provided quality medical services. No compromise should be made with the quality. National academy of science USA defines quality medical care as: "the degree to which health services for individuals and population increased the likelihood of desired health outcomes and are consistent with current professional knowledge."

16. Good governance

Hospital administration must be efficient. The issue of good governance is hammered again and again as an essential to element to solve existing and emerging problems of hospitals. Good governance is about providing an efficient and effective administration that is committed to improving the quality of life of the people. It is about what people expect from the administration, and the willingness and capacity of the administration to fulfil their expectations. The main tenents of good governance can be enumerated as: (i) improved delivery systems for services, (ii) increasing simplicity and accessibility of systems and procedures, (iii) increased fiscal responsibility and efficiency of expenditures through sound financial management, (iv) higher level of accountability and transparency in governance, and (v) stringent anti-corruption measures. Good governance enables a citizen-friendly, citizen-caring and responsive administration, and in the process, results in the exercise of public authority for the common good.

Good governance is about providing an efficient and effective administration that is committed to improving the quality of life of the people. It is about what people expect from the administration, and the willingness and capacity of the administration to fulfil their expectations.

Components of good governance are:[8]

(i). Improving service delivery

- To provide services to the people in accordance with specified standards, devoid of harassment or corruption, minimising waiting time or inconvenience to the members of the public;
- To ensure cost effectiveness in the provision of services by adopting the most appropriate system;
- To adopt participatory mechanisms in public service delivery, involving the people, people's institutions, civil society groups, community based organisations, and self-help groups;
- To develop the appropriate cost time and Quality benchmarks for service delivery outcomes;
- To develop, implement and monitor performance measurement and management systems by developing performance indicators for service delivery;
- To promote decentralisation and strengthen rural and urban

local bodies in order to deliver services by empowering them with devolution of functions, finances and functionaries, and undertaking capacity building programmes; and

- To undertake objective assessments of programmes and obtain feedback in order to improve policy contents and implementation mechanisms.

(ii) System Improvement

- To take steps to simplify government procedures, reduce costs and improve interface with citizens;
- To improve systems in order to improve transparency, cut red tape and ensure better performance management;
- To modify complicated and rigid government processes so as to reduce and eliminate delay, duplication and redundancy and improve the speed and Quality of public service; and
- To reform processes dealing with citizens and those which breed corruption, such as procurement and tenders

(iii) Financial management

- To ensure fiscal responsibility and sanctity of the budget process;
- To move away from expenditure targets to performance-related measures and milestones which can be defined and are measurable; and
- To institute effective budget formulation, execution, monitoring, reporting and asset management in order to ensure that public money is made available quickly and without delay for the purpose for which it is meant and utilised properly for the benefit of the people.

(iv) Accountability and transparency

- To develop and implement Citizens' Charters and Service Charters so as to obtain feedback on implementation and take corrective action with the involvement of citizens;
- To develop and implement a grievances monitoring and redressal mechanism to ensure sensitivity of the administration to the problems faced by the citizens;
- To end secrecy and opacity in administration and bring about transparency so that the administration is seen as just and fair, especially in matters relating to public procurement;
- To ensure that citizens have maximum access to governmental information, by making transparency the rule and official secrecy the exception; and

- To establish citizen evaluation mechanisms such as citizen report cards, social audit, user groups monitoring and independent evaluation by professional agencies.

(v) Anti-corruption measures

- To declare zero tolerance for corruption, strengthen vigilance and anti-corruption machinery, eliminate duplication in enforcement functions and to promote measures to prevent and combat corruption more effectively and efficiently.

(vi) Accreditation

Hospital accreditation means "A self-assessment and external peer assessment process used by health care organisations to accurately assess their level of performance in relation to established standards and to implement ways to continuously improve" as per Dr. Chandrima B. Chatterjee and Dr. Sudha Sheth. Accreditation is not just about standards-setting: there are analytical, counselling and self-improvement dimensions to the process. Hospitals and healthcare services are vital components of any well-ordered and humane society, and will indisputably be the recipients of societal resources. That hospitals should be places to safety, not only for patients but also for the staff and for the general public, is of the greatest importance. Quality of hospitals and healthcare services is also of great interest to many other bodies, including governments, NGOs targeting healthcare and social welfare, professional orgnizations representing doctors, patient organisations, shareholders of companies providing healthcare services, etc. However, accreditation schemes are not the same thing as government-controlled initiatives set-up to assess healthcare providers with only governmental objectives in mind—ideally, the functioning and finance of hospital accreditation schemes should be independent of governmental control.

WHO, South Asia Regional Office organised a workshop in "Hospital Accreditation" at Bangkok, Thailand from 7-11 Dec. 1998. The group found the following advantages of accreditation:[9]

- Stimulates improvement of care.
- Strengthens community confidence.
- Reduces unnecessary costs.
- Increases efficiency.
- Promotes personnel training.
- Provides credentials for education.
- Can protect against lawsuits.
- Provides comparative data.

The Indian government proposed to take the following measures to introduce accreditation:

(1) Initiate the process for setting up a core group in the Ministry of Health.
(2) Sensitization of policy-makers by organizing national-level workshop by January 1999 for generating awareness about the need for hospital accreditation.
(3) Sensitization of professional bodies, service providers, and consumer groups by organizing regional workshops.
(4) Organize discussions on proposed legislation for compulsory registration of hospitals.
(5) Set-up expert groups to suggest minimum conditions for hospital registration.
(6) Set-up expert groups to suggest standards for hospital accreditation.[10]

Accreditation is going to be beneficial to both the providers and receivers of the services. Providers would be clear as to what standards are to be maintained and the receivers would know what to expect from the particular hospital. In this way, there can be a race among hospitals to get accreditation for better marketing of their services. Even in Universities and colleges accreditation is being done in a big way by National Assessment and Accreditation Council (NAAC), an Inter-University Centre of University Grants Commission. Health Departments of the Union and State governments can set-up such accreditation council for hospitals under the auspices of Medical Council of India. We have to take care that this work should be done in association with professional associations, research institutes, so that there may be less resistance at the implementation level. This would promote medical tourism as they would be aware of the standards.

(vii) Efficient and cheap hospital services for promoting medical tourism

Medical tourists are coming to avoid higher charges in their own country. Therefore, we must run our hospitals efficiently and economically so that our hospitals can provide them quality services at cheap rates.

The new millennium, the hospitals should be run on scientific lines. This would require research and in-depth study of various administrative issues impinging on the medical services. Some of these areas may be mentioned here:

- the effective use of hospital services, e.g. X-rays, beds and of imaging and other services;
- staff issues such as job satisfaction and the retention of staff members, particularly nurses and other highly trained personnel;
- patient satisfaction;
- clinical data, such as readmission rate, length of stay for various illnesses, and the effectiveness and efficiency of referral to and from the hospital and health centres;

- cost-benefit analysis of different programmes;
- the incidence, etiology, and prevention of infection;
- design of new aids and gadgets for the care and comfort of patients, especially the disabled;
- management of human, financial, and material resources;
- quality assurance in hospitals;
- cost accounting of various services;
- utilization time of different categories of persons; and

Besides, in the new millennium, the hospitals should attend to maintenance of buildings, equipment, dietary services, security services, registration services, etc. to maintain the prestige and dignity of the hospital as well as ensure quality health care in new millennium. In this great venture, hospital authorities may seek the involvement and co-operation of the people to make the medical services, patient-oriented. Hospitals in the new millennium should provide an environment of extended family where the patients can get professional and expert medical care and homely environment. Patients should be welcomed in this extended family type hospital services.

A spirit of service and dedication must pervade among the providers of the health care as they are considered second God on earth by the receivers of health care. In the new millennium, we must empower the patients by looking after them carefully and making them feel important.

The progress and achievements of the past 50 years are solid foundations for a healthier and better world. It is already time to build on them. Life in the 21st century could and should be better for all. We can pass no greater gift to the next generation than a healthier future. That is our vision. Together, the people of the world can make it a reality.

(viii) Cost Containment

Foreign nationals should be charged less as his main purpose of coming to India is to get treatment at low cost. In the new Millennium, the cost of hospital services would increase beyond the capacity of the hospital resources. The expenditures on salary, equipment and drugs would be an ever increasing pressure on the capacity of the hospitals. The result would be either dilution of quality of services or limiting the hospital services. In both situations, hospital services and prestige would be affected.

What can be done to keep the hospital services in operation in the new millennium? We suggest here some facts and suggestions:

(i) Hospitals should set-up an economy committee which should scrutinize the current activities, their mode of financing and their utility. An examination would indicate a great scope for curtailment of unwanted expenditure.

(ii) The Director/Medical Superintendent through financial experts apply the modern management techniques like performance budgeting, zero-base budgeting, cost accounting, etc. to ascertain the genuineness for expenditure and its utility, e.g. what is the cost per patient admitted to an emergency? What is the cost per operation? In this way, we can locate where expenditure can be controlled without affecting the delivery of quality health services.

(iii) Hospital staff should be made cost-conscious so that they should use hospital resources judiciously and economically. They should use only those services which are essential.

(iv) Since a large part of the hospital expenditure is on the salary of medical and supporting personnel there is a need to ensure optimisation of their services.

(ix) Absence of any legislation for the organisation and functioning of hospitals

Patients coming from other countries must be ensured that the government would support them if the hospital authorities do not attend them properly. They must know whom to complain and what to do in case of poor services.

At present there is no comprehensive legislation to guide the organisation and management of hospitals. There is need of a hospital legislation to ensure maintenance of standards, to define rights and duties of the hospital staff and to ensure the efficient functioning of hospitals. It is suggested that the Government of India may set-up a body, i.e. Development Council for Hospitals with its branches in the States like the Medical Council of India, to lay down policies to ensure that the hospital have requisite facilities and provide efficient services to the patients. It has become a common practice to set-up nursing homes in the private sector. These so-called 'nursing homes' are often huge money-making projects devised by the specialists in league with one another. All these nursing home must be under the control of the proposed council. It should be the duty of the council to see that the specialities like the private industry do not fleece the people and provide medical care of right quality and at a reasonable price. Besides, the proposed council may attend to the complaints of the patients to ensure smooth relations between the hospital authorities and the beneficiaries and thus help in the building of a 'Welfare State', a cherished ideal in the constitutions of most of the states in the world.

We must attend to all these problems to ensure efficiency of the hospitals. These problems also emanate from a number of constraints on hospital authorities, e.g., shortage of staff at all levels, absence of proper accommodation to provide space to the ever increasing number of patients, shortage of funds, shortage of medicine, shortage of equipment, political and administrative inference, etc., which need to be attended to by the governments at the Union and State level to provide satisfactory hospital services. Besides, the patients and their relatives must cooperate with the hospital authorities to make the best use of the available resources. Thus, we shall have to have a three-pronged attack-increasing internal efficiency, mobilising government support and enlisting people's cooperation to ensure the reputation, prestige, credibility and viability of the hospital services.

CONCLUSION

There is a need of good marketing system to promote medical tourism. Before doing that, we must ensure that all the facilities are available before the arrival of foreign patients. One satisfied patients would create a chain in positive ways. Therefore, the success of medical tourism would depend upon the satisfied patients going after treatment. They will become our publicity agents. Therefore, what is needed to attract medical tourists is to ensure decent care to them and their excellent stay.

Tourism is an important component of demand in the services sector which has shown considerable dynamism in recent years and is poised for even more rapid growth. It is difficult to estimate the full contribution of tourism to the economy since much of it shows up indirectly in sectors such as hotels and restaurants, transport, handicrafts, etc. but there is general agreement that the sector has great potential and needs to be encouraged.

To fully benefit from natural, cultural, business, leisure, spiritual, religious, ecological, adventures and medical tourism, the 11th Plan should focus on creation of adequate tourism infrastructure like modernization and expansion of airports, increase in accommodation facilities under star and budget category and improved road connectivity to tourist destinations. At the same time it is important to ensure the upkeep and preservation of historical sites, lakes and rivers—all of which attract tourists. Measures need to be devised to enhance India's competitiveness as a tourist destination by *inter alia* reducing luxury tax and sales tax on ATF and by providing for hassle-free inter-state movement of passenger vehicles. Hotel management and catering education programmes need to be widened and hitherto undeveloped archaeological sites opened up for development and maintenance through public-private partnerships.

A Case Study of Chandigarh

While ill-health looms constantly on us, Chandigarh and even SAS Nagar have begun to offer world-class medical facilities. The list that finds its way in reads: PGI, GMCH-32 and Forties and Silver Oaks in SAS Nagar promising medical services have promoted the Chandigarh Administration to develop medical tourism in the City for which the Administration is working in collaboration with leading hospitals which provide state-of-art medical facilities.

The idea is to promote Chandigarh as a destination for Medical Tourism. Facilities and services of various hospitals would be compiled and posted on to the website and the same would be publicized through mass media. Further, the low pollution levels here compared to the other cities and the ample green space in here will be major USP. Vivek Atray, Director, Tourism, Chandigarh Administration, says, "We have hospitals providing the best medical services and infrastructure and medical tourism has great potential here since these hospitals have JCI certification that enables tourists to claim insurance back home."

"The medical services here come at a lower budget as compared to metros and the expertise of the doctors is creditable," informs Akhil Bharadwaj, MD, Fortis, SAS Nagar who tells: "We have the whole infrastrucuture and state-of-art services besides the JCI certification wherein our foreign patients don't have to bother with insurance formalities and can claim it back home. And then, the rates here are 20% less as compared to Delhi and Mumbai." But on deterrents, Akhil points pertinently, "Absence of international flights here is a big deterrent because when tourists land in metros, they opt for treatments there itself.

Public hospitals still need more resources and facilities before to be in the fray. Manju Wadwalker, PRO, PGI, says, "even though we have all facilities and infrastructures, we need more because if we are treating a foreign tourist then we also have to offer him a good accommodation with modern day facilities. Yes we provide services with economy but for medical tourism, public hospitals have to go a long way and that can take a lot of time." The Chandigarh Administration has its sights set on selling Chandigarh as a medical tourists' destination.

Notes and References

1. Ministry of Health and Family Welfare, GOI, Annual Report, 2006-07, p. 292.
2. Francisco Vilardell, "Organ Transplants: are they ethical, *World Health*, June 1988, p. 20.
3. Jawaharlal Nehru and Public Administration, Ed. By Prof. V. Jagnadham, I.I.P.A., New Delhi, 1975.
4. Mary D. Shanks and Dorothy A. Kennedy, The Theory and Practice of Nursing Service Administration, McGaw-Hill, London, 1965, p. 95.
5. John W. Gardner, Excellence, New York, 1961, Harper and Brothers, p. 154.
6. K.G. Agarwal, "Managing Patient Satisfaction in Hospitals", in the *Indian Journal of Public Administration*, Vol. XXII, No. 2, April-June, 1976, p. 277.
7. K.K. Kaul, "Hospitalisation of Children", Health and Population—Perspective and Issues, 2(1); 49-53, 1979.
8. Karnataka Human Development Report, 2005, *op. cit.* pp. 269-70.
9. WHO: SEARO, Hospital Accreditation Report on Inter-Country Meeting, Bangkok (Thailand), Dec. 7-11, 1988.
10. *Ibid.*, pp. 41-42.

7

CHAPTER

Health and Travel

INTERNATIONAL TRAVEL

In the 21st Century, International Travel has increased many folds, as the world has become a small globe. The recent policies of Globalization, Liberalization and Privatization have accelerated international travel. Every New Year is adding to this phenomenon.

The health problems of travel are very diverse, but they tend to be most often of an infectious or parasitic nature, such as diarrhoea, hepatitis A and malaria. Diarrhoea, afflicts around two-fifths of all international travellers, of whom 30 per cent of suffers may be confined to bed, and 40 per cent may be compelled to change their travel plans. Some people accept diarhoea as an inevitable part of travel, but that is plainly not so. Hepatitis A remains the most common serious infectious illness in travellers continue to rise, drug resistant malaria continues to spread, and the choice of effective drugs available for prophylaxis is now seriously limited by toxicity.[1]

Maintaining good health while traveling is not just something that matters to affluent visitors from wealthy developed countries. It is of vital concern to many developing countries, which are in the process of building up a tourist industry as part of their economic infrastructure. This is a labour-demanding industry, providing employment for many people in all walks of life, and is also an important source of foreign exchange for some developing countries.[2]

In addition, people are traveling as tourists, treating diseases, sexual pleasure, International exchange programme, pilgrimage, etc. International travel can be done by airliners, ships, buses or cars. What are the health consequences of this mass travel? How can we make travel safe? How can we protect the people from health hazards? We shall discuss the issues and problems of travel to other countries in the context of health.

We can think of international travel as a four-sided arrangement between the travellers, the travel organisation, the transport company and the host government.[3]

I. Traveller is the main person who has to bear the consequence of any health hazard

Travellers should ensure that all precautions are taken against any preventable disease by immunization, drugs and careful behaviour.

It they fall ill on their return, they should advise their medical practitioner where they have been. Unfortunately doctors in many countries are frequently ignorant of health hazards elsewhere. From time to time there are reports in the newspapers about returning tourists dying of malaria because the disease has not been diagnosed when they reached home. This is not altogether surprising, probably fewer than a quarter of total doctors in the world have ever seen a case of malaria. Appalling examples occur of travellers who have been bitten by rabid dogs but who are advised neither by local doctors in the country they are visiting nor by their doctor back home to have antirabies vaccine; the result is an agonizing death.

Lets us discuss the likely diseases that the travellers can encounter.

(1) Insect Pests and Insect Borne Diseases

These are fully dealt within three separate articles—on the insects and methods of protection, on the virus diseases transmitted by insects, and on malaria. Apart from carrying disease, insects have a great nuisance value, particularly for people who react in a hypersensitive manner to such bites and may become quite ill as a result.

Biting insects occur all over the world; in some areas of the far northern tundra, black flies may cause severe loss of blood in unprepared travellers. But vector-borne diseases are mostly prevalent in the tropical zone. The risks are quite different in urban and rural areas. In the towns, malaria, dengue, sand fly fever and possibly yellow fever may occur, but in the countryside all these are more likely and there is the additional risk of sleeping sickness (in Middle and South America), Chagas' disease (in Middle and South America), filariasis (including river blindness), plague and various virus diseases. Of the virus diseases, only yellow fever and equine and tick-borne encephalitis can be prevented by immunization. Further articles in this issue deal with dengue and dengue-related diseases, and also with the one virus disease that is found all over the world-viral hepatitis (though this is not normally insect borne).

Another contributor deals with malaria, that bane of residents and travellers alike wherever there are the appropriate species of mosquitoes in the tropics and sub-tropics. It is easily prevented by prophylactic drugs, if these are taken regularly and continued for at least a month after leaving a malarious area. The main danger for tourists is that the disease may not be recognized by physicians back in their home countries who have not previously encountered it.[4]

Drugs used for individual protection against malaria

Drug or combination	*Dosage for 60-kg adult*	*Frequency of administration*	*Remarks*
Chloroquine	300 mg (base)	Weekly	Tablet bitter: overdose can be dangerous. Some side-effects reported.
Amodiaquine	300-400 mg (base)	Weekly	As for chloroquine
Sulfadoxine	500 mg	Weekly	For use in areas of resistance of falciparum malaria to 4-aminoquinolines.
Pyrimethamine	25 mg		Not recommended for prolonged use or for pregnant women.

(A pregnant woman who is obliged to visit malarious areas where P. falciparum is resistant to 4-aminoquinolines should seek specialist medical advice about the most appropriate form of prophylaxis for her).

From Vaccination Certificate Requirements for International Travel and Health Advice to Travellers (WHO), 1982.

Self-protection

As a traveller, how can you protect yourself against malaria? Information on whether there is malaria risk in a certain area at a certain time, as well as advice on protective measures, should be sought from the national health administration of the traveller's home country, which can call on the medical profession, tourist agencies, shipping companies, airline operators and other bodies for aid.

The following measures are also recommended:

- Choose rooms with screens on windows and other openings so as to prevent mosquitoes from entering;
- Use "anti-fly" spray containing pyrethrum insecticides to kill any mosquitoes that may have entered in spite of screening; but the effect is rather short-lived, and the spraying must be repeated frequently if mosquitoes continue to enter;
- If the entrances to bedrooms are not screened, the use of cloth

mosquito nets around the beds at night is advisable, especially for babies and young children; it is essential to tuck in the net carefully under the mattress, and the net should have no holes;
- After sunset, all persons staying in the open should wear sufficient clothing to protect the body from mosquito bites (long sleeves, long trousers and so on); smear uncovered parts of the body with an insect repellent, such as dimethylphthalate; but the lasting effect of these products is only two to three hours and they must be reapplied.

Bear in mind that in many countries where there is malaria, the main towns are often free of the disease, though this is not necessarily true of the outskirts. While there is usually much less risk of malaria at altitudes greater than 1,500 metres above sea level, the disease can occur in certain climatic conditions at much higher elevations. The degree of risk of infection varies with the season.

If you are in any doubt about malaria, it is wise to take precautions anyway and equip yourself with the recommended drugs. And on your return home, if you feel ill, don't forget to tell you doctor about any recent international traveling you have done.[5]

Yellow fever is another important mosquito-borne disease in tropical Africa and parts of South America; visitors to countries where the disease may occur are advised to have a prior inoculation against yellow fever if there is the slightest possibility of traveling outside the main towns.[6]

While the average traveller may be assured of a good night's rest in well-run hotels, less salubrious and less hygienic accommodation may on occasions be unavoidable. Bed-bugs or fleas rarely cause diseases, but may give rise to a sleepless night. Bed-bugs are thin, flat, nocturnal insects capable of running rapidly over exposed skin without being felt; their bites made at random, usually on or near the feet, develop into large red weals. Fleas, as is well known, are very small insects, which jump when disturbed. Their bites characteristically occur three in a row, where clothing fits tightly to the body, and generally result in small raised spots. A bed infested with bed-bugs requires professional disinfection and should be abandoned as soon as possible. But a flea-infested bed can be rendered serviceable by hunting out, handcatching and destroying as many fleas as possible, and then applying insecticide powder between the sheets; unlike bed bugs, fleas are very susceptible to most insecticides.

Besides these personal precautions that the treaveller can take, governments and municipalities can apply a number of public health measures to protect visitors from insects pests and vectors of disease.

These include: siting tourist recreation areas away from large natural breeding places of mosquitoes; installing and maintaining a good water supply and solid and liquid waste disposal systems, so as to minimize the formation of breeding sites for pests; checking on, and insisting on, high standards of hygiene in hotels; applying mosquito abatement measures;

ensuring that game parks are free from serious vector-borne diseases, or at least present a minimal risk to visitors; notifying travellers of seasonal health risks and providing appropriate advice.

And, of course, in view of the tremendous growth in international travel that has taken place in the last two decades, governments and airlines share a responsibility for ensuring that harmful insects are not transported by aircraft into countries where they did not previously live.[7]

Strange Food

Many travellers blame strange food and a change of diet for their diarrhea, and there is good reason for this. After all, as we have mentioned, food and water may carry the infecting agent, especially where hygiene is poor. But in addition travellers in strange places may relax their own code of cleanliness and take risks they would not take at home. In a holiday environment, people tend to drink too much alcohol and eat large heavy meals that they are not used to. All this may dilute the acid in the stomach, which acts as a natural defence against infection and, with the defences down, the infection can gain entry to the intestine and start its painful work.[8]

Under conditions of poor hygiene, foods most likely to be safe include—

- food that must have been freshly cooked-for example, a fried egg, or an omelette;
- freshly boiled food, such as rice or sweetcorn;
- fresh fruit or vegetables that are easily peeled or cut open—such as bananas, citrus fruits, melon and papaya;
- food from sealed packs or cans; and
- food that one has prepared, or watched cooking, oneself.

When travelling in areas with low standards of environmental sanitation, hands should be washed at every opportunity. Food should only be handled with hands that are scrupulously clean.

Plates and cutlery need to be washed with detergent, rinsed with hot water, and protected from flies. The risk from contaminate plates can be reduced by rinsing with hot weak tea or boiling water or an alcohol-soaked cotton swab. Alternatively, paper plates and one's own cutlery should be used.

Cups and glasses should be swilled out with hot tea or boiling water before use. Flies often settle on rims—the rim of a teacup can be rinsed by pouring away a little tea. Bottled drinks should be taken direct from the bottle. Alternatively, one's own cup or water bottle should be used.

Hospitality poses a difficult dilemma; not traveler likes to give offence to a host who has taken great trouble to prepare a meal. Personally, I believe that one should never relax one's own standard of food hygiene when travelling, under any circumstances.[9]

The best way of preventing travellers' diarrhoea is to avoid exposure to the infective agent. To do that, food and water must be clean and standards of personal and environmental hygiene must be adequate. Public health authorities in countries with a high incidence of diarrhoea should ensure that a good standard of food and water hygiene is maintained in establishments serving travellers. To support this, it is necessary to have adequate laboratory facilities, so as to be able both to perform the necessary checks on food and water, and to identify the causative agent when any outbreaks of diarrhoea occur.

What can the individual do to prevent diarrhoea while traveling? First and foremost, it is prudent to reduce the risks as much as possible: eat clean food, drink clean water. This means in fact drinking only water that is boilded or bottled (be sure it is carbonated), tea or coffee made with boiled water, or other carbonated beverages, and eating only food that has either been well cooked immediately before serving, or is protected from tins). Beware of salads and avoid them if at all possible.

There is some evidence that taking prophylactic antibiotics may be of some value. However, if they are used at all, they should be used only by adults traveling for a short period (less than three weeks) to high-risk areas where it is impossible to obtain safe water and food. This would especially apply to persons with conditions associated with decreased gastric acidity or other serious conditions.

Moderation in all things is a good motto, and this applies to traveling: eat and drink sensibly, do not take risks, and—if the worst happens—then be prepared and have some oral rehydration mixture handy.[10]

Jaundice has been a familiar disease since classical times. Today three main forms of viral hepatitis are recognized, which threaten the health of travellers all over the world.[11]

Tourists are not the only travellers for whom food safety is a vital concern. The mass travel of pilgrims to holy places, the international coming and going of millions of workers in search of employment, the routine passage of thousands of merchant seamen between ports in every continent-all these involve food and hygiene risks that have to be kept to a minimum by the responsible authorities.

Two of the key provisions of the International Health Regulations, to which virtually all countries of the world are signatories, are that:

- Every port and airport shall be provided with pure drinking-water and wholesome food supplied from sources approved by the health administration for public use and consumption on the premises or on board ships or aircraft. The drinking water and food shall be stored and handled in such a manner as to ensure their protection against contamination. The health authority shall conduct periodic inspections of equipment, installations and premises, and shall collect samples of water and food for laboratory examinations to verify the observance of this Article. . .

- Every port and airport shall also be provided with an effective system for the removal and safe disposal of excrement, refuse, waste water, condemned food, and other matters dangerous to health.
- Finally, what can travellers themselves do to protect themselves from gastro-enteritis and other food risks? Firstly, where possible eat foods that have been freshly cooked and served hot—and if you have any doubt about their safety, avoid such foods as ice cream, soft cheeses, cold meats, shellfish and other sea-foods, salads and soft skinned fruits. Secondly, avoid drinking or cleaning teeth in cold water unless it is known to be chlorinated. Thirdly, avoid using ice unless you know safe water was used to make it.[12]

Regional distribution of some arboviruses that may threaten the traveller

	Dengue and pseudo-dengue	*Haemorrhagic fever*	*Encephalitis*
North Africa	Rift Valley fever (Egypt), Sandfly fever, West Nile, Sindbis		West Nile
Tropical Africa	Chikungunya, O'nyong-nyong, dengue, Zika, Rift Valley, Orungo		Eastern equine, Western equine, St. Louis California
North America	Colorado tick fever		
Central America and tropical, South America Yellow fever	Dengue, Mayaro, Mucambo, Sandfly fever, Murutucu, Oropuche	Yellow fever, Crimean and Congo haemorrhagic fever*	St. Louis, equine encephalitis of Venezuela, Ilheus, Rocio type
Tropical Asia	Chikungunya, Sindbis, Dengue, Sandfly fever, Zika	Chikungunya, Dengue Haemorrhagic fever	Japanese B encephalitis

* Under this heading come the Lassa, Marburg and Ebola fevers.[13]

	Dengue and pseudo-dengue	*Haemorrhagic fever*	*Encephalitis*
Central Europe and Mediterranean	Sandfly fever, West Nile	Crimean and Congo haemorrhagic fever	Tick encephalitis
Middle East	West Nile, Sandfly fever		West Nile
Western Pacific	Sindbis, Ross River fever, dengue	Dengue haemorrhagic fever	Japanese B encephalitis, Australian encephalitis.

Sexually transmitted diseases lie in wait for the traveller who is too casual about casual sex. Every effort of health education must be made to ensure that our potential traveller is both more prudent and better informed about STD.

All the evidence shows that information about STD is much more convincing, particularly among youngsters, when they are bluntly warned about the possible consequences, namely the risk of sterility in both men and women. It should also be brought home to them again and again that dormant cases of salpingitis in young girls may result in irreversible sterility.

An all-out effort is required to overcome the widespread ignorance of STD. The objective should be to ensure that our potential travellers, on the threshold of some exciting new adventure, should be both more prudent and better informed when tempted by the siren-song of seduction.[14]

2. Traveling Organisation or Travel Agency

They should be able to tell the traveller in detail about the health conditions in the countries to be visited. A useful book is published by WHO to help health administrations to advise those concerned, and is of particular value for travel organisations. This is Vaccination Certificate Requirements for International Travel and Health Advice to Travellers, 1982 (obtainable from Distribution and Sales, World Health Organisation, 1211 Genevea 27, Switzerland. Price: 12 Swiss francs). It lists some health risks to which travellers may be subject in different parts of the world, and suggests the precautions that they can take against certain diseases and injuries.

Travel Organisation are too busy and they never inform the traveller. There is a need of legislation, which can ascertain that some literature about the likely health problems to be encountered may be given along with the ticket. In addition, the Airport authorities must ensure the availability of health literature of different countries is available at the Air Port.

3. Transport Companies

These have two distinct responsibilities. Firstly, to advise travellers if a particular health risk exists in the country of disembarkment, especially malaria—some airlines even supply the traveller with a small pack of an anti-malaria drug. Secondly, they must ensure that their own food hygiene is impeccable. Codes of recommended practices and recommendations on the application of specific procedures for monitoring sanitary food and water standards have been established by such bodies as the International Air Transport Association (IATA) and the International Civil Aviation Organisation (ICAO). These are available to their members' airlines and to related multinational hotel groups. Similar standards should be maintained on passenger liners and in all establishments used by land transport operators. (WHO has also published the following: Guide to Hygiene and Sanitation in Aviation, by J. Bailey; Guide to Ship Sanitation, by V.B. Lamoureux, and Guide to Sanitation in Tourist Establishments, by J.A. Salvato, Jr.)

WHO has a collaborative role in this four-sided arrangement through its liaison with IATA, ICAO and the Inter-governmental Maritime Consultative Organisation (IMCO), as well as with the World Tourism Organisation. In addition, it is a sounding box on international health, receiving information from member-countries and disseminating it in a journal called the Weekly Epidemiological Record. It also advises governments on precautions to be adopted when disease outbreaks occur, and draws their attention to health regulations when they are too stringent or are in excess of the requirements of the International Health Regulations.[15]

4. Host Country

Failure on the part of governments, local authorities and caterers to maintain adequate sanitation can mar a holiday or a business trip completely. One effect of inadequate food and water hygiene, as well as of carelessness by the traveller, is diarrhoeal disease. Travellers' diarrhoea is extremely common and takes many forms, but all are caused by an infection. As another of our articles shows, drugs play little part in curing this condition, but in high-risk areas certain prophylactic antibiotics may be of value for short visits, particularly for people who are not in full health. The most dangerous and debilitating effect of diarrhoea is dehydration. This can be overcome by drinking dissolved oral rehydration salts, which are readily available in most countries.

SUGGESTIONS

1. Carrying a First Aid Kit

Let us take it for granted that—whether you are going on business, for family reasons or on holiday—you will carry a small first aid kit: antiseptic cream, wound dressings, aspirins, travel sickness pills, sun cream to prevent sunburn (for those with fair skins), insect repellent and an ointment to relieve irritation from insect bites and stings, Depending on where you are going, you may need some other pharmaceutical preparations, but your doctor will advise you on this.

2. Immunization against diseases prevalent in the host country

As soon as you know where you are going and when, ask your doctor about the possible health risks in the places you are planning to visit, and whether you will need any immunizations.

For visits to tropical Africa or parts of South America, yellow fever vaccination is essential if you are going outside the main towns even for a day. This can only be obtained on certain days at special clinics in the bigger cities.

Chad still requires a small pox vaccination certificate although this disease no longer exists in the world. The following countries require a certificate of cholera vaccination in certain circumstances: Albania, Angola, Brunei, Cape Verde, Chad, Dominican Republic, Egypt, Iran, Lesotho, Libyan Arab Jamahiriya, Madagascar, Malawi, Maldives, Mali, Malta, Mozambique, Niger, Pakistan, Paraguay, Pitcairn, Republic of Korea, Somalia, Sudan, Swaziland, Tuvalu, United Arab Emirates, Viet Nam and Zambia. However, vaccination does not offer you much protection and should not be regarded as the only precaution you need against this disease.

Other immunizations which may be advisable are tetanus and diphtheria which each last about 10 years and typhoid lasting 3 years. Where there is a high risk of poliomyelitis, make sure you are immunized. Most of these protective vaccines are normally given in childhood, but the doctor will assess their present effectiveness. Gamma globulin can provide some protection for 3 months against the form of jaundice (infectious hepatitis) to which are most likely to be exposed. If your children are going to visit a country where tuberculosis is rife, their BCG vaccinations status should be checked.

If you are going to an area where malaria occurs, your doctor will advise you on which drug to take and how often you should take it. For certain countries you may be advised to carry a few sachets of an oral rehydration mixture to restore you fluid balance if you have diarrhoea, and possibly an antibiotic drug incase you get a severe attack.

If you normally have to take certain medicines (after all, chronic illness is usually no barrier to travel), make sure you have more than enough of these to cover the time you are away. Pharmacies in other countries may not stock the same preparations.

Have you thought that a sudden toothache might spoil your visit? It is worth having a dental check-up before you leave.

In case of accidents, you may wish to carry what may be termed a health passport. This records your blood group, any idiosyncrasy or allergy to drugs, a copy of the optician's prescription of your glasses if you use them, and information about any chronic disease you have and what drugs you use to keep it under control. This is particularly important if you are a diabetic.

The travel agent will probably advise you about health insurance-but make sure it is enough. Costs are particularly high in Europe and the USA; for these areas US$ 25,000 should be the minimum coverage for each person.

3. Dirty Travel

Travelling itself involves an abrupt psychological change of lifestyle, and subjects even the most experienced travellers to certain stresses. Many people may find difficult in sleeping; a few may suffer from seasickness or airsickness.

A change of time zone will affect your appetite. You may be inclined to help yourself to too much food and liquid (particularly alcohol); on the other hand, in some circumstances you can easily suffer from dehydration.

At stopovers, it is wise in some airports to wear long sleeves and use an insect repellent on the neck and face.

If you live in a country with a warm climate and travel to a cold one, remember to have a supply of warm clothes and strong footwear available on arrival.

4. At the place of stay

If you have been traveling from east to west, you will probably have trouble sleeping at the usual hours; avoid staying up late until your <<mental clock>> has adjusted, otherwise you will suffer from <<jet-lag>>.

If you have gone to a hot and humid area from a cooler or dryer one, you should take care not to overdo exercise at first. Too much sun can be very dangerous; if you have a fair skin, only sunbathe on the first day for 10 to 15 minutes at the most, then gradually increase the exposure until you build up a good tan. The sun is at its strongest between 10 a.m. and 2 p.m.

A change of diet in itself can cause stomach upsets; but in addition, food and drink are the most common sources of germs entering the body and causing food-borne and water-borne diseases.

All raw food is a potential source of infection. In places where you have any doubts about cleanliness and kitchen hygiene, avoid vegetable salads and other uncooked vegetables and thin-skinned fruits.

Undercooked and raw meat, fish and shellfish may carry various disease organisms. All these foods, if left to cool without refrigeration, may also be dangerous. Better to avoid re-cooked foods.

Unless you are very sure about the purity of the water provided, don't use it for drinking and cleaning your teeth unless it has been boiled or treated with water purification tablets. These can be obtained from a chemist before leaving on you trip. Carbonated beverages are safe to drink, but non-gaseous waters (even if bottled) and fruit drinks may not be. Milk and its by-products, including ice-cream, may be risky in some areas.

Far away from home, some people may be tempted to embark on casual sexual relationships. If so, the use of a condom or diaphragm would be a wise precaution, and so would careful washing after intercourse. But there are no prophylactic drugs to prevent all venereal diseases, and their initial signs are very often so slight that they may be overlooked; thus the more dangerous and painful secondary and tertiary forms of certain sexually transmitted diseases can develop without previous warning. If you do suspect venereal disease, don't delay before telling you doctor, or have a check-up at one of the special clinics that are found in most cities.

In many tropical areas, it is wise to reduce the risk of insect bites by wearing long trousers and long sleeves at night, and better to stay in the hotel area rather than go into the town. In East and West Africa, don't picnic in the shade of trees near ponds or stream; these are favourite places for the tsetse files that cause sleeping sickness.

Avoid petting stray dogs and cats. Rabies is a serious danger in many countries. This is a killer disease which is generally transmitted by the bite—or even the lick—of a rabid animal. If you are bitten, even by what looks like a harmless puppy or kitten, wash the area carefully with plenty of soapy water, pour strong alcohol on it, see a doctor and make sure you get a course of anti-rabies serum or vaccine as soon as possible. It could save your life.

Be careful where you swim. Avoid muddy ponds, and remember that in some tropical countries, dykes and canals are infested with the freshwater snail, carrier of the parasite, which causes schistosomiasis (bilharziasis). Seawater bathing too has its hazards-sharks; the jellyfish called Portuguese men-of-war, poisonous fish and sea snakes, or infected cuts from sharp coral. Not every country ensures that its beaches are free sewage pollution. Young people particularly like to go barefoot on the sand, or even in the street. But they should be warned about such parasites as hookworm, or insect pests like chigger fleas.

Snakes are rarely a danger, since most species slither away when they hear a human approaching. If anyone is bitten, a light tourniquet should be immediately applied to the affected limb (but only for a short period of time) and medical attention should be urgently sought so that anti-venom can be given if needed. Scorpion and spider stings can be extremely painful and some are quite dangerous too. Remember to shake out your clothes and shoes in the morning before dressing.

5. After return fun travel

Remember to go on taking the anti-malaria pills for at least a month. The most dangerous form of malaria usually causes severe illness within two weeks, but other forms may not affect a person for weeks or even months. Similarly, sleeping sickness may take several months to become obvious, and other diseases may not develop for as long as a year after the return home.

One form of jaundice (infectious hepatitis) may take up to two months to appear, and rabies up to one year if no post-bite immunization has been given. Anthrax, which causes a dangerous boil and is acquired from handling infected untanned leather goods, appears after several days. Syphilis may not become apparent for three months.

Be sure to tell your doctor about any international journeys you have made during the previous 12 months if you have to see him for any sickness after your return.

The simple precautions outlined here should enable you to plan your trip, to travel, and to return home—without undue anxiety about endangering your health.

Be prepared before you travel. Find out what health risks may exist in the countries you will visit, and what precautions you can take. Be a healthy traveller.[16]

A case studies: (1) The author went to Bangkok to receive as award from Economic and Social Commission for Asia and Pacific (ESCAP). I stayed in the house of my fried as he accompanied me from India. He did his Ph.D. with me. He provided me a good independent room on the 1st floor of the house. However, he did not tell me that water coming from taps is sanitary water. I drank water is the morning from the tap and got ill after 2 days. I had to cut short my visit and hospitalized in India.

(2) The author visited Dubai recently. The temperature outside was 47°C. It came to my mind that I must walk outside for 10-15 minutes. After walking I came back. When I reached India, there was a serious skin problem, which continued for more than a year. This was after getting treatment—

(a) All passengers whether travelling abroad or in India must give priority to their health as without good health, purpose of travel defected.

(b) Travellers much check whether the medicines, which they are taking are stocked in sufficient quantity as these may not be available in other countries.

(c) Travellers must move or visit places only to the Extent that one is not Exhausted.

(d) Travellers must not be tempted for commercial set as this can lead to many complications.

(e) Travellers must be careful in taking food and water as these can contain harmful germs.

(f) Proper rest and sleep must be taken to avoid any stress/steam.

(g) Travellers must take alcohol, etc. as per one's capacity and not as per the capacity of host or friends.

(h) Government must ensure cleanliness, availability water and food at all the places—Bus Stands, Railway Stations, Ports, Air Port, etc.

(i) Self-care is the best care and most reliable.

CONCLUSION

We should now be done that will have the greatest impact on the challenge of travellers' health? Only one single measure is capable of accomplishing the dramatic change that is needed, and that is health education. Until now it has received insufficient priority, yet it costs little and depends upon no major new technological break-through.

To be effective, it must be broad, comprehensive and detailed. Health precautions for travel are not complicated. The objective should be to give prospective travellers enough information to convince them to observe precautions even when these may seem unreasonable; lists of do's and don'ts, to be taken on trust, are simply not enough.

Everyone needs health education for travel-even doctors, who are often as unfamiliar with hazards that occur outside their own environment as anyone else. People from developed countries with a sophisticated public health service and high general safety standards rarely have to think about such things at home, and are particularly in need of health education. We are all travellers now, and at different times will travel for pleasure, on business as pilgrims, as refugees or as job-seekers. Health education should focus on general principles that apply anywhere. Reliable information about hazards abroad is often most lacking from the countries with the greatest risk, and advice should not be too closely oriented to specific destinations; it is better to travel in a general state of preparedness.

We often see people in the airport preparing for foreign travel who seem far removed from the robust young people featured in travel ads. They are in wheelchairs, supported by oxygen, and many require considerable physical assistance. Yet they are traveling long distances and may be entering a truly alien landscape of medical response, relative to the one that has cared for them thus far. These intrepid travelers are not rare. This chapter does not address the issues of the medical traveler coming to the United States seeking health care. That broad topic is related but is not the subject of this section. The medical evacuation and medical assistance programs available for repatriation will be given only short coverage. The focus of this chapter is the emerging resources of electronic information and telecommunications to support the traveler with regard to health care define telemedicine. No matter where you are, you should be in an electronic continuum with familiar, competent, and interactive health care.

Health needs abroad are usually thought of as traveler's diarrhea, other infectious diseases, and injuries. However, our infirmities travel with us, and we travel with increasing frequency. Unexpected health challenges may arise in travel. However, many people are also engaged in vigorous programs of disease management, and they bring along not only the imponderable risk of accident but also the daily need to manage a chronic condition. What risks do those with health issues really take in international travel? What risks do those with health issues really take in international travel? What are the resources that might help them? What

CHART 7.1

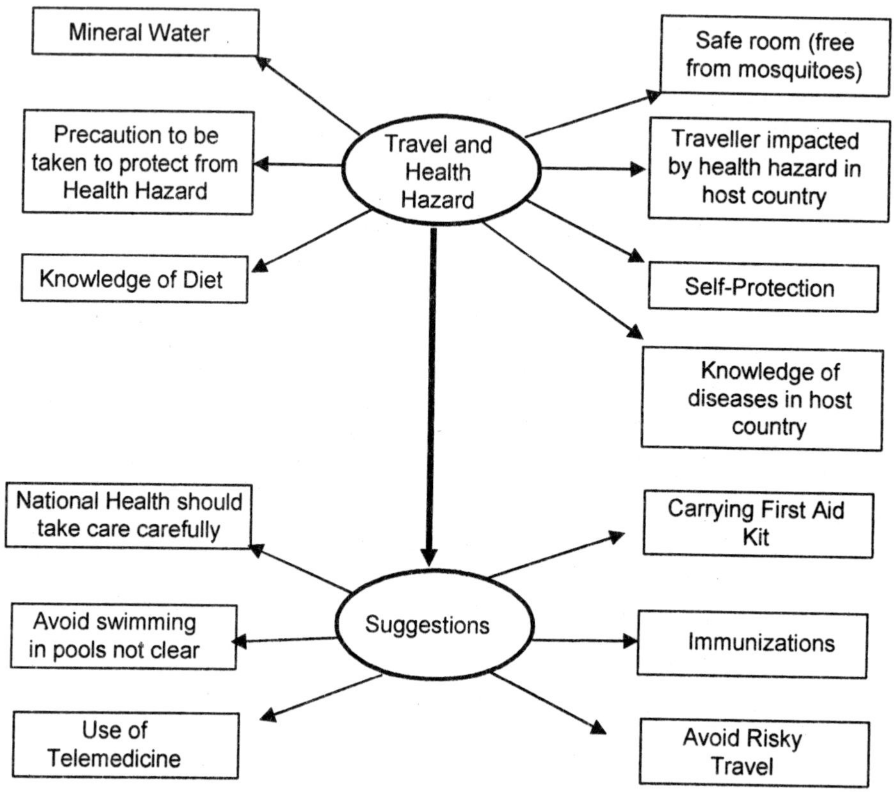

preparations before travel are prudent and practical? In this brief chapter, the scope of medical issues in travel will be considered along with the comparative anatomy of health services in the United States and abroad. Most important, the excellent resources in telecommunications and electronic information will be reviewed along with those services that the public demands and the steadily improving technology may bring to bear in the near future. Ideally, our medical care should be as portable as our medical conditions.[17]

Learning to stay healthy abroad takes a little effort, and the necessary information is sometimes difficult to obtain. Ultimately, travellers have to take responsibility for their own health abroad, and have to look after themselves; they cannot afford to do otherwise. Experts who have knowledge of the hazards of travel should develop the skills and the means to communicate this knowledge to the travelling public, as effectively and as widely as possible.[18]

National Health Travel

It is not only International health travel which is responsible for health hazards, even the National health travel especially in India is prone to health disorders. The following are the problems:

1. Buses are loaded, carrying persons beyond capacity. A truck carrying more than one hundred people resulted in an accident causing 85 deaths on the spot and large number of inured. Government must ensure that the vehicles carry only passengers who can sit comfortably.
2. During travelling, buses, trains, cars stay on the way for food which is not worth consuming even at restaurants opened directly by the Government. It is a common phenomenon that the people go on vomiting on the way and ultimately get food poisoning. Bust Stops must provide the ideal food so that people can get health education. Government Authorities allot booths at the bus stand but never check the quality of food because of corrupt practices.

In addition, Trains, Buses, Airlines are not in time. People are huddled in small areas at airports, bus stands, railway stations where they can catch infectious diseases. We suggest the following to improve national travel:

1. Bus Stands/Railway Stations/Airports should be clean and well managed.
2. Food at these places must be of high quality so that people get health education.
3. Buses, Aeroplanes, Railway Stations must be clean.
4. Behaviour of management people should be courteous.

National travel like International level can cause many infectious diseases and other health problems, which need the attention of the authorities. Traveling should be enjoyable and enlightening rather thus a dull experience.

Notes and References

1. Richard Dawood, Traveller's Health, *World Health*, 1987, p. 3.
2. Alec Smith, Keeping Insects at Bay, *World Health*, April 1982, p. 11.
3. James Haworth, Travel and Health, *World Health*, April 1982, p. 3.
4. *Ibid.*, pp. 4-5.
5. J.H.G. Malaria, "King of Diseases", *World Health*, April 1982, pp. 9-10.
6. Alec Smith, Keeping Insects At Bay, *World Health*, April 1982, p. 11.
7. *Ibid.*, p. 13.
8. R.H. Herniman, Travellers' Diarrhoea, *World Health*, April 1982, p. 15.

9. Richard Dawood, The art of defensive eating, *World Health*, December 1987, p. 20.
10. R.H. Herniman, Travellers' Diarrhoea, *World Health*, April 1982, p. 17.
11. Arie J. Zuckerman, Viral Hepatitis, *World Health*, April 1982, p. 19.
12. John Bland, "Is it safe to eat", *World Health*, April 1982, pp. 22-23.
13. P. Bres, Viruses transmitted by insects, *World Health*, April 1982, p. 25.
14. A. Siboulet, The siren-song of seduction, *World Health*, April 1982, pp. 28-29.
15. Travel and health by James Haworth, WHO, April 1982, p. 4.
16. *World Health*, Division of Public Information, 1211, Geneva, 27, Switzerland.
17. Ronald C. Merrell, The Medical Traveler Abroad: Implications for Telemedicine, Consumer Informatics, pp. 143-44.
18. Richard Dawood, Travellers' Health, *World Health*, December 1987, p. 5.

8

CHAPTER

Appropriate Technology for Health

Appropriate Technology for Health is a concept that has launched thousand of projects and programmes all over our planet, initiated by governments, non-governmental organisations, small local voluntary groups and private individuals.

Generally abbreviated as A.T.H. or A.T., it has been defined by WHO as "technology that is scientifically sound, adaptable to local needs, and acceptable to those who apply it and those for whom it is used, and that can be maintained by the people themselves in keeping with the principle of self-reliance with the resources the community and the country can afford." So from the start, the accent has been put on people's participation, and on their appropriate means to provide and use health care.

A.T. does not mean cheap, second class technology, nor is it a fashionable that can be used to sell cheap devices to developing countries. Although sometimes scornfully dismissed as "bamboo-technology", this is to overlook the fact that, in some places, bamboo can indeed be a better adapted and more appropriate choice of material than, say, corrugated iron. One basic characteristic of A.T. is that it entails the choice of the best locally available produce, irrespective of whether it stems from the indigenous culture or from the latest high technology. Indeed, the pioneers of A.T. emphasized the need in today's world for "appropriate science and technology by and for the people."[1]

Healthcare is an important sector in the vision of developed India. This vision can only be realized if we harness the technological strength and academic brilliance into a cohesive manner, integrating the bio-diversity with value addition.

KNOWLEDGE POWERED SOCIETY

Human resources particularly with large young population are the unique core strength of the nation. This resource can be transformed into skilled manpower through various educational and training programmes and makes them creative manpower for wealth generation. Knowledge intensive industries can be generated out of our existing industries by injecting demand for high-level software/hardware, which would bring tremendous value addition. It is said that "the precious asset of the country is the skill, ingenuity and imagination of its people." With globalization this will become more important because everybody will have access to the world class technology, and the key distinguishing feature will be the ability of people to use their imagination to make the best use of technologies. Indeed development and innovative use of multiple technologies with mission projects and transparent management, structure will transform India into a developed nation. The changes in India have been more profound than one could have imagined. Over the past five years alone, more than one hundred IT and science-based foreign firms have located their R and D bases in India. High tech companies are coming to India to find innovators, the bright Indian minds, whose ideas will take the world by storm. "When other countrymen live in India they become rich. When Indians live in other countries, those countries prosper.[2]

When WHO's constitution was written by its founding fathers, they made it quite clear that the Organisation was to have both a technical and a political mandate. To carry out this total mandate, a continuous search for new and improved technical solutions has been and continues to be essential. But it is also necessary to arrive at the right decisions regarding health and social policy for the application of the appropriate technology.

Carrying out this mandate through different forms of technical cooperation and international coordination in the field of health, WHO's Member-states and the WHO Secretariat are constantly involved with this interplay between the technical possibility and the political feasibility of various techniques and methodologies.

The political aspects include the establishment of a policy for health and social development based on the needs of the population. Availability and allocation of resources are essential elements in implementing such as policy. This is where the technical aspects become closely related to the political realities.[3]

Since 1981, Dr Hakan Hellberg has been the WHO Director responsible for the coordination of strategy aimed at Health for all by the year 2000. He was based at the Organisation's headquarters in Geneva.

But there is often a gap between what one would like to do and what one is able to do. With an abundance of technical solutions available in the world, the temptation to aspire to, or to acquire, more technology than one is able to afford is great.

Some countries of the world, or some parts of country, obtain for themselves a disproportionate amount of what is available, while others may lack even the most essential technical solutions.

Technical Solutions

Decisions concerning the health technology that is necessary and affordable should be made after evaluating the basic procedures to be carried out in the fields of medicine, surgery, paediatrics, obstetrics and so forth. There is no point in training "Cadillac-mechanics" if they are to work on "motor scooters and bicycles."

But man is not a machine and technology does not only mean "nuts and bolts." We need improved technologies and abilities to undertake health advocacy, to inform and communicate about health. We have to create social awareness about appropriate decisions about the use of resources that will result in relevant technical solutions. But for all of this, we need to build a sound scientific and technological base in order to give credibility to our persuasion.[4]

Vision for Healthcare

Technology will play a significant role in the field of healthcare as evident from the sophisticated technology-*cum*-devices, equipment, which are being used today in the treatment of various ailments. India is a vast country with diverse climatic conditions and a very large population. Due to inadequate healthcare facilities, lack of awareness about hygiene and malnutrition, a wide spectrum of diseases occur. India however had a rich tradition in the field of medicine. About 2500 years ago Charaka consolidated the Ayurveda and Sushruta conducted complicated surgeries. The knowledge remained largely confined and did not get disseminated, which was further weakened by successive invasions and foreign rule. There has been a transition in the 20th century. As we have presently moved to the knowledge society the present developments are well known. In order to meet the growing demand of healthcare. The Technology Vision 2020 has suggested the methods for improving healthcare with an objective of providing affordable, accessible and quality health care to the entire cross-section of our society. The specialist team of TIFAC (Technology Information Forecasting and Assessment Council) identified the imperatives for eradication of three major diseases—tuberculosis, HIV/AIDS, and waterborne diseases by the next decade. There are several others like cancer, cardiovascular diseases, which also would require our attention. We have to generate cost effective knowledge products in order to cope up with such problems. There is an urgent need for a unified approach to the planning of healthcare delivery in our country. Besides traditional medical education and research programmes, emphasis must be laid on polyclinic-level training programmes in clinical technologies. Indigenisation of expensive diagnostic and curative equipment, to make them cost-effective, and the establishment of a nationwide maintenance mechanism of medical equipment using indigenous skills and spares is equally important. One of the challenges of healthcare is the growing cost. Therefore, it is imperative to reduce the cost of drugs through scientifically innovative techniques and by developing alternative form of treatment through the new herbal formulations and validating their effectiveness through clinical database. Our hospitals—some of them are world class, therefore patients from rich and advanced countries like the medical treatment offered by these hospitals. India should become the hub of super-specialty hospitals in the world.[5]

Innovation as a way of Life

R.A. Mashelkar, Director General, CSIR, and Former Secretary to the Government of India, Department of Scientific and Industrial Research, New Delhi delivered the Convocation Address at the 12th convocation of Maharshi Dyanand University, Rohtak on 10th April 2005. He said, "Innovative India of the future must be compassionate. It should continuously look at the problems of the poor. If the problems that affect millions of people every day do not get solved through the use of existing scientific models, new innovative India of our dreams must carry that compassion so that the problems of the poor can be solved. We must harness the talent of the scientists so that value can be added to the local, indigenous ability." Excerpts.

Everyone recognizes that 21st century is the 'century of knowledge'. Nations, which have developed mastery in the production of knowledge, its dissemination, its conversion into wealth and social good, and its protection, have assumed a leadership position in the world today. But it must be recognized that knowledge without innovation is of no value. It is through the process of innovation alone that new knowledge can be created. It is also innovation alone, which converts knowledge into wealth and social good. In fact, innovation must become a way of our life. Why do I say this? India was a leader in innovation several centuries ago. Indeed, since the Indus Valley Civilization of about 5000 years ago, innovation has been the part of the Indian culture and the basis of its civilization. Our innovation was characterized by scientific thought, capabilities and techniques, at levels far more advanced than others.[6]

Health Information Technology provides technological solution to improve patient care by offering data support and remote monitoring services. The advent of modern communication technology has unleashed a new wave of opportunities to the delivery of health services. Telemedicine, a broad umbrella term for delivery of medical care at a distance, has reached around the world, and now health professionals can communicate faster, more widely, and more directly with clients and colleagues, no matter where they are. Telemedicine and telehealth has brought hope to developing countries and their remote areas. Advanced technology such as computers, diagnostic imaging, robotics, voice activated machines, and remote controls have changed the hospital and operating room theaters around the western world. Thanks to telemedicine, geography and distance are loosing their meaning in healthcare. With the internet come email, websites, chat lines, multimedia presentations, and occasional opportunities for synchronous communication via internet phones and videoconferencing. This connectivity allows greater flexibility in consultation, whether it is on health policy for hospitals or unique therapy for rare autoimmune diseases.

Space satellite technology is being used for mosquito control tracking of vectors using Geographic Information System (CIS). Software is also being developed for PARAM computer, which will provide vital information for vector control.[7]

Let us discuss some areas:

1. Basic radiological system

Medical students everywhere are taught the need for x-ray examinations for most of their patients. This may be to find out if a bone is fractured or, if a joint has been dislocated, to see the exact position of the bone fragments and, after the injury has been treated, to make sure the final position of the bones is correct and that eventually they have healed well.

Yet these same students, when they have become qualified doctors, often go to work in rural areas or the suburbs of big cities and find that there is no x-ray set available. Even more upsetting, there may be an x-ray machine but it does not work, or there are no films or no chemicals to develop them: quite often there is no one who knows how to take the pictures properly. WHO estimates that over two-thirds of the world's peoples cannot ever have an x-ray examination, and that in most developing countries at least one-third of all the available x-ray machines are likely to be broken. The doctors may well wonder how they can deliver proper health care.

Professor Philip E.S. Palmer is Professor of Radiology at the University of California, USA, and is at present visiting professor at the Kenyatta National Hospital in Nairobi.

Faced with this dismal situation, WHO a few years ago called together a small advisory group of radiologists, all of whom had many years' personal experience of radiology in developing countries. They are helped as necessary by experienced radiographers (x-ray technicians). Their terms of reference were straightforward: "Devise an x-ray system for developing countries. It must be able to x-ray all parts of the body easily and efficiently. It must be reliable and strong. It should work even where the electrical supply is unreliable, and even when there is only a small hospital generator to provide the power. It must be easy to use by relatively untrained operators, yet it must be radiation-safe so that neither patients nor operators are at risk of too much x-radiation. The system must include a method of developing the x-ray films after they have been exposed, and it would help if the doctors could have some guidance in interpreting the radiographs (the x-ray pictures) when they are ready."

This was quite a challenge for the group, who started by looking at many existing x-ray machines and many different ways of producing the final image. Was photographic paper better than film, for example? Could power be produced by solar panels, from small nuclear units, or from other ways of storing energy? None of the existing units was satisfactory, but there were some good ideas available. Some of the manufacturers of x-ray equipment already had units running from batteries or storing power by charging up condensers.

The Pan American Health Organisation, the Regional Office of WHO for the Americas, held a week-long international meeting in Washington, D.C. in 1974, which focused on some preliminary and very basic concepts. The participants discussed the minimum power of the x-ray generator, the sizes of films, the methods of film-processing, the minimum acceptable safety requirements, and some suggestions for the size of the x-ray rooms.

It was with all this information that the WHO advisory group started to work, and after many meetings, and correspondence all over the world, the final specifications for the WHO Basic Radiological System (BRS) were produced. Then the major x-ray manufacturers, following these design requirements, started to produce the actual units, while the BRS group went on to devise the Radiographic Technique manual, the Darkroom manual, and the Diagnostic manual for the doctors.

The BRS is the equivalent of those small, simple but really very sophisticated cameras and has been so designed that, even for x-rays, it is almost possible to point the x-ray tube and press the button. Yet there will always be the need for that expensive and complicated x-ray machine, with highly skilled professional radiologists and radiographers to help with the very difficult and often unusual illness. Not least, they are needed to train the x-ray operator for small hospitals.[8]

2. Simple Handbooks Contains use of Appropriate Technology

The handbook acknowledges the importance of parasitic diseases and other particularly severe problems that exist in many areas of the world. Similarly, it enumerates animal bite and insect bites, including snake and scorpion bites. In the field of pediatrics, neonatology and infancy, preschool and school-age children are dealt with separately, with emphasis on important problems such as neonatal tetanus, and jaundice in the newborn. The section on medical and paediatric therapeutic and diagnostic procedures contains about 20 individually described procedures, which are tackled step-by-step so that they can be carried out by a qualified doctor who has had little practice. Simple procedures from setting up an intravenous drip and giving an enema to laryngoscopy and intubation, pleural aspiration and tapping an ascites form part of an illustrated section. This will provide enough guid-nce to enable a doctor to handle many medical problems with confidence, whether in an emergency room in a hospital or at the patient's home.[9]

3. Oral Dehydration Therapy

Few health technologies have as great a potential as oral rehydration therapy (ORT) to make an impact on childhood mortality in developing countries. Simple, inexpensive and effective, ORT can be used not only throughout the health system but at home as well.

Perhaps the most important achievement is the dissemination of this technology outside the formal health structure. Community health workers (CHWs) can effectively deliver ORT services, bringing about dramatic reductions in diarrhoeal disease mortality rates. In one community in India, a drop of 75 per cent has been achieved. Treatment of children in the home also allows CHWs to discuss with the parents other important topics such as domestic hygiene and better nutrition for sick children. In many settings, ORT has provided a stimulus for the accelerated development of primary health care programmes, and has become a vital element in the overall strategy to improve child health in developing countries.[10]

4. A new use for yeast for hepatitis B

Plasma-derived vaccines against hepatitis B cannot satisfy the needs of less affluent areas of the world where the disease is endemic. But vaccines produced in yeast by recombinant DNA technology seem likely to fulfil all the needs on a global scale.

To ensure the consistency of hepatitis B vaccines produced in yeast by DNA technology, testing will be required to show that the synthetic gene insert does not change when the yeast grows and reproduces and that the plasmid possessing the synthetic gene is retained by the yeast. Vaccine purification procedures must also be shown to remove host cell proteins and nucleic acids.

So far, untoward responses attributable to residual yeast proteins in the vaccine have not been seen in man, and the synthetic gene appears to be stable in the yeast plasmid. Only time will tell if yeast-derived hepatitis B vaccine will live up to its advanced billing. No doubt, there will be unexpected problems as yeast-derived vaccines are injected into larger number of persons, but these vaccines should be free from infectious viruses. At present, they appear well on their way to eventually replacing plasma-derived hepatitis B vaccines for the prevention of the disease worldwide and perhaps for the prevention of hepatocellular carcinoma as well.[11]

5. International Insulin Pump Study

One of the best examples of medical technology intended for home care of the patient is the miniature insulin pump. No larger than a pack of playing cards, it is usually secured by a belt to the chest or thigh of a diabetes sufferer. An implanted "shunt" (Valve) releases insulin into the patient's vein in quantities that he or she can regulate according to need. Insulin is essential for diabetes victims to maintain their blood-sugar level, and without it they risk falling into a coma. The pump can be recharged manually from an external source, or by inserting a cartridge containing fresh insulin.

In the early 1980s, it became clear that, while many countries were interested in developing these devices, there was no international coordination on evaluating them. The potential world market was estimated at some US $ 10,000 million, and more than 15 competing instruments were being manufactured, each with different optional features and costs. So managers of health care systems were faced with questions about the general medical efficacy of the pump, which pump to use, the possible side effects, patient acceptance, relative costs, maintenance and reliability. Costly and time-consuming trails tended to overlap with each other, and there were no plans to coordinate findings or to share costs and expertise.

Eventually WHO forged an agreement between the health ministries of seven European countries—Finland, France, Federal Republic of Germany, Hungary, Norway, Spain and the United Kingdom—to jointly pursue the evaluation and development of this potentially important instrument. The international programme that then evolved was assisted by a group of distinguished experts from different medical specialties and also engineers, economists and sociological psychologists. Not only has the programme provided an unusually detailed and multi-disciplinary analysis of a new medical system for the international evaluation of biotechnology.[12]

6. Appropriate Technology for Birth

There is no more crucial passage in life than birth. Yet 60 per cent of the world's women do not have access to pregnancy care and safe delivery care, which would dramatically reduce the risk of maternal and newborn mortality. Making available to them the appropriate technology that is required would be a decisive step towards Health for All.

The basic kit is simple, inexpensive and can be made from locally available materials. It supports three essential factors that will dramatically reduce the risk of infection in mother and child: a clean delivery surface, clean hands (soap and a nail stick), clean cutting of the umbilical cord (a razor blade and cotton for tying off the cord.) A tape measure enables the health worker to monitor the growth of the uterus regularly, in order to detect conditions that require special care. Newborn babies and infants can lose as much as 25 per cent of their body heat unless they are well wrapped up; a simple cap made from several layers of cloth can conserve a large part of their body heat, and thus make them less vulnerable to sickness. This is another example of Appropriate Technology for Birth.[13]

7. Medical Diagnostic Ultrasound

New technologies in the field of radiology have sprung up like mushrooms after rain in the last decade, a Japanese professor of radiology told a recent meeting on the use of new technologies in medicine.

Indeed, within the last ten to fifteen years medical technology has evolved with a sometimes bewildering rapidity, improving and creating new diagnostic tools which complement, or even compete with, each other. The difficult task for the doctor, health administrator and policy-maker is that of informed choice. Even the richest countries cannot possibly provide the total range of available technology, so high is the cost to patient and society.

But the routine use of ultrasound is something different! May obstetricians have found this diagnostic tool so beneficial that they recommend its routine use for all their patients, even in the absence of any clinical indications. This has led to a heated debate in medical and public health circles as to whether it is ethically acceptable to use routinely a method which, in theory at least, could harm the patient, and whether it is economically advisable to increase the already high cost of medical care by the routine use of any technique or medical device.

Professor H. Abrams, one of the most prominent radiologists in the United States, concluded his presentation at a symposium on the impact of the new imaging technologies on health care by stating:

> "In summary, we simply cannot afford the new technologies. They will cost a great deal and be overused. They will take resources from the poor and have little impact on the health of the sickest segment of the population. A paradox thus unfolds. On the one hand, a nation with high unemployment may well have better things to spend its resources on than computer tomography scanning, nuclear magnetic resonance and digital radiography. On the other hand, the individuals who constitute the nation and are subject to illness want nothing less than the best and the newest, if there is the faintest possibility that it may affect their health."

The key surely lies in the cost, benefit, risk equation in its broadest sense. And until we truly view health care and the medical technologies, not in isolation but as part of a total pattern of social and economic development, we shall be unable to use to real advantage the extraordinary advances in knowledge which make the present age so challenging and stimulating.[14]

CONCLUSION

One of the founding fathers of A.T., Dr. E.F. Schumacher, was famous for his saying: "Small is beautiful." It is equally true that "Small is useful." Modern miniaturization of electronic systems enables us to reach such unfortunates as leprosy sufferers. A "leprosy pencil" has been developed by WHO's Leprosy Unit with the assistance of CERN, the European Nuclear Research Centre in Geneva, Switzerland. Only about five million of the estimated eleven million leprosy cases in the world are registered, because of the difficulty of detecting the disease. Control of the disease depends to a large extent not only on adequate treatment but on starting treatment as early as possible.

The new pencil permits diagnosis at a very early stage. Nerve dysfunction is characteristic of leprosy, and one of its early symptoms is the impairment of thermal sensation. Hitherto, clinics tested for this by asking the patient to differentiate between one test tube containing warm water and the other containing water at room temperature. The new pencil consists of an electronic sensor that fits into a pencil-shaped holder and is powered by two small batteries. A person should easily be able to distinguish between the warmth of the sensor and the cooler part of the pencil—unless he or she is suffering from early leprosy. The device makes it possible for health workers to test for the disease under all field conditions.

So here too, the A.T. principle of "acting locally" is invoked, and modern technology in an appropriate form makes it possible to reach people where they are bringing health care to where it is needed is one of the most pressing preoccupations of health authorities in developing countries; no device or method that makes this more possible is to be despised.

The accent on people's participation is reflected in the concepts that are related to the A.T. approach; self-development, self-efficiency, self-reliance. A.T. appeals to people's sense of responsibility. And at the same time it is a process of continuous education, of conscious adaptation to the evolving needs of any developing country or community.

For far too long, it was thought that only university-trained people could become qualified health personnel able to cope with modern technologies. The emphasis that the A.T. approach puts on indigenous values has relegated such an attitude to the history books. It is now readily accepted that people who have not grown up in a highly literate culture are not at all automatically deprived of learning capacity.[15]

Technology stimulates science and science acts as a spur to new technology. Social progress depends on both technology and science, but both of these again depends on man's basic desire to live a life that is both physically and intellectually richer and fruitful. A piece of technology may be regarded as appropriate for a community if its design is related to the real needs of that community and its use fulfils these needs. Its use and promotion are based on that community's economic viability and technical competence to support, service, maintain and even improve upon it to suit local conditions. Appropriate technology is thus an approach in which technical innovation and adoption go hand in hand with social and cultural integration.

As stated in a WHO document, appropriate means: besides being scientifically sound the technology is acceptable to those who apply it as well as those for whom it is used. This implies that the technology should be in keeping with the local culture. It must be capable of being adapted and further developed if necessary. As stated in a WHO document, health technology has been defined as "an association of methods, techniques and equipment, together with the people using them." The use of appropriate technology is an important factor that will contribute to the success of health care. The following are some examples of these technologies:

1. Biogas generation for cooking, lighting and refrigeration.
2. Use of plastic mouds for water-sealed latrines.
3. Indigenous cooling system using running water to help maintain the cold chain.
4. Use of bamboo to fortify concrete-based hand pumps and community maintenance of these hand pumps.
5. Organisation of community maintenance of hand pumps.
6. Rain water storage tanks.

It is not defined in terms of the high level of technology used, but by the attention given to the local conditions and environment. Thus, appropriate technology, depends on the local skill, resources and talent. Appropriate technology is the only answer to promote primary health care. These were also reiterated by Alma Ata Declaration.

Ashok Khosla in his article, "Technology and Development" in *IJPA*, July to September 1989, pp. 531-32 rightly defines appropriate Technology as: "Technology which serves the goals of development is defined as appropriate technology. Appropriate technology springs from creative, in response to local needs and possibilities. It is relevant and ready for use by the common people, and aims directly to improve the quality of their lives. It derives maximum leverage from the local cultural environment, by drawing upon the existing managerial and technical skills and providing the basis for extending them. It uses the physical potential of an area and maintains man's harmony with nature.

It has become highly difficult to decide on the use of appropriate technology keeping in view the various factors—need, finances, nature of disease, etc. It has become a fashion to use complex technology for simple health problems thereby increasing costs and non-availability to majority of the people.

Sidney Nickhe in his article, "Money for Health" in *World Health*, May 1989, writes based on his experience in Kiteto district hospital. The costs incurred in running a district hospital are often high because the technology used in providing health services is neither sustainable nor effective. An affordable technology could be helpful to district health managers especially in the areas of support services and energy use.

To cook for the 50 or so patients admitted each month to the Kiteto district hospital requires seven truckloads of firewood, each weighing seven tons. This does not only mean deforestation and destruction of the environment, but is also an expensive and inefficient use of resources.

Cooking is done on an open fire where three stones serve as a stove.

Money could be saved by using an improved energy-saving stove, which also burns firewood. Such stoves are produced at an appropriate technology center in Arusha (CAMARTEC) and are sold to institutions, which use firewood for cooking purposes. The stoves reduce fuel wood consumption by more than 50 per cent compared to the three-stone fireplace. Where energy problems prevail, health services are inevitably adversely affected. For example, refrigerators for preserving vaccines use kerosene but practice shows that the unreliability of fuel supplies may result in spoiled vaccines. The use of kerosene for refrigerators, lighting and sterilizing purposes is too expensive for most district hospitals. Alternative sources of energy are available but capital investments are forbidding. A biogas plant could be more efficiently and effectively used at a district hospital than wood-burning systems.

Biogas is produced when bacteria break down organic material under airless conditions. It is a simple technology and when carefully used in rural hospitals where human and livestock dung is easily available, it would come cheaper than using kerosene, firewood or charcoal, with their added labour and transportation costs. Although capital costs are relatively higher—about US 1,000 dollars for material, labour and accessories—biogas is cheaper in the long-run.

Other technological innovations which could be used to reduce running costs in health care delivery include:

- use of solar energy for refrigeration, lighting and heating;
- water "harvesting" during the rainy season for hospitals and dispensaries in areas where water is scarce; underground storage of water has been found to be relatively cheap;
- Use of Ventilated Improved Pit (VIP) latrines in areas where water supply is unreliable and where resources are inadequate for installing and maintaining flush water toilets; and
- Avoiding recently introduced brand name drugs and relying instead on cheap generic products.

Dr. Nashara's five-year experience at the district hospital underline the importance of preventive rather than curative measures. He has seen a steady drain of the resources needed to treat patients suffering from preventable diseases.

> "If the environment is kept clean, swamps are sprayed and water is treated, the incidence of diarrhoea can be kept low," he says confidently, since experience has shown him that diseases prevalent in the area have a devastating impact on the community and on available resources."

Health care is gaining acceptance as a strategy for bringing basic health services to all the people. Such programmes can have a significant impact on health by focusing on a carefully selected number of health problems that are preventable by means of simple, and relatively low cost, interventions.

There is the knowledge to prevent cancer pain, derived from several decades of clinical experience and research, and there are simple inexpensive methods to ease pain. There are, as well, drugs to provide relief for patients, and to allow the incurably ill to die with dignity.

Yet despite the best intentions, what is known is not applied, and even though pain relief is the only human therapeutic alternative, it is not offered adequately to millions.

- Advocate campaigns through mass media to inform patients, and particularly their families, that pain is not inevitable, and is almost always controllable.
- Ask that a global network be established to help disseminate knowledge about what can be done to relieve pain.
- Call for more education in pain management at both graduate and under-graduate levels.
- Set as a goal the treatment of cancer pain not only in specialized cancer centers, which is the case now, but in hospitals and homes, it is estimated that only 10 per cent of cancer patients have access to centers. There is the need to reach the other 90 per cent.
- Urge governments to ensure that legislation controlling the use of opioids do not prevent patients from getting the pain-relieving drugs that they need.

The purpose of these and other measures is to change attitudes about cancer pain management, to dispel fears about medications that relieve pain, to make drugs available, to encourage their proper use, and to increase awareness that there are drugs and therapeutic approaches for pain relief.

Pain relief therapy already exists. The goal must be to share this knowledge with all, and to make realistic "Freedom from Cancer Pain" as quickly as feasible, certainly by the year 2000, but as immediately as is possible. Appropriate technology is available. It is now a question of putting it to use. Those who are in pain cannot wait.[16]

K. Ramamurthy, in his Article, "Environment and Development" some issues in G.S. Monga rightly states: "Excessive technological growth has created an environment in which life has become physically and mentally unhealthy. Polluted air, irritating noise, traffic congestion, chemical containments, radiation hazards and many other sources of physical and psychological stress have become part of everyday life for most of us. These manifold health hazards are not just incidental by products of technological progress, they are integral features of an economic system obsessed with growth and expansion, continuing to intensify its high technology in an attempt to increase productivity." This passage from the best seller, "The Turning Point by Fritijo Capra" admirably sums up the effects of so-called 'development' of the Western countries. Development without regard for ethics and environment has produced many harmful effects. The last hundred years have seen whole families of previously unknown diseases: new infections, genetic disorders that frustrate any attempts at prevention, endocrine disorders, allergies, toxic diseases, including the radiation and toxic allergic sickness gaining momentum with growing mass of synthetic materials totally alien to natural human environment; the notorious AIDS is but the latest addition to the list. Further, the development has the effect of making the developed countries richer and developing countries poorer, besides the mindless exploitation of valuable natural resources.[17]

Sustainable means meeting the needs of present generation without compromising the abilities and opportunities of future generation. It thus, implies both inter-generational and intra-generational equity. Sustainability is an important dimension of human development. Human development is a process of enlarging people's choices. But such enhancement must be for both present and future generations without sacrificing one for the other. Thus, sustainable development is a technique of eating the portion of bread and butter by the present generation in such a way that it must last long so as to enable the future generations to enjoy over it.

The last decade witnessed a heightened awareness of the detrimental environmental impacts associated with high industrial growth and economic progress. There was also a growing appreciation of the fact that sustainable development cannot be achieved in a climate where socio-economic development and environment planning are pursued as independent activities. This environmental concern is reflected in the various measures as are mentioned below:

- Developing a set of standards for regulating emissions and effluents from polluting industries.
- Periodic monitoring of the status of polluting industries. This resulted in a significant increase in the number of units that installed pollution control equipments.
- Seeking to control the discharge of effluents into water bodies by identifying the 851 grossly polluting industries and directing them to install effluent treatment systems or face closure. This resulted in 829 out of the 851 industries adopting effluent treatment plants. The remaining plants were forced to close down.
- Setting up of Common Effluent Treatment Plants (CETP) for Small Scale Industry (SSI) clusters.
- Preparing Zoning Atlas to help locate industries in areas where minimum environmental damage can take place.
- Encouraging research and development of clean technologies for use in various types of industries.

- Introducing and actively encouraging industry to adopt internationally accepted environmental management systems like ISO 14001 (launched in 1996).

The mind of man today both in developed and developing countries, more in developed countries, is prone to limitless desires in all areas whether industrialization, mining, construction activities, means of conveyance and communication, resulting into exploitation of environment beyond its capacity leading into frequent calamities in the form of earthquakes, floods, cyclones, health hazards, etc. All these make the life of the people poor, nasty and restless. Every nation must create a culture of service and not accumulation as it can induce positive vibrations in the environment.[18]

> "The miseries of the world cannot be cured by physical help only. Until man's nature changes, these physical needs will always arise and miseries will always be felt, and no amount of physical help will cure them completely. Ignorance is the mother of the evial and of the misery we see. Let man have light, let them be pure and spiritually strong and educated; then alone will misery cease in the world."[19]

From times immemorial, our seers and guides have made our society believe that the man only needs three basic things to tread on the path of human-graphs in ones life. They had been also guiding us to observe penance and perseverance in all spheres of our activities.

The three basics, they had enumerated as "Horne, Hearth and Helmet." No doubt, all these three are subject to their maintenance, through money and money only. For the achievement of this motive, they had also given us a set pattern of human endeavours, fixed, in certain parameters, and had advised the human race not to contravene those parameters, otherwise the man would suffer from the mental as well as physical disorders.

Now with the passage of time, the old perceptions have between rendered totally redundant by the man-made short-cuts and selfish tendencies, and a sort of rat-race is going on, on all sides of the world, in which the only object of life seems to be collection of money. With the new innovations, the new trade laws have come up in national and international arena and to opt these practices has (to some extent) become a necessity. The moral content of our culture and traditions has now taken a back seat, and the driving force is the unethical and unprincipled tendencies, which are sprouting and multiplying everyday, in these fast changing conditions.[20]

The Earth Summit 1992 is widely regarded as being one of the most important events of the century to address issues of global environmental degradation, inequalities between nations and possible strategies to protect the future of life on earth. Agenda 21, which emanated from the earth summit, effects a global consensus and political commitment at the highest level on development environment cooperation. It provides a framework for governments in their endeavour to seek a balance between population and pathways of development. It strives to formulate plans of action that meet the needs of people while providing for the ecological security of natural systems.

The main policies and programmes contained in Agenda 21 provide a major re-affirmation of a number of traditional values inherent in the Indian culture. It is also in conformity with all those values that are enshrined in the Indian constitution. The notion of sustainable developments is not a new one. The history of the country is replete with innumerable initiatives undertaken by people that demonstrate not just concern for environment, but also the awareness of the need to balance it with livelihood resources. This 'tradition' of care, conservation and preservation of environmental resources is also reflected in the spirit of the constitution of India, which has acted as the guiding inspiration of the nation now for over half a century. The strength of the Indian Constitution lies in the fact that it does not advocate any new or imported principles, instead it builds on the deep-rooted and therefore, resilient practices of sustainable development that have evolved over time in the country.

Thus, the congruity of Agenda 21's objectives of sustainable development with India's own traditional values provided renewed thrust to several initiatives in the country. It also provided new direction in sectors that have merged as areas of global concern.

From the beginning of time people have heard the still small voice of obligation and brotherhood. When they have listened society has worked. Why they have refused to listen, society has broken.[21]

The Stockholm Declaration (1972) on the human environment, said to be the "Magnacarta" on human environment proclaimed: "The natural resources of the earth, including air, water, land, flora and fauna are especially representative samples of natural eco-system. These must be safeguarded for the benefit of present and future generation through careful planning and management, as appropriate. The state should take all possible steps to prevent pollution of seas by substances that are liable to create hazards to human health, to harm living sources and marine life, to damage amenities or to interfere with other legitimate uses of the seas. The man and his environment must be spared against the nuclear weapons and all other means of mass destruction.[22]

"Carl Sagan in his magnificent, awe inspiring work Cosmos has described human predicament and dilemmas that surround us in the most thought provoking manner."

"The earth is a lovely and more or less placid place. Things change, but slowly. We can lead a full life and never personally encounter a natural disaster more violent than a storm. And so we become complacent, relaxed, unconcerned. But in the history of Nature, the record is clear. Worlds have been devastated. Even we humans have achieved the dubious technical

CHART 8.1

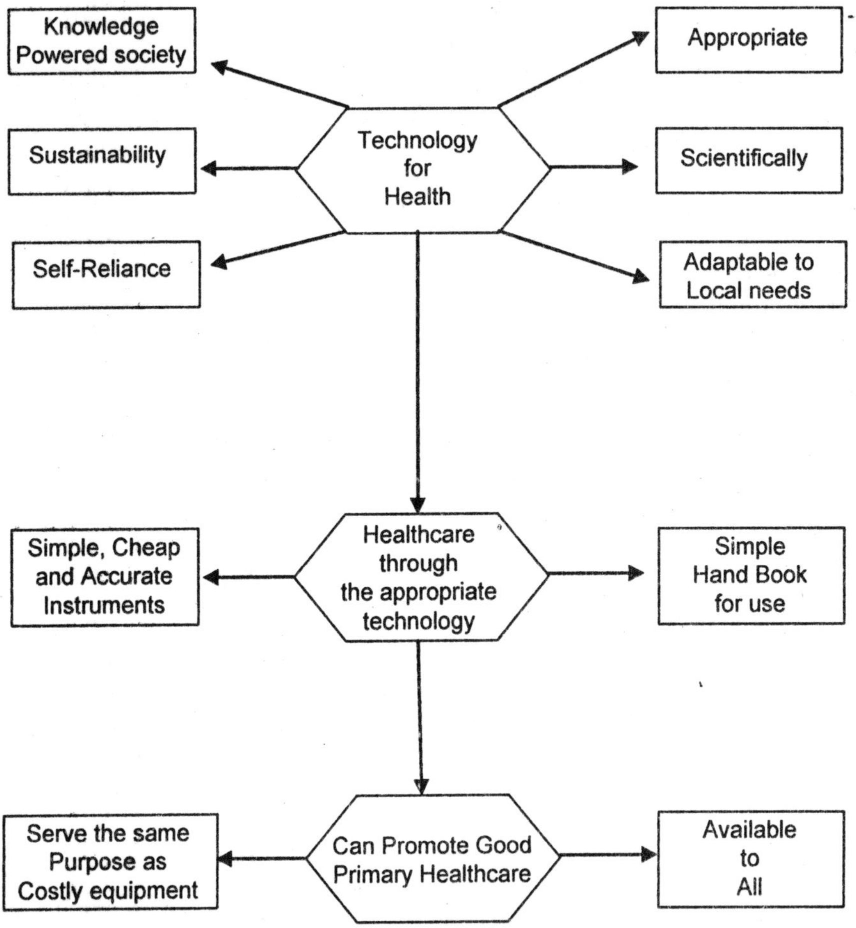

distinction of being able to make our won disasters, both intentional and inadvertent. On the landscapes of other planets where the records of the past have been preserved there is abundant evidence of major catastrophes. It is all a matter of time scale. An event that would be unthinkable in a hundred years may be inevitable in a hundred million."

Our lovely blue planet, the Earth, is the only home we know. Venus is too hot. Mars is too cold. But the Earth is just right, a heaven for humans. After all, we evolved here. But our congenial climate may be unstable. We are perturbing our poor planet in serous and contradictory ways. Is there any danger of driving the environment of the earth towards the planetary Hell of Venus or the global ice age of Mars? The simple answer is that nobody knows. The study of the global climate, the comparison of the Earth with other worlds, is subject in their earliest stages of development. They are fields that are poorly and grudgingly funded. In our ignorance, we continue to push and pull, to pollute the atmosphere and brighten the land, oblivious of the fact that the long-term consequences are largely unknown.[23]

Indeed, within the last ten to fifteen years medical technology has evolved with a sometimes bewildering rapidity, improving and creating new diagnostic tools which complement, or even compete with, each other. The difficult task for the doctor, health administrator and policy-maker is that of informed choice. Even the richest countries cannot possibly provide the total range of available technology, so high is the cost to patient and society.

The key surely lies in the cost benefit risk equation in its broadest sense. And until we truly view health care and the medical technologies, not in isolation but as part of a total pattern of social and economic development, we shall be unable to use to real advantage the extraordinary advances in knowledge which make the present age so challenging and stimulating.

Professor H. Abrams, one of the most prominent radiologists in the United State, concluded his presentation at a symposium on the impact of the new imaging technologies on health care by stating:

> "In summary, we simply cannot afford the new technologies. They will cost a great deal and be overused. They will take resource from the poor and have little impact on the health of the sickest segment of the population. A paradox thus unfolds. On the one hand, a nation with high unemployment may well have better things to spend its resources on the computer topography scanning, nuclear magnetic resonance and digital radiography. On the other hand, the individuals who constitute the nation and are subject to illness want nothing less than the best and the newest, if there is the faintest possibility that it may affect their health."

There has been a great revolution in technology in medical sciences. Complicated machines to be handled by experts are available. 21st century is going to be more explosive as far as the innovations in new technology are concerned. However, there is a need to simplify this highly complicated technology, which only a few can afford. We must develop simple technology, which people can afford and sustain, e.g. Oral Dehydration therapy.

Appropriate technology in health is going to be the greatest challenge of new millennium because of the following reasons:

1. Technology is becoming highly sophisticated with the passing of time.
2. It is highly costly to afford by developing countries on a large scale.
3. Manpower to make use of new technology is not available as it costs in their retention and training.

4. There are many inherent dangers in the new technology to have negative effects on health of the people.
5. Very less attention is being paid to develop appropriate technology to suit the needs of millions of people suffering from abject poverty and illness.
6. Complicated machines go out of order and we need highly trained specialists to maintain them.

Therefore, in the new millennium, we should focus attention on providing appropriate technology to suit majority of the population.

Notes and References

1. Claudine Brelet, Appropriate Technology for Health, *World Health*, June 1985, p. 21.
2. *University News*, 43(52), December 26, 2005-January 01, 2006, p. 18.
3. A. Sivathanu Pillai, Integrated Health Care Management.
4. Hakan Helberg, Technology for health, *World Health*, June 1985, p. 3.
5. A. Sivathanu, Integrated Health Care Management, *University News*, 43(52), December 26, 2005-January 1, 2006, pp. 15-16.
6. R.A. Mashelkar, Innovations as way of life, *University News*, 43(28), July 11-17, 2005, p. 14.
7. N.K. Ganguly, The magic neurotechnology for medical sources, *University News*, 43(17), April 25-May 01, 2005, p. 23.
8. Philip E.S. Palmer, Basic Radiological System, *World Health*, June 1985, pp. 4-6.
9. Balu Sankaran, Basic Medical Procedures, *World Health*, June 1985, p. 8.
10. Denise Ayres, Oral rehydration therapy, *World Health*, June 1985, pp. 9 and 11.
11. Robert J. Gerety, A new use for yeast, *World Health*, June 1985, pp. 12 and 14.
12. Kirsten Staehr Johansen, International Insulin Pump Study, *World Health*, June 1985, p. 15.
13. Appropriate Technology for Birth, *World Health*, June 1985, pp. 16-17.
14. Eero Lehtinen and Daphne Fresle, Medical Diagnostic Ultrasound, *World Health*, June 1985. pp. 18-20.
15. Claudine Brelet, Adaptable and Acceptable, *World Health*, June 1985, pp. 21-22.
16. Jan Stjernsward and Peter Ozorio, Why not "Freedom from Cancer Pain"? *World Health*, June 1985, pp. 23-25.
17. Mathur (ed.) ETMG, p. 4.
18. Swami Lokeswarananda: Practical Spirituality, the Ramakrishna Mission Institute of Culture, Calcutta, Calcutta, 1995, p. 6.
19. J. Mishra, Address of the General President, 38th Session, All India Oriental Conference, January 28-30, 1997, Jadavpur University, Calcutta, 1997, pp. iv-v.
20. Gurcharan Singh, "Pollution to Purity of Enviornment", Deep & Deep Publications, 2000, p. 4.
21. *Ibid.*, p. 632.
22. *Ibid.*, p. 4.
23. V. Suresh and Tranjot K. Gadhok, Sheler, Dec. 13, 1999, p. 110.

9

CHAPTER

Health and Research

Health research is indispensable for the growth and development of medical sciences. The control and eradication of communicable diseases has been possible by inverting vaccines and chemicals, which helped the control of diseases. All institutions develop with health are engaged in research in one field or the other. Medical science has developed the technique of organ transplant, which has made people hopeful. Through research medical institutions are progressing to solve the problems of patient. Doctors based on research have got the power to do miracles. However, in India we are not devoting time and money for research, rather we are depending on research in developed countries. There is a need that medical research may be given priority to make the people of India lead a healthier life. More money may be devoted for research in indigenous system of medicine, which has great potentialities. We have to do medical research in the areas, which are important to us and within our means.

From times immemorial researcher have been engaged to find better methods to keep human beings healthy. Human machinery is highly complex as health depends upon physical, social, mental and spiritual happiness. Human beings come in contact with plants, animals' human beings and environment daily. He affects and is affected by all these factors. From the last two hundred years, scientists are engaged to find medicines to keep human beings healthy. Mental health, which is most important, remained most neglected as physicians treated the body from outside but not his mental ailments. The mental phenomenon is becoming of greatest importance as most of the people today are suffering from tensions, stresses and other problems inspite of the availability of all physical facilities.

There are millions of people who seek medical care as a result of behavioural process, and millions more whose behaviour interferes with or is tragically untouched by the care they receive. There may be germs or viruses involved, and lesions, fevers, and pathogenic tissue changes. But the real cause of their problems is nothing a pathologist could see under a microscope and nothing a doctor can cure with a pill. Koch or Pasteur would have less technical understanding of the basic causes than would such behavioural scientists as Pavlov, Mead, or Parsons.

These millions are made up of sufferers from coronary heart disease, ulcers, asthma, migraine or allergies, who lead stressful, pressure-filled lives. They include chronically-ill migrants literally working themselves to death for slim pay which supports dozens of kin. Among them are counted those with pulmonary disease who yet continue to smoke heavily; those who know that they drink too much yet continue to drink too excess; obese people who cannot stop over-eating. Others need care because they or someone else has been careless or violent.

The problems of these people make up what T.A. Lambo has called "the other side of medicine." Many of them show no sign of physical disorder yet they constantly turn to doctors for help. Often the questions to which they desperately need answers concern serious (or for that matter trivial) personal problems, yet those answers now lie outside the province of most health care providers.[1]

When it comes to prevention of behavioural health problems, the need is among other things for application of knowledge of ways in which social change can be made more congruent with health and well-being. In some respects we have too much information on social alienation and lack of job satisfaction pursuant to industrialization, and not enough information on how planners, policy-maker and government officials can be made more responsive to the human squalor revealed by this information. Some governments are supporting research on what facilitates and impedes utilization of behavioural research results by responsible officials, and this shows that even specifically commissioned research runs little risk of being read. Until we learn more about this rather incredible impasse, the development of broadly based systems for identifying and preserving social practices beneficial to health will remain a dim possibility.

Even when governments are agreed on the need to improve the well being of their citizens through increased benefits such as new towns or settlements, little understood behavioural resistances contribute to the failure of costly projects with potential human benefit. The role of health care providers in increasing the successful adaptation of new communities can undoubtedly be a more significant factor in the future than it has been heretofore.

All these suggestions are another way of affirming that health is part of life and that medicine is part of society. We know that our success in the future will depend on working out, practicing, and mastering "the other side"—the behavoural side of medicine.[2]

In addition, the knowledge has been made available by great scientists as to keep oneself physically healthy but the Government have become ineffective especially in developing countries to make these available to people. One factor responsible for this is the rising cost of medical treatment. High cost of investigation by complicated machines has made the poor people not to avail of the benefits of health facilities.

We must also carryout research as to how the benefits of medical science can reach the people.

HEALTH SECTOR REFORM

According to a recent definition (WHO, 1995), health sector reform is a sustained process of fundamental change in policy and institutional arrangements, guided by government, designed to improve the functioning and performance of the health sector and ultimately the health status of the population. Health sector reform is concerned with defining priorities, refining policies and reforming the institutions through which those policies are implemented. As with health policy, there is increasing awareness that the process of reform and the difficulty of implementing policy and institutional change has been relatively neglected, compared with the debate about the content of reform (Walt & Gilson, 1994; Cassels, 1995).[3]

Survey Research

Survey Research is an indispensable tool to help the managers in the analysis of human behaviour. Cohen and Nagel have rightly stressed the need for Survey Research. "Most of our daily activities are carried on without reflection, and it seldom occurs to us to question that which generally passes as true. We cannot, however, always remain in a state of unquestioned belief. For our habitual attitudes are frequently challenged by unexpected changes in our environment, if they are not challenged by our own curiosity of the inquisitiveness of others."[4]

We must, therefore, understand the process of survey research *vis-a-vis* organisations, as it would enable us to be more effective in: (a) solving problems in organisational contexts, (b) understanding and applying results of research performed by others; (c) assessing the validity of claims made by others concerning the benefits of new practices, equipments, etc.; (d) evaluating; and (e) infusing scientific attitude among the administrators and managers to enable them to look at facts and events critically.[5]

Thus, we must introduce scientific research to design our organisations to make them efficient. Kerlinger has rightly defined survey research as "systematic, controlled, empirical and critical investigation of hypothetical propositions about the presume relations among natural phenomenon."[6]

Wolf says that research is "investigation or experimentation aimed at the discovery and interpretation of facts, revision of accepted theories in the light of new facts, or practical application of such new or revised theories of laws."[7]

We may keep in mind that research is a costly exercise; therefore, we must prioritize our research issues so that the outcome of the proposed research can be utilized meaningfully. The outcome of research should be widely disseminated to the concerned users.

Meaning

According to P.V. Young, "Social Research may be defined as a scientific undertaking, which by means of logical and systematized techniques, aims to: (1) discover new facts or verify and test old facts; (2) analyze their sequence, inter-relationships and causal explanations, which were derived within an appropriate theoretical frame of reference; (3) develop new scientific tools, concepts and theories which would facilitate reliable and valid study of human behaviour."[8] As stated in the Encyclopedia of the Social Science, "Social Research is systematic method of exploring, analyzing and conceptualizing social life in order to extend correct or verify knowledge, aids in construction of theory or in the practice of an art."[9]

The purpose of research is to discover answers to questions through the application of scientific procedures, i.e., Research Method. There is no guarantee that any given research undertaking actually will produce reliable, relevant and unbiased results. But scientific research procedures are more likely to do so than any other method known to man. According to Young, "A researcher's primary goal, distant or immediate is to explore and gain an undertaking of human behaviour and social life."[10]

Even though research cannot provide any final answer to the questions with which it is concerned, there has been a constant effort to devise procedures that will enhance the probable accuracy of research results. Why its necessary to be familiar with these research methods? For a student, teacher or any other interested person, who is preparing for a career in research in social sciences, the answer is clear: Research methods/ techniques are the tools of this trade. He needs not only to develop skill in using them but also to understand the magic behind them. The familiarity with research methods brings satisfaction of acquiring a new intellectual tool. The person who really understands the basic steps of research methods is in a better position to ask, with respect to every statement he reads or hears: What is the basis for that view? Is it supported by evidence? Under what conditions is it likely to hold true? And so on and so forth. According to Seltiz, "The research process consists of a number of closely related activities that overlap continuously rather than following a strictly prescribed sequence. These activities are so much interdependent that the first step of a research procedures have not been taken into account in the early stages, serious difficulties may arise and prevent the completion of a study. Frequently, these difficulties cannot be remedied at the time they become apparent because they are rooted in the earlier procedures. They can be avoided only by keeping in mind, at each step of research process, the requirements of subsequent steps."[11]

CONTENTS OF RESEARCH DESIGN

A research design should give detailed information about the following aspects:

1. The Topic of Research

The Researcher should be very clear regarding the topic of his research. It should clearly mention the scope and its limitations. He should review the existing literature on the subject.

2. Introduction and Background

It is necessary to introduce the topic of the research and its background so that the reader may be able to appreciate the framework in which research is carried out.

3. Objectives

The purpose of research must be very clear to the researcher, i.e. he should know as to what is the relevance of the research he is undertaking.

4. Concepts

Concepts in research must be communicable in a definite sense. They should not arouse a vague feeling. Working definitions are adequate if the instruments or procedures based on them collect data that constitute satisfactory indicators of the concepts they are intended to represent.

5. Variables

The research design must clearly mention as how to measure the concepts. This should be pointed out, in unmistakable terms.

6. Reference and Survey Period

The research design should indicate the period during which survey was conducted and the areas to which it pertains.

7. Time and Money

The research design mentions the time required for completion of research and the cost involved.

8. Schedules and Questionnaires

These should be prepared in a comprehensive manner so that the research design is pursued in right earnest, and the right amount of information is solicited from the target group.

Modern medicine studies man in detail,.but man is an indivisible whole of such enormous complexity that, at the present state of our knowledge and without present crude techniques, it is impossible to grasp the whole truth about him. There is a tendency to separate a part of the truth from the web and present it for the whole. This is the unsatisfactory state in which the social and biomedical sciences is equally true of the whole body of knowledge from which it has not yet been possible to deduce any consistent laws of life.

It is now apparent that a more balanced consideration of the biological, social, and cultural aspects of health is needed. Life is a process and not a substance—a living system based upon the primacy of continuity and interrelatedness throughout the universe. The history of human culture is not an evolution but continuous development, which is not broken at each generation as organic evolution is.

In most of these cultures there is a more unitary concept of psychosomatic interrelationship, i.e. a reciprocity between mind and matter. Health is not an isolated phenomenon but it is part of the entire socio-religious fabric; it is more than the absence of disease. When analyzed closely, the concepts of health and disease in non-Western cultures can be regarded as constituting a continuous transition with almost imperceptible gradations.[12]

SCIENTIFIC ADVANCES

Only in the past ten years has there been an awakening interest in biomedical research as an indispensable arm of health services. Health services research has become a critical issue and, in addition, an instrument for the enhancement of health and for the guidance of choice amid a multitude of health models. There exists today what one can call the ideal of science and of scientific research that has no frontiers, that speaks all "civilized" languages, that has no racial prejudices or ethnocentricity, and where scientists are the citizens of the world rather than of any particular nation. It is gratifying that there are still in our society men of science who are of broad human sympathy, deep sensibility, and deep compassion. Some of them have contributed to this issue of *World Health*, others are involved in different aspects of the Organisation's programme.

During the first two decades of the life of this Organisation, serious research was insignificant as compared with the exciting and dynamic advances now in progress. Many members of our Advisory Committee on Medical Research understand that a new world is in the making, a world shaped by that spirit that lives in communion with all men and women of science. It has now become virtually impossible for a scientist, a center, or a country, isolated from his or her associates, from other centers or from other parts of the world, to contribute to the progress of research. The history of scientific discovery has clearly shown that it has always been due to the labour of teams, working in centers scattered all over the globe and exchanging the results of their scientific work.[13]

Science and technology in the health sciences have provided some remarkable tools in the forms of vaccines and chemotherapeutic agents, while the latest advances in physics, chemistry and engineering have resulted in highly sophisticated diagnostic and surgical techniques, best epitomized by such "break-throughs" as open heart surgery or heart transplants. But to think that these great advances alone will have the desired impact on the total condition of man is to harbour a mistaken view. I hold this view to be false and suspect that its baneful influence has led to the cultural and social destruction of vast regions of Europe and America, and is beginning to spread confusion through all countries.

These very advances in the knowledge and application of high-level technology have resulted in:

- — a domination of human life by technology;
- — an over-emphasis on curative care to the detriment and at the expense of preventive and rehabilitative practices;
- — an increasing dependence by people throughout the world on technology and science developed and practiced in the most developed countries; and
- — soaring expenditures in health services and rises in the cost of health care which only the most affluent minority can afford.

The habit of comprehending and apprehending a technology in its completeness—"the essence for the technical humanism"—is an essential for the technologist. The scientist must not forget the history of medical progress and the invaluable part played by favourable social and economic conditions. Thomas McKeown, in his challenging article, "The Direction of Medical Research" (1979), reminded us of some of the fundamental issues. He wrote: "The most fundamental issue confronting medical research is evaluation of two approaches to the control of disease, one through knowledge of disease origins, the other through an understanding of disease mechanisms. And as both are needed, what is wanted is a decision about the distribution of effort between them and, if possible, recognition of the kinds of problems with which each is likely to be rewarding." Without undermining the achievements of medical research, he added, "the conclusion which seems inescapable is that with due regard for the invaluable contribution which immunization and therapy have made in some diseases, we owe the decline of the infections essentially to control of the conditions which led to them, rather than to knowledge of their mechanism applied through clinical practice."

We do however need, and we are seeking, new knowledge and new technology to ensure that there is health care available to all who need it, to ensure that there are health services at national and local level which meet health care needs in curative, preventive and rehabilitative areas.

We must foster a better knowledge of how health services can be organized to meet these ever-changing needs, how one might set the necessary priorities, how efficiency and effectiveness can be achieved with a reasonable amount of resources. Yes, and even how national authorities can be weaned away from the "disease palace" syndrome, that is, hospital-oriented medical services.

As long as the world's Research and Development capacity remains an exclusive prerogative of the industrialized societies in whose hands this capacity is highly concentrated, the focus and emphasis will continue to be largely on the problems of the affluent countries, and the developing world's potential capacity will continue to be eroded. The latter will never attain any substantial degree of self-reliance and, consequently, will remain dependent on imported—and frequently inappropriate—technology for their overall development. What is even more tragic, and perhaps criminal, is that the few active centers of excellence in the developing countries will continue to be funded by big centers from affluent countries to work exclusively on affluent society problems.[14]

ASSESSING HEALTH POLICY AND SYSTEMS RESEARCH PRIORITIES

A framework for setting research priorities will have to take into account at least three sets of factors:

Firstly, there is a need to assess the perceived importance of the topic. If this cannot be judged in terms of impact on health status, then the assessment must be based on potential impact in relation to other policy objectives, such as efficiency, equity or responsiveness to users. In addition, priority topics for health policy and systems research will necessarily already be on the policy agenda, nationally or internationally. In other words, there must be an expressed interest and a client who has a stake in addressing the policy issue concerned.

Secondly, even if the topic is perceived as being important, there is a need to decide whether the research proposed will advance the current state of our knowledge about the issue-either globally or locally. To receive priority, a research initiative must have the potential to tell us something new, and add to the "state of the art" in relations to the topic concerned. In this respect, international and local priorities may conflict. Locally, for example, it may be politically important to support research that documents the problems associated with introducing national health insurance in the context of a specific country. In terms of adding to the global picture, however, a research study that provides further confirmation of the difficulty of insuring a population with a large informal sector may receive much lower priority.

Thirdly, there is a need to consider the extent to which there is an appropriate match between the issues to be investigated and the research methods to be used. Returning to the problem of methodology discussed earlier in this paper, there is little to be gained by studies that focus on important health system problems if the research methods proposed are unlikely to generate information that is useful to policy-makers. Even if experimental studies are rigorously designed, they have limited value if they do not take adequate account of the context in which the change is taking place. In assigning priority to competing claims for research funding, it is essential to take into account the need for methodological development in the area of health policy and systems research.[15]

APPROPRIATE RESEARCH FOR COMMON HEALTH

W.A. Hassouna[16] in his article, "Solving People's Problems" has rightly said that, "Health services research is a relatively new field of scientific endeavour which achieved recognition in the 1960s. It seeks to identify ways and means of taking medical knowledge, expertise and technology out of laboratories, academic institutions and pilot projects, and applying it in order to solve the health problems of the people. It is an interdisciplinary approach, which is mainly concerned with action involving all the factors that affect health status through the use of health resources. It assists decision-makers at various levels in making accurate assessments of the health services delivery system and in identifying and testing the changes that can be made so as to lead towards more effective and efficient methods of meeting people's real health needs."

George C. Salmond[17] discuss the need, meaning and scope of research for Primary Health Care.

To many people the word "research" conjures up visions of laboratories, mathematical formulas and scientists in white coats. The work is thought to be complex, difficult to understand, and of little interest or concern to ordinary people. Health services research is not like this at all. It is best characterized by relatively simple studies of practical health problems, carried out in the community with the wide involvement, not only of those who organize and provide care, but also of those who use it.

Health services research can be defined as the systematic study of the means by which basic medical and other relevant health knowledge is brought to bear on the health of individuals and communities under a given set of conditions. Its aims is to provide new information and insights which will:

- permit a better understanding of health problems and the role and influence of health services;
- assist in more rational health planning;
- result in more effective and efficient health care, which at the same time is better attuned to the cultural and emotional needs of people; and
- by actively involving people in the study of their own problems, will encourage greater personal, family and community self-reliance in health matters.

Research has a particular contribution to make towards the development of strategies for primary health care. If systems are to be designed providing the essential care that people need, wide coverage and the people's full participation, all at a cost the community and country can afford, then research is needed to explore the possibilities, and to cost and test the various options. It is important for research efforts to focus on all points of the spectrum of services provided, and therefore, the effectiveness and efficiency of the whole referral system up to the big and specialized hospitals must also be considered.

The scope of the research is very wide, and may involve scientists and health workers from many disciplines. Research projects may range in size from major multinational collaborative studies to small studies involving one or two workers in a village or urban neighbourhood. But, regardless of the size and type of operation, the success of health services research must be measured not by the mere production of results but by whether those results are used to good effect to promote health and improve health services.

Incorporating community interests in health services research has brought benefits to both the researchers and the community. From the researchers' viewpoint, the priority health problems were identified and studied, and the results used to promote health and improve health services. Some compromises did have to be made. 'The research design was changed on a number of occasions to meet the requirements of the steering committee. The researchers grew .in their understanding of the ways of communities, and in their sensitivity to people's need for well definition. Without these insights such research must be limited in its success.

Huge sums of money are poured out annually on clinical hospital-based research 'in most States of India. One would not under-estimate the importance of this type of research because it adds to knowledge. However, one has to think in terms of defining the priorities of research. A State where the bulk of people are living in the rural areas, should normally involve the greater number of doctors doing researches in community health. India is one country, which cannot boast of even a single good epidemiological study of such communicable diseases as tuberculosis, from which a sizable number of people suffer every year. In fact, the area of community health research does not encourage clinicians to work in the rural areas. The problems of community health, no doubt, are vast and intriguing. Yet, the state cannot afford to ignore them. India lives primarily in the villages and it is the villagers who are the recipients of probably the poorest quality of medical care. The future of the state also depends on the progress made in the villages, particularly in the area of health. One has to watch and see how different States plan and administer their health programmes so that their rural beneficiaries are not outnumbered by their urban beneficiaries. Thus, the present trend of our spending on curative medicine research has to change in favour of community health research particularly in the rural areas. This is a challenge, which no State of India can afford to ignore.

B.O. Osuntokun[18] has rightly said, "We already know that health services research can produce impressive innovatory advances in health care services and a significant improvement in the health care of populations. The infectious disease yaws was eliminated from the forest belt of West African countries not by doctors but by "yaws scouts"-young illiterate men trained over periods of three to six weeks to recognize the early lesions, and armed and empowered to use the syringe, needle and penicillin-based drug. In Bangladesh, young women trained in a few weeks to carry out tubal ligation on women who chose this as a means of contraception achieved results as good or even better than those recorded by doctors. A glorious achievement of WHO's immunization programme is the worldwide eradication of smallpox, inspite of the various constraints including man-made ones such as wars."

Finally, epidemiological and health services research imply the establishment of a template of primary health care which is unchallengeably the ideal *modus operandi* by which WHO's goal of an acceptable level of health for all can be achieved. Developing countries must however bear in mind in supporting medical research that-as Daniel Coit Gilman, first President of the Johns Hopkins University, in Maryland, USA, expressed it, "Those ventures are not always most sagacious that expect a return on the morrow. It sometimes pay. . .to make investments with an eye to slow but sure returns."

Sir Gustav Nossal[19] in his article "Global and regional strategy has rightly said, "The great strength of these expanding national efforts has been the fact that local experts, knowledgeable in the cultural traditions and practical constraints pertaining to particular regions, are addressing and solving local problems. This brings solutions adapted to the situation and applicable in the given socio-economic framework."

The weaknesses will differ from country to country, but four constraints are sufficiently widespread, and sufficiently soluble in principle, to warrant drawing to the attention of decision-makers.

- Career structures for full-time medical research are nonexistent or inadequate in many countries. In some countries where adequate number of posts do exist, the remuneration is so far below that available in private medical practice as to represent a serious disincentive.
- Specialized consumable supplies, such as enzymes, chemicals and biologicals, which require foreign currency and importation, are difficult to obtain on a regular basis, while maintenance of equipment represents a great problem.
- Training programmes available for younger scientists, are poorly adapted to their needs, and to their future tasks. On many occasions, the researcher receives his training in a highly sophisticated overseas institution specializing in a complex line of fundamental experimentation. He soon becomes dependent on a vast infrastructure, and skilled in that ultra-specialized field. Returning home, he finds the simpler working conditions and the more applied nature of the problems frustrating.
- Communication links between scientists in developing countries and their counterparts in the developed nations are still far less evolved than they should be. Medical research is quite

> essentially international in character, depending on a network of communication and scholarship, each component part complementing every other one like the pieces of a huge and ever-growing jigsaw puzzle. Frequently the scientific literature cannot keep up with the pace of progress, and the chief operational tool guiding research consists of informal communication between members of a peer group (constituting an "invisible college"), or a small, specialized conference or symposium with participation by invitation only. It is vital that academics in the Third World be embraced in this network.

W.A. Hassouna[20], has pointed out that, "It is my conviction that health services research should form the core of the WHO strategy to develop primary health care as a means of achieving Health for all by the year 2000. What will be essential will be to develop a clear understanding of the practical aspects of primary health care, and to support research activities that demonstrate the cost-effectiveness of this approach as an essential and integral part of a pyramidal health services system. It will be necessary to support the development of national capabilities in health services research, and to concentrate on small-scale activities at country level. An information education communications programme will have to be developed."

Some areas for research are mentioned below[21]:

(a) Health manpower—their training, development, utilization, availability, needs and demands, etc., including experimentation with the development of various categories of health manpower.
(b) Primary Health Care—their availability, utilization, needs and demands.
(c) Organisational and management process in health and family welfare services, their linkages, etc., including referral systems.
(d) Perception, attitude, utilization factors (promoters and barriers) effecting utilization, etc., of population towards health and family welfare services.
(e) Problems and bottlenecks in the existing organisational systems and redesigning of existing systems to eliminate the same.
(f) Cost-benefit and cost-effectiveness analysis of health and family welfare services, programmes and projects.
(g) Development and testing of technology suited to the Indian health scene and needs.
(h) Studies focused on the interphase between community and health services organisations.
(i) Studies on health status and social and economic development.
(j) Enlisting of community participation.
(k) Identification of goals and priorities of the health services.

In the past, there has been little progress in the areas of research in vital areas affecting the health of the people. There has been research in high technology and sophisticated fields benefiting few people. In the new millennium, health research should become an indispensable part of other socio-economic research being carried out in universities and research institutes. In a WHO document, it has been realized that the universities can play a great role in conducting community researches.

Today, the universities must have a wider vision. Its three functions of teaching, research and service have to be reviewed in the light of a world blemished with gross inequalities and glamours with need. The winds of change must blow away the cobwebs of learning for its own sake (and of course Oxford itself is changing).

In the particular field of health, teaching is vital; but it must be directed towards all categories of health workers, including those in primary health care, not merely towards the medical specialist. And then research too is vital; but it should seek to resolve real problems, rather than being "pure research." And the service function of a university should surely rate top priority; in any country, whether developing or developed, there are serious gaps in the public health services which can only be filled through the efforts of well motivated people who are keen to apply their talents and their hard-earned skills to serving the community.

Problem-based learning is seen as a powerful educational strategy to maximize students' achievement of relevant knowledge, skills and attitudes. Specific considerations include the following:

- The systematic selection of problem and population-based concepts, which represent health needs of the community. This will require a balanced understanding of scientific, technological advances and social systems;
- The definition of relevant skills, including skills in problem solving, independent learning, critical appraisal of evidence and teamwork;
- The strengthening of teaching staff capacities related to community-orientation and problem-based learning;
- The development of curriculum design methods and learning tools appropriate to a community-oriented and problem-based educational system;
- A system of selecting health professional students, if feasible;
- The design of procedures and tools for assessing student and graduate performance; and
- The evaluation of innovative programmes including their contribution to the development of effective, efficient and human health care, and the commitment to Health for All.

The Network attempts to establish health research programmes that include basic, applied and operational research that is relevant to health and health care problems of the community to be served.

In the new millennium, we have to explore researches in health, which can raise the quality of life of the people living in rural areas, urban slums and tribal areas.

Despite the remarkable advances in medical science over recent decades, parasitic diseases still affect or threaten more than a thousand million people in the tropical countries, taking a heavy toll in human lives and gravely impeding economic development.

To stimulate and coordinate goal-oriented research leading to the development and application of new and improved tools to combat these diseases, the Special Programme for Research and Training in Tropical Diseases has been planned and initiated by WHO, with the assistance and co-sponsorship of the United Nations Development Programme (UNDP) and the World Bank.

This Programme's two principal objectives are:

- research and development for better tools to control tropical diseases; and
- training and strengthening of institutions to increase the research capability of tropical countries.

The six diseases initially selected for attack are malaria, schistosomiasis, filariasis, trypanosomiasis (both African sleeping sickness and the American form called Chagas' disease), leishmaniasis and leprosy.

Intimately related to the search for new tools is the equally important and interdependent objective: the development of manpower and the strengthening of research institutions in the endemic countries of the tropics.

While the Special Programme is especially concerned with training leaders in research, it is not neglecting the training of supporting workers in the laboratory, the clinic and the field, in the hope that within the next five years some of the new tools will be ready for extensive trails within the national health services of those countries that most need them.[22]

The pure and applied aspects of medical research, never as far apart as would be critics would have us believe, have come together surprisingly well to form balanced programmes with a judicious mixture of short, medium and long-term goals. WHO has managed to galvanize the biomedical research community into taking a new look at its global responsibilities, and has given a new reason for living to many scientists. The speed with which this has happened has been breathtaking. Now we must have the courage and the patience to stick with the programmes for the long haul, because, even with the expanded budget, progress will be slow and unpredictable. But WHO is in medical research to stay, using its special moral force in the most creative of ways.[23]

Health services research is a relatively new field of scientific endeavour which achieved recognition in the 1960s. It seeks to identify ways and means of taking medical knowledge, expertise and technology out of laboratories, academic institutions and pilot projects, and applying it in order to solve the health problems of the people. It is an interdisciplinary approach, which is mainly concerned with action involving all the factors that affect health status through the use of health resources. It assists decision-makers at various levels in making accurate assessments of the health services delivery system, and in identifying and testing the changes that can be made so as to lead towards more effective and efficient methods of meeting people's real health needs.[24]

Last but not least, health services research capabilities will need to be strengthened within WHO at country, regional and global levels. This may require some organisational changes but it is most important to involve WHO staff in field activities so that they acquire a practical understanding of the realities that influence health services in various countries.[25]

WEAKNESS IN POLICY ANALYSIS

While we believe that policy analysis has much to offer as both a research and planning tool, we are aware of the arguments that are marshaled against this view. For example, it is said that:

- all policy is decided on political grounds, therefore is unique in time and place, and cannot be generalized;
- the policy process is so complex that the social sciences cannot offer sufficiently specific tools to be precise about outcomes;
- the complexity of the research process makes it too long to be of use to policy-makers;
- information needed for policy analysis is sensitive and delicate, so that researchers may not get access to it, and even if they do, they may not be able to use it;
- information may become outdated because of changes in policy environments, especially in the uncertain and unstable current conditions affecting many countries;
- policy analysis is based on Western concepts that are not appropriate or applicable in developing countries; and
- information is qualitative, and is subject to bias from many different quarters; much will depend on the sensitivity of the researcher.

While many of these statements have some basis, they do not dismiss the case for policy analysis. Policy analysis is increasingly being used as a tool to analyze past policies, and as part of a process to change current policy. With growing interest in using methods of policy analysis will come a refinement and development of theories and methods, which will begin to meet some of the limitations mentioned above.

The benefits of policy analysis can be summarized as:

- providing in-depth explanation of why how policy outcomes were or were not achieved;
- providing tools to make future policy development and implementation more effective;
- providing a process which itself involves those making and implementing policy and which is therefore likely to lead to more workable policies; and
- providing mechanisms that open the policy process to a broader array of stakeholders.[26]

There has been an abiding interest in bio-medical research as an indispensable arm of health services. There exists today what can call the ideal of science and scientific research that has no frontiers and is useful for all the people living in this universe. The history of scientific discovery has clearly shown that it has been collaboration among scientists all over the world through World Health Organisation.

At present in India, we have good potential of research through specialized institutions like Indian Council of Medical Research, Tertiary Hospitals like AIIMS, PGI, and tertiary hospitals in particular areas hospital for mental health, cardiology, communicate diseases, etc. in addition Universities and Medical Colleges also conduct researches for their doctor degrees. Ten students have worked under the author in different aspects of health and hospital administration for their doctoral research. Inspite of all these research, we have not been able to provide decent care to people in India especially in rural, tribal and backward areas. The author conducted research in Himachal Pradesh and found that health facilities do not reach tribal to rural areas. We formulate one scheme after another but what is the result? The result is no improvement.

We need in India application of research to people through good work culture and dedication, i.e. we need good governance to provide services to people. Until and unless doctors do not provides existing health care to the people, him the system can be improved through good governance.

Good Governance is an essential ingredient for socio-economic development to the country. The Government of India and State Governments come out with new ideas and approaches but these do not succeed when put to action because of lack of good governance. Good Governance is of paramount importance in these times of far reaching changes. In this backdrop of major changes, we need to re-orient ourselves to deliver ways and means to promote good governance. No government of course can hope to survive without a strong and effective good governance nor can an administrative system exist without the support of those it was established to serve.

S.G. Barve feels that Good Governance is more an art than a science and there can be very few esoteric principles about it. It is a question of performance rather than theory or action. There are no sensational short-cuts to good governance. There are no spectacular solutions. What is wanted is a long and patient siege. Another outstanding deficiency is failure to locate definite responsibility at different points and levels of the administrative hierarchy. This location of responsibility has to be finally carried down to the level of the individual functionary.

The issue of good governance has, in recent times, emerged at the forefront of the agenda for sustainable human development. It is imperative that this process while being sustainable in terms of resources over generations and across space recognizes the legitimate claim of each person in a society to be an active and a productive participant. Empowering people for meaningful participation in this development process is one of the key interventions of the government of India in its attempt to usher in sustainable development.

Good governance implies utmost concern for people's welfare wherein the government and its bureaucracy follow policies and discharge their duties with the deep sense of commitment; respecting the rule of law in a manner which is transparent, ensuring human rights and dignity, probity and public accountability.

In the new millennium, the greatest challenge before the largest democracy of the world, is to steer the overall growth in the country along the lines of fairness, equality, justice and sustainability especially when the role of the Government itself is being redefined. Good Governance is of paramount significance in these times of far reaching changes and ushering in an era of globalization, liberalization and privatization.

The Prime Minister had announced during the National Conference of District Collectors in May 2005, the institution of awards for excellence in Public Administration. Accordingly, the Department of Administration Reforms and Public Grievances has instituted Award Scheme titled, "Prime Minister's Award for excellence in Public Administration" during the financial year 2005-06 for the recognition of the meritorious and outstanding contribution made by Civil Servants in the following areas:

- Implementation of innovative schemes/projects;
- Bringing about perceptible systemic changes and building up institutions;
- Making public delivery systems efficient and corruption free;
- Showing innovation and adaptation to meet the stake-holder's requirements;
- Extraordinary performance in emergent situations like floods, earthquakes, etc.; and
- Setting high standards of services and continued improvement, showing high leadership qualities and improving employees motivation, etc.

Indian administration is certainly the core of all human affairs. India is certainly on the cross roads of her national destiny, facing a serous challenge to our politics and administration, i.e. chronic delays, lack of sympathy and humane approach, time consuming meetings, corrupt practices, lack of work culture, criminalization of politics, insensitive and callous, etc. All these are the obstacles in the part of good governance, which can be removed by personnel in government both political and administrative to reassure good governance.[27]

CONCLUSION

All countries, East, West and Third World, have an urgent need to acquire competence in health services research. Some "developed" countries already have considerable competence in this area; but the topics selected for study are often unrelated to the priority health problems. And often the strategies adopted do not ensure that the research results will be sued to improve the delivery of care. Despite the increasing expenditures on health services in "developed" countries, health status is not improving and in some instances may be on the decline. National research efforts need to re-focus on the effects on health of environmental change and changing lifestyles, on the changing nature of health problems, and on the changing role of health services.

In Third World countries, the problems are different. Here the potentials of health services research need to be better exploited so as to make an efficient use of the scarce available health manpower, to mobilize and involve those additional health manpower resources that exist in the communities and, by strengthening the cadres of research workers, to minimize the dependence on external support.

The thrust of WHO's initiative in primary health care is mainly directed at the needs of the developing world, but the principles apply elsewhere. An obvious failing of the health care system in most developed countries is the unsatisfactory balance among the different components of the health system and the exaggerated attention being paid to expensive hospital care. Health services research is one of the strategies which may be used to promote healthy and the balanced development of health services in the community.[28]

Lack of Community Health and Health Administrative Researches

Huge sums of money are poured out annually on clinical hospital-based research in most States of India. One would not under-estimate the importance of this type of research because it adds to knowledge. However, one has to think in terms of defining the priorities of research. A country, where the bulk of people are living in the rural areas, should normally involve the greater number of doctors doing researches in community health. India is one country, which cannot boast of even a single good epidemiological study of such communicable diseases as tuberculosis, from which a sizable number of people suffer every year. In fact, the area of community health research does not encourage clinicians to work in the rural areas. The problems of community health, no doubt, are vast and intriguing. Yet, the country cannot afford to ignore them. India lives primarily in the villages and it is the villagers who are the recipients of probably the poorest quality of medical care. The future of India also depends on the progress made in the villages, particularly in the area of health. One has to watch and see how different States plan and administer their health programmes so that their rural beneficiaries are not outnumbered by their urban beneficiaries. Thus the present trend of our spending on curative medicine research ahs to change in favour of community, health research particularly in the rural areas. This is a challenge, which no State of India can afford to ignore.

Further, the health administration at the State level is poorly equipped. Most of the health administrators have got no training in the modern knowledge of management. There is no effort on the part of the personnel working in health departments to use modern to improve health care delivery. Moreover, the health departments, training institutions, medical colleges, nursing colleges do not seriously concern themselves with finding methods for optimum utilization of resources. Health services research should be multi-disciplinary, involving not only medical professionals and experts but also system analysts, operational researchers, social scientists, health economists, public administrators, anthropologists, etc. The State health department may encourage research inconsonance with priority problems of its health care delivery system. The health department may encourage researches, which affect programme delivery. Some areas mentioned below:

(a) Health manpower—their training, development, utilization availability, needs and demands, etc., including experimentation with the development of various categories of health manpower.
(b) Equipment, materials, etc., their availability, utilization needs and demands.
(c) Organisational and management process in health and family welfare services, their linkages, etc., including referral systems.
(d) Performance and impact of health and family welfare services.
(e) Needs and demands of population for health and family welfare services.
(f) Perception, attitude, utilization factors (promoters and barriers) effecting utilization, etc., of population towards health and family welfare-services.
(g) Problems and bottlenecks in the existing organisational systems and redesigning of existing systems to eliminate the same.
(h) Information systems for health and family welfare.
(i) Cost-benefit and cost-effectiveness analysis of health and family welfare services, programmes and projects.
(j) Cost-analysis of health and family welfare services programmes and projects.

(k) Development and testing of technology suited to the Indian health scene and needs.
(l) Studies focused on the inter-phase between community and health services organisation.
(m) Studies on health status and social and economic development.
(n) Materials Management in a hospital.
(o) Working of intensive care units.
(p) Cost of running hospital services.
(q) Staffing of emergency services.
(r) Utilization of operation theatres.
(s) Enlisting of community participation.
(t) Development of planning and management techniques.
(u) Identification of goals and priorities of the health services.

Research Policy and Cooperation

The thirtieth session of the WHO South-East Asia advisory committee on health research (SEA-ACHR), held in Jakarta from 14 to 16 March 2007, reviewed WHO's work on health research in the SEA Region for 2004-05 and 2006-07. The issue of national health research capacity was discussed in the context of strengthening of human resources for health research, improving health research management and promoting the utilization of evidence-based research results. The implementation of recommendations of the thirtieth session of SEA-ACHR included the establishment of a regional task force for research on avian influenza and strengthening of research management for better utilization of research findings.

According to the World Health Assembly (May 2007) resolution WHA 60.15, Member-countries should invest at least 2% of their national health expenditures in research capacity strengthening and 5% from health development programmes. In 2006, the average allocation for research in countries of the Region was 5.12% of the total allocation. However, the distribution of resources for research in individual countries indicated distinct disparities. Research budgets ranged from 2.7% to 9.4% of the total country allocations.

India, Indonesia, Nepal, Sri Lanka and Thailand participated in the Sixth International Conference on "transparency and accountability in health research" which was held in Ayutthaya, Thailand, in November 2006, and was conducted by the Forum for Ethical Review Committees in Asia and the Western Pacific Region (FERCAP). In 2006, training activities on international standards for good ethical review practice were conducted in India, Indonesia and Thailand.

The updated country profiles on helath research for assessing and strengthening national health research systems were received from 9 of the 11 Member-countries. These country profiles will be complied in the form of a book depicting the current scenario on health research systems.

During 2006, meetings, were conducted by the Regional Office to

CHART 9.1

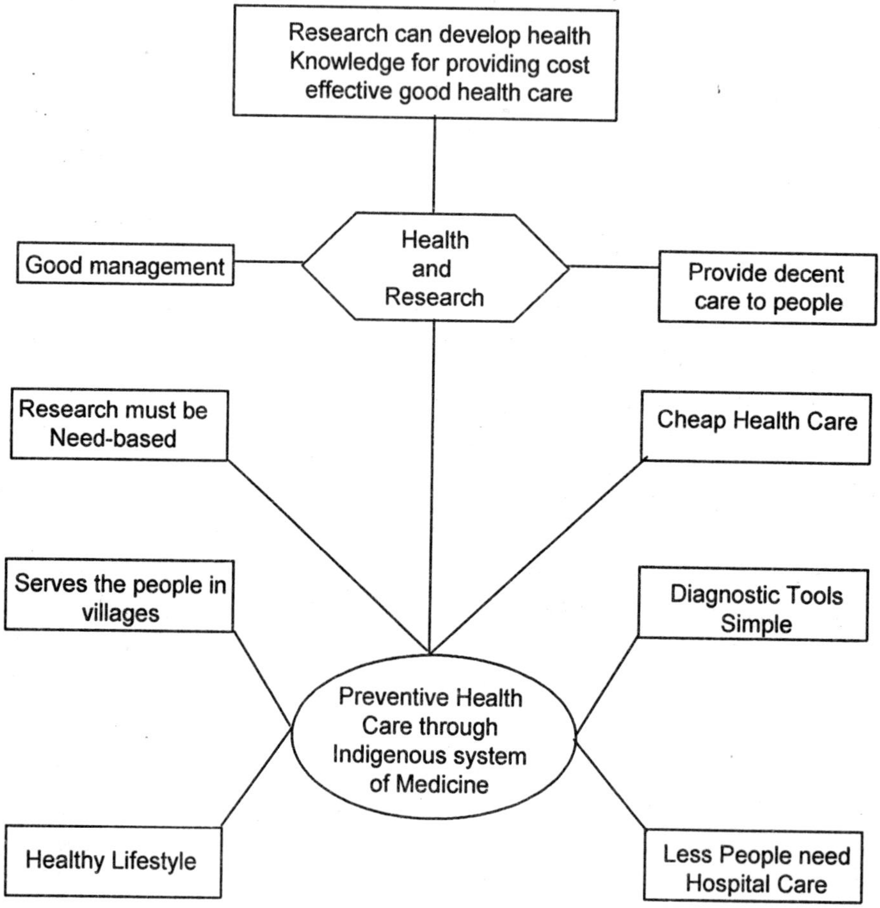

review research proposals under "the small grants research programme" of the Special Programme for Tropical Disease Research and Training of WHO (TDR/HQ). Ten out of 16 research proposals reviewed were supported in the area of leprosy, malaria and tuberculosis in Bhutan, DPR Korea, Indonesia, Myanmar, Sri Lanka and Thailand.

Indonesia took the lead to conduct orientations using the modules developed by WHO with guidance from research experts. It formed core groups of trainers, identified target audience for training and selected the appropriated modules and their relevant sections for developing the course package. Besides Indonesia, other Member-countries also used these research modules for training in research management. Output received from countries in this regard will be reviewed at a regional consultation and utilized for research management strengthening.

CHART 9.2

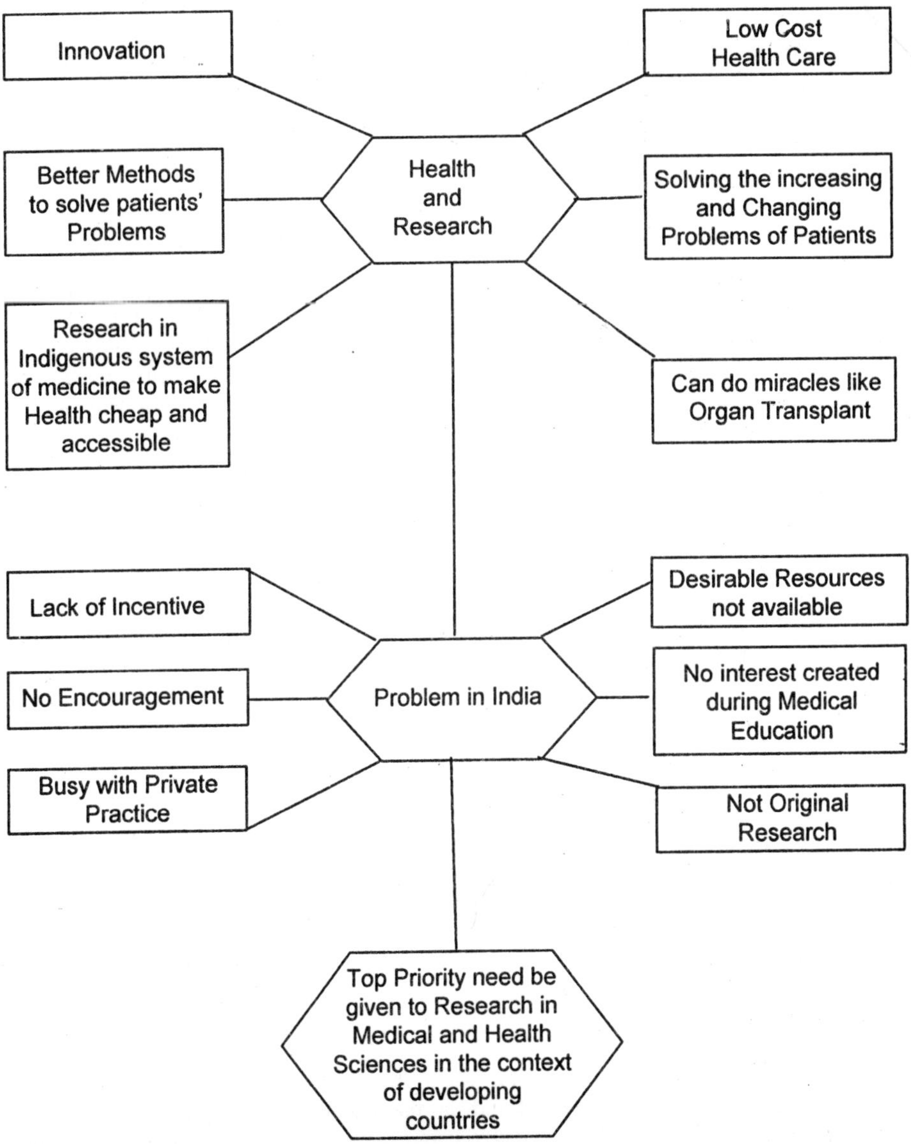

WHO collaborating centers and expert advisory panels

As of May 2007, the total number of active WHO collaborating centers (CCs) in the Region was 84, while two new proposals for designation of WHO CCs were undergoing the approval process. The country distribution of WHO CCs is summarized. There is a need to identify WHO CCs in un-represented countries.

The network for national WHO CCs and national centers of expertise (NEW-CCET) in Thailand was supported technically by WHO.

The newsletter brought out by the network secretariat was widely disseminated in all Members countries.

Furthermore, the managerial guidelines for designation/re-designation of WHO CCs were revised, printed and disseminated in March 2007.

Expert advisory panels

WHO has been working closely with the scientific communities of Member-countries to identify experts to be selected and appointed as expert advisory panel/expert advisory committee (EAP/EAC) members. In May 2007, 72 experts represented 38 areas of expertise as compared to 69 experts in 2006. There were 42 male experts and 30 female experts on the panels. The majority of members were from India and Thailand. Four member-countries in the Region did not have representation on any of the WHO expert advisory panels.[29]

Notes and References

1. Maureen A. Bailey, "The Human Side", *World Health*, December 1975, p. 4.
2. *Ibid.*, p. 9.
3. Katja Janovsky and Andrew Cassels, "Health Policy and Systems Research: Issues, Methods, Priorities," World Health Organisation, Geneva, 1995, p. 13.
4. M. Cohen and F. Nagel: An Introduction to Logic and Scientific Method, New York: Harcourt, Brace and Co., 1934, p. 3.
5. Eugene F. Stone: Research Methods in Organisational Behaviour, Good Year Publishing Company, Inc., California, 1978; p. 2.
6. F. Kerlinger: Foundations of Behavioural Research, 2nd Ed., New York: Holt Linkert and Winston, 1973, 1973, p. II.
7. H.B. Woolf: (ed.), Webester's New Collegiate Dictonary, Springfield, Man, G. and C. Merrian Company, 1975, p. 984.
8. Pauline V. Young: Scientific Social Surveys and Research, New Delhi, 1973, p. 30.
9. Donald Slessinger and Stevension, "Social Research", *Encyclopedia of the Social Sciences*, Vol. IX, p. 330.
10. Young: *op. cit.*, p. 30.
11. *Ibid.*
12. T. Adeoye Lambo, Total Health, *World Health*, December, 1975, p. 3.
13. T. Adeoye Lambo, A New World in the making, *World Health*, April, 1980, p. 2.
14. *Ibid.*, pp. 4-5.
15. K.atja Janovsky and Andrew Cassels, Health Policy and Systems Research: Issues, Methods, Priorities, World Health Organisation, pp. 21-22.
16. W.A. Hassouna, "Solving People's Problems", in *World Health*, April 1980, p. 27.
17. George C. Salmond, "New Problems New Strategies", in *World Health*, January 1980, p. 15.
18. B.O. Osuntokun, "Third World Needs", in *World Health*, April 1980, p. 9.

19. Sir Gustav Nossal, "Global and Regional Strategy" in *World Health*, April 1980, p. 20.
20. W.A. Hassuna, "Solving People's Problems", in *World Health*, April 1980, p. 27.
21. S.L. Goel, Public Health Administration, New Delhi, Sterling, 1984, p. 312.
22. The burden of the tropics, *World Health*, April 1980, p. 16.
23. Sir Gustav Nossal, Global and Reginal Strategy, *World Health*, April 1980, p. 24.
24. W.A. Hassouna, Solving People's Problems, *World Health*, April 1980, p. 27.
25. *Ibid.*, p. 29.
26. Gill Walt, Policy Analysis: An Approach, Health Policy and Systems Development, World Health Organisation, Geneva, pp. 236-37 and 239.
27. S.L. Goel, Preface, Good Governance: An Integral Approach.
28. George C. Salmond, New Problems—New Strategies, *World Health*, January 1980, p. 15.
29. The Work of WHO in the South-East Asia Region, 1st July 2006-30th June 2007, World Health Organisation, Health System Development, pp. 62-64.

10

CHAPTER

Health and Peace

> Science and technology have been employed to produce nuclear weapons in such quantities that nobody, anywhere in the world, would be secure if they were used. Even a small part of the stockpile might produce serious climatic changes, in addition to the devastating immediate effects from blast, heat and radiation, followed later by the effects of the radioactive fallout.[1]

NUCLEAR DISASTER

Nuclear emissions are very dangerous. Many countries of the world have nuclear power, which can create disaster of unbelievable nature, as there is a possibility of finishing life on this earth. The world leaders must come forward to ban nuclear power and made use of nuclear power to make the life of people disaster free. For example, India and Pakistan are busy in nuclear war preparation dangerous to both beyond imagination.

The introduction of nuclear weapons has added entirely new dimensions to warfare. Quantitatively it has brought an enormous increase in explosive power over that of conventional weapons. Whereas atom bombs of the type used in Hiroshima and Nagasaki represented an increase from tons of TNT to the equivalent weight of thousands of tons (kilotons), hydrogen bombs, developed about a decade later, represented an increase from kilotons to millions of tons (megatons). During the last two decades nuclear weapons have been amassed to an estimated total of nearly 20,000 megatons. Such is the increase in destructive potential that a single thermonuclear bomb can have an explosive power greater than that of all the explosives used in all wars since gunpowder was invented. The explosive power of the nuclear arsenals of the world is now about 5000 times greater than that of all the explosives used in the Second World War.

The weight of nuclear material needed to produce a 20-megaton bomb

CHART 10.1

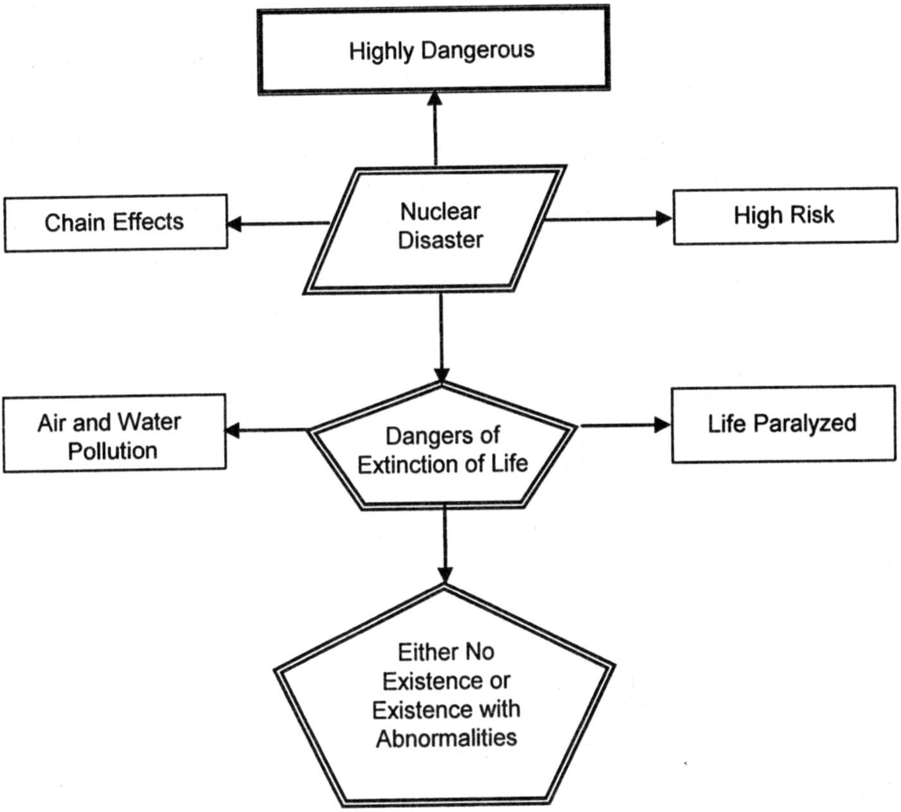

is less than 10 tons. With present day technology nuclear bombs can be projected to any place in the world. To produce the same blast effect with dynamite would require material weighting more than the Great Pyramid of Egypt.[2]

The potential for the release of radioactivity to the environment is a serious concern for the future generation. The wastes from nuclear fuel processing plants are endowed with a hazard life of 600 years. One may visualize the magnitude of the problem in that half life of plutonium is 24,350 years and its potential for causing hazards may persist for several times this period. With even low levels of exposure, the induced mutations may wreck several generations. This long-term effect, leading to abnormally and lethality, is responsible for regarding radiation hazards as the most severe of all other hazards so far known. Somatic damage induced in irradiated embryos as noted in the uranium miners from Colorado plateau and the survivors of Hiroshima, are too well-known to be recounted. The number of deaths from leukemia, following a continued radiation exposure even at the guideline dosage of 170 mrem per year, ranges from 160 to 32,000 per year in the United States.[3]

It is imperative that the health consequences of nuclear war become common knowledge. There exist today national societies of physicians against nuclear war in about 50 counties. The aim of these societies is to study and spread knowledge about the expected results of a nuclear conflagration.

Yet, at the same time, conventional weapons are being developed and produced in such numbers that a large-scale war using only such weapons would itself have terrifying consequences.

It is therefore self-evident that the most important approach to peace is to try to eliminate sources of conflict and work actively to increase trust between nations. This is a process in which increased scientific cooperation should be of great importance-even in areas where peace at present prevails.[4]

An acceptable level of health for all the people of the world can be attained through a fuller and better use of the world's resources, a considerable part of which is now spent on armaments and military conflicts. A genuine policy of independence, peace, détente and disarmament could and should release additional resources that could well be devoted to peaceful aims, and in particular to the acceleration of social and economic development of which primary health care, as an essential part, should be allotted its proper share.[5]

War Casualties

Detailed prediction about the number of casualties in a nuclear war cannot be made with any claim to accuracy. But estimations show that the detonation of a one-megaton bomb over a large city would kill more than one and a half million people and injure as many. A "limited" nuclear war with smaller tactical nuclear weapons, totaling 20 megatons and aimed at military targets in a relatively densely populated areas, would exact a toll of about nine million dead and seriously injured, of whom more than eight million would be civilians. And an all-out nuclear war using at least half of the estimated present stockpiles of nuclear weapons (an approximate total of 10,000 megatons) might result in more than 1000 million deaths and 1000 million injured people.

Rule-of-thumb procedures have been developed for dealing with the injured in conventional warfare and civilian disasters, but it is difficult to see how they could be applied in situations where the number of casualties could run into millions, hospitals and other care centers would be mostly reduced to rubble, fires rage, survivors be panic-stricken or, as in Hiroshima, reduced to a state of stupor, and help, if available at all, be prevented from reaching the people who needed it by the omnipresence of radiation.

Under such conditions, with facilities and supplies reduced, the capacity of the surviving medical personnel to provide adequate treatment for causalities or even merely to provide first-aid and keep the victims alive, would be next to nil. Moreover, entering the fallout area would present considerable hazards. Rescue teams would have to be monitored and, if possible, decontaminated, and personnel would have to be rotated to prevent them from being subjected to too much radiation. In the prevailing disorganisation such measures would probably be impossible. And the proportion of health personnel dying would probably continue to be greater than that of the general population, because of their exposure to radiation, disease and other hazards.

It is obvious that no health service in any area of the world could cope adequately with the hundreds of thousands of people seriously injured by blast, heat of radiation from even a single one-megaton bomb. Even the death and disability that could result from an accidental explosion of one bomb from among the enormous stockpiles of weapons could overwhelm national medical resources.

The World Health Organisation has its own contribution to make to a peaceful and equitable world, as its member-countries work towards the agreed goal of Health for all. But WHO is also active in drawing public attention to the fearful consequences of war.

The 36th World Health Assembly in 1983 received a first report on the effects of nuclear war on health and health services, and it approved a resolution, which emphasized "the role of physicians and other health workers in the preservation and promotion of peace as the most significant factor for the attainment of Health for all." The WHO Management Group formed by the Director-General to follow-up that resolution is for convenience known as WHOPAX; it consists of six scientists specializing in this field and meets regularly to draw up progress reports for submission to subsequent World Health Assemblies.

In May, for instance, WHOPAX submitted to the 39th Assembly the first results of specific studies on acute radiation mortality in a nuclear war, the impact of fires on casualties, the immunological consequences of a nuclear conflict, the possible climatic effects, including "nuclear winter", problems with food supplies and starvation in the aftermath, and the biological effects of pre-natal irradiation. More details of these studies will be made available in a second report on the effects of nuclear war on health and health services, which will be presented to next year's 40th World Health Assembly. A small working group is also examining, on behalf of WHOPAX, the psycho-social aspects of the nuclear threat, especially its impact on children and adolescents.

In its work, the Management Group continued its collaboration on individual issues with scientists, organisations and institutions specializing in the subjects concerned. These included the Committee on Environmental Consequences of Nuclear Wars (ENUWAR) of the Scientific Committee on Problems of the Environment (SCOPE), the erstwhile USSR Academy of Sciences, the Institute of Medicine of the National Academy of Sciences of the USA, the International Physicians for the Prevention of Nuclear War (IPPNW), the Greater London Area War Risks Study, meetings on the Red Cross and Peace, the International Symposium on "Medical implications of nuclear war" (Washington) and the Fifth International Congress of the IPPNW (Budapest). Discussions on areas for future collaboration were held with PPNW, a non-governmental organisation now in official relations with WHO. Specific issues for cooperation were agreed upon, such as the exchange of technical information and elaboration of curricula for medical schools on nuclear war and its effects on health and health services.

It was the General Assembly of the United Nations, which solemnly proclaimed 1986 to be the International Year of Peace, and called on all peoples to join with the UN in resolute efforts to safeguard peace and the future of humanity. WHO is playing its part in making the world aware how unthinkable warfare is today when, as Alfred Nobel foresaw, "armies are able to destroy each other in one second."[6]

Short-term Effects

In the first few days and weeks after a nuclear attack a great many health problems would appear, not only for the injured but also for the uninjured survivors, as a consequences of the collapse of the existing framework of society, the lack of food, the disruption of the health services, and the damage inflicted on the environment. These problems would be aggravated by the dislocation of the administrative structure, the destruction of sources of energy, the breakdown of communications and, possibly, social disturbances. Since the supply of water would undoubtedly be interrupted, water would be of crucial importance. Rain could concentrate the fallout in some localities, producing high levels of radioactive contamination, and fresh water would be contaminated above safe levels for drinking. Fresh food would also be contaminated with radioactivity, the only safe food being canned or food stored so as to prevent contamination.

Long-term Effects

The long-term effects of a nuclear war are more difficult to predict but may be just as devastating to human health as the short-term effects. Among them are the effects on the social and economic structure—the destruction of industry and agriculture, the uprooting of people, social disorder, and secondary warfare; on water supplies; on sanitation and public health; on the incidence of cancer and genetic effects; and on the climate and the environment.

With the destruction of public health and sanitary facilities the way would be open for the spread of disease. Water supplies would be contaminated not only by radioactivity but also by pathogenic bacteria and viruses, sewage treatment and waste disposal facilities would have disappeared, and lack of refrigeration would have led to spoilage of food supplies. The survivors emerging from shelters would not find conditions outside much better than those inside. Millions of putrefying human and animal corpses and mounds of untreated waste and sewage would provide an effective breeding ground for fillies and other insects that are more resistant to radiation than man. The uncontrolled growth of insect populations would favour an increase in the number of insect vectors of disease. Contaminated water and food would spread the enteric diseases.

Adequate food for the survivors would be an acute problem. Fertile agricultural lands would have been laid waste by fire and residual radioactivity. Erosion by wind and weather would lead to desertification of some areas of at present arable land, rendering it unfit for agriculture or even animal husbandry. Many millions of survivors from the immediate attack would die of starvation and malnutrition during the ensuing few years. It is a tragic irony that, whereas the warning time and action and reaction in nuclear warfare have shrunk to hours and minutes, the detriment to health it could cause would continue for years, decades and generations.[7]

The appearance in 1956 of the first sizeable nuclear reactor (at Calder Hall, in the United Kingdom) threw the glove into the world energy ring, at that time dominated by the heavyweights of the coal and oil industries. Thirty years later, there are now 26 countries which are members of the still somewhat exclusive nuclear energy club, comprising 406 reactors worldwide. In real terms, the figures speak for themselves: 70 per cent of all energy produced by France, nearly 50 per cent in South Korea and a quarter in energy-hungry Japan. The nuclear power stations are cheaper than coal or oil in the long-run, and emit no acid rain or industrial smog.

Provided nuclear waste in buried deep under the sea bed, the "worst possible scenario" has shown that it would take between 300,000 and 500,000 years for the most potent radio nuclide to get back to the surface. In many coal-mining areas in the world coal-tips are important emitters for radiation that are bound to stay on the surface forever. So much for ecologically sound fossil fuel.

Our age saw the introduction of several hundred "man-made" radio nuclides used in medicine, the production of energy, prospecting for minerals, treating cereals, and fire detection, to name just a few of their applications. Modern medicine alone has drawn heavily on these. Today, practically every hospital features at least some kind of radiation medicine equipment, whether for diagnosis or for treating diseases. Its uses range from the familiar x-ray machines to computerized tomography for detecting cancerous tissues. However, paradoxical it may seem, radiation treatment is one of the principal means of fighting cancer.

To sum up, it may be said with reasonable assurance that low-level radiation poses a relatively minor public hazard. Many people habitually accept the much greater risks of, for instance, smoking or driving. According to a UN publication, "a citizen of a developed country receiving an average dose from both natural and man-made sources of radiation is five times more likely to die on the road and more than hundred times more likely to perish from smoking 20 cigarettes a day, than he or she is to contract a fatal radiation-induced cancer."

The workings of modern science and technology in general, and of nuclear science in particular, are way beyond comprehension by the non-scientific community. When one is bombarded with rems, becquerels, millisievert, grays, it takes a lot of time and patience to be able to see the light in this terminological maze. With time, the paths of the two groups seem to be drifting further and further apart. Therefore, at least some of the blame for the general public's reluctance to accept the nuclear age should be placed at the feet of those ivory tower scientists who have been unwilling to translate the realities of their highly sophisticated world into language understandable by the non-specialists.

Knowledge is power—but not only for the few![8]

Professor Sune Begstrom, a Noble Laureate was the Chairman of an International Committee of Experts in Medical Sciences and Public Health who was invited "to study the contribution that WHO could and should make to facilitate the implementation of the UN resolutions on strengthening peace, détente and disarmament and preventing thermonuclear conflict." In May, the report of that Committee was put before the 36th World Health Assembly, held in Geneva.[9]

> "As doctors and scientists, the members of the Committee feel that they have both the right and the duty to draw attention in the strongest possible terms to the catastrophic results that would follow from any use of nuclear weapons. The immediate and the delayed loss of human and animal life would be enormous, and the effect on the fabric of societies would be either to impede its recovery or make recovery impossible. The light of survivors would be physically and psychologically appalling. The partial or complete disruption of the health services would deprive survivors of effective help.
>
> The Committee is convinced that there is a sound professional basis for its conclusions that nuclear weapons constitute the greatest immediate threat to the health and welfare of mankind. It is not for the Committee to outline the political steps by which the threat can be removed; but mankind cannot be secure until that is done."[10]

The basic issue, then, is not the cost of the nuclear weapons or the nuclear shelter but the treat the nuclear war systems pose to our biological existence. The credible nuclear deterrence would deter whom? And what would they defend? And if the concerned scientists' warnings about the nuclear night and nuclear winter are correct nuclear weapons pose a potential threat to the entire civic society.

For us Indians, therefore, the question is not of our national security but the survival of entire life-support eco-system on the Indian sub-continent. A nuclear conflict would lead to irreversible calamity for the whole SAARC region, a clear possibility of total obliteration of the great civilization extended all the way from the Hindukush of the Karakoram

CHART 10.2

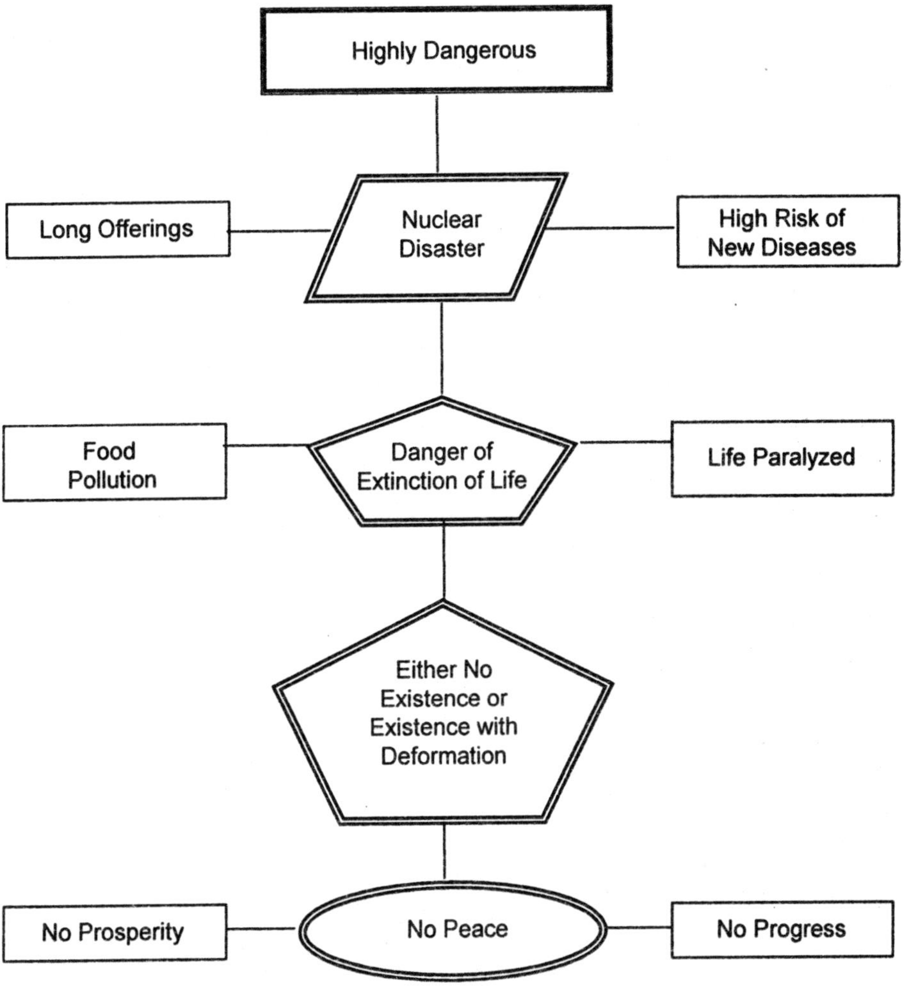

Range of the Himalayas to Kanyakumari and Rameshwaram. It would be practically impossible for any life to escape the unprescedented eco-devastation. "Traveling the slippery slope towards a nuclear arms race will keep us perpetually on the edge of a nuclear abyss," says retired Air Marshal Brijes Jayal.

From any scientific analysis, the credible nuclear deterrence is an obsolete paradigm. In the 1950s the nuclear-weapon states had built shelters to ride and fire the missiles with nuclear warheads. Americans had constructed tens of thousands of underground shelters and even homes were stocked with essential supplies of food and fuel. When 9/11 took place, President George Bush was taken inside such a shelter equipped notwithstanding, their efficacy in a nuclear theatre had never been tested.

The nuclear Non-Proliferation Treaty (1968) had received widespread popular support and many countries, including Japan, Germany, New Zealand and South Africa, have constitutionally declared themselves nuclear-free. Efficiently, there is strong popular appeal for creating a nuclear-free world orders in the 21st century. There is still time for us to cease the mad nuclear arms race.[11]

The term "safety" is however relative and cannot be absolute as, even at a very low level, continued exposure may lead to genetic damage. Most of the radiation standards are devised on the basis of harmful effects on taken into account, which affects the overall food chain in our ecosystem. In order to set a proper standard against radiation hazards, the entire ecosystem and the food chain in nature require to be considered. Absence of such a standard may cause irreversible genetic damage to life on earth and its environment.[12]

Social Effects

The social and economic effects of war on children are more subtle to discern, more difficult to measure and, consequently, even less known to the public and policy-makers than the physical effects of war.

War disrupts the economy of the country that it involves, interrupts development and progress, contributes to poverty unemployment and inflation, destroys natural, human and established resources, increases despair, decreases creative initiative. Children in the war zone, when they are not targets of shelling, suffer from the death of parents and providers, from homelessness, malnutrition, insufficient medical care, interrupted formal education and stunted growth.

While military expenditures throughout the world continue to grow, global productivity has not kept pace. The poor, the malnourished and the illiterate in the world exist in ever-increasing numbers, as do those who lack adequate housing, medical care and safe environments. Furthermore, the financing of the military has brought about neither peace nor security; arms spending can be directly linked to the worsening economic and social conditions worldwide which, in turn, increase the likelihood of war in the Third World.

Just as poverty, ignorance, disease and malnutrition cripple a developing country and inhibit the appearance within it of motivated, creative, capable individuals who can help it to attain the national goals of health, food and education for all, so too does war. Children brought up in war, made to view violence as acceptable behaviour in resolving problems, will be unlikely to forswear violence as adults.

Rather, they may no longer regard killing as an immoral act. And their generation, when faced with some regional dispute, may be more likely to opt for, and support, the financing and waging of war. The vicious cycle of militarism leading to poverty and despair, in turn leading to further militarism, would thus become firmly established.[13]

NOTES AND REFERENCES

1. Battle for Peace, *World Health,* July 1986, p. 3.
2. WHO: Profenor Bergstorm, Nuclear War, *World Health,* July 1983, p. 26.
3. The Shaping of Indian Science, Indian Science Congress Association Presidential Addresses, Vol. II, 1948-81, p. 1248.
4. Battle for peace, *World Health,* July 1986, p. 3.
5. Alma-Ata 1978—Primary Health Care, HFA Series No. 1, Battle of Peace, *World Health,* July, 1986, p. 4.
6. Alma-Ata 1978—Primary Health Care, HFA Series No. 1, *World Health,* July 1986, pp. 4-5.
7. WHO: Nuclear War, *World Health,* July 1983, p. 29.
8. WHO: Valery Abramov, One man's meat, another man's becquerel, *World Health,* June 1988, p. 13.
9. WHO: Nuclear War, *World Health,* July, 1983, p. 27.
10. WHO: Nuclear War, *World Health,* July, 1983, p. 29.
11. Dhirendra Sharma: Fallacy of Nuclear Deterrence: Very Biological Existence in Peril, *Tribune,* Chandigarh, Saturday, November 6, 2004.
12. The Shaping of Indian Science, Indian Science Congress Association Presidential Addresses, Vol. II, 1948-81, p. 1249.
13. Amal Shamma, Children in war, *World Health,* July 1986, pp. 7-9.

11 CHAPTER

Health and Disaster Management

Disasters of all kinds affect the health and well-being of people which make the life of people miserable, troublesome and unproductive. Until and unless, we take care of the health of the people, they cannot perform their daily routines. Health is the first important area which need to be restored during and after disasters.

Disasters cause mortality, diseases, disabilities, psycho-somatic problems and morbidity in their wake. The potential for transmission of communicable diseases increases manifold. It has been observed that transmission of water and food borne diseases occur within two weeks of the disaster. This is often due to faceal contamination of food and water. Other contributory factors are endemic level of disease, population density, population displacement and disruption of public health programme.

A disaster is a level of disruption which cannot be absorbed by the adjustment capacity of affected community within its own resources. Modern day construction, automobiles and fast moving trains, as well as air travel make the potential for getting many trauma cases at one time, due to a natural or man-made disasters. Any action to minimize the impact on the community consists of increasing the adjustment capacity of the community by way of training and contingency planning. During disasters it becomes a big struggle to cope up with the health problems that ensue, and the systems tends to collapse, especially in under-staffed or under-trained institutions. Usually the resources for health management are limited and already over-stretched. Thus, it becomes difficult to have set-up at local level, ready for disaster management.

The response to disasters usually starts as a primary health care problem. It needs collaboration at local level between sectors, the involvement of community and the resources of people and services. Many health problems follow in the wake of disasters, viz. diarrhoea, acute respiratory infections, vaccine-preventable diseases and malaria, etc.

CHART 11.1

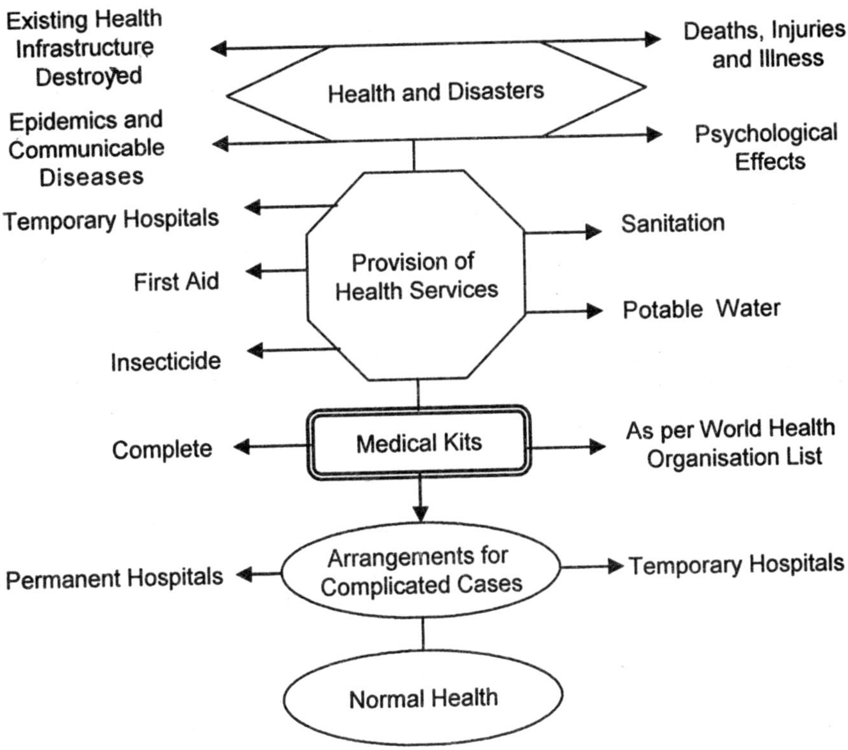

The population most seriously affected are poor, isolated, women and children. These problems however, are late squillae, and the present chapter deals with the problems related to the health and trauma caused by the disasters. Personal visit to many disaster affected areas would reveal the following:

(a) Lack of supply of potable drinking supply causing the spread of water borne diseases.
(b) The area or temporary camps created for the flood affected people are not clean resulting into many diseases caused by unsanitary environment.
(c) Food available or supplied is polluted.
(d) There is lot of congestion as many people are huddled in small areas.
(e) Children and women are the most sufferers as their need is not attended to effectively.
(f) People on duty are generally callous and try to make money through corrupt practices.

Therefore, Government, NGOs and community must provide safe drinking water, sanitation, safe food till the normal situation arises. Any planning for health preparedness has to be considered at local, district level or at central level. Many cases will definitely present at one stage, with all types of surgical trauma. Axial and appendicular injuries are perhaps the most common presentation. The element of chance exists in disasters, and most decisions need to be made quickly so as to minimize the potentially grave complications associated with spinal and limb trauma. There is need for rapid and appropriate response at a time when there is often great deal of political, medical and other pressures for immediate actions.

The district health plan should have in place a good system for mass causalties management and evacuation, continued management of common acute and chronic conditions, maternal, pediatric and other emergencies. Sufficient to say, that from the trauma point of view sufficient supply of resources in disaster prone areas is needed especially stretchers, splints, emergency lights, torches, pop, etc. Their ready availability and access are important. For emergency light smaller generators should be available in large numbers, so that the teams can work properly even in darkness

Let us classify the impact of disasters on health of the people.

(1) Mortality caused by Environmental factors—
  (i) Burying in debris,
  (ii) Drowning,
  (iii) Hunger,
  (iv) Fear psychosis, stress, anxiety and depression,
  (v) Famine,
  (vi) Electrocution,
  (vii) Accidents, and
  (viii) Poisonous gases.

(2) Morbidity and Mortality from Communicable diseases—
  (i) Lack of safe drinking water,
  (ii) Lack of sanitation,
  (iii) Improper Nutrition,
  (iv) Food Shortage, and
  (v) Failure of Electricity.

(3) Injuries—many people suffer injuries mainly fractures (orthopaedics), hemorrhages, Laccrated wounds and burns.

(4) Psychiatric Diseases born out of sudden shock, e.g. depression stress, social disharmony.

An important aspect of efficient management is to learn from the experiences of the past. Previous experiences at the local level can tell what works and what does not work in disasters, especially in third world countries, where the resources are always limited. It is important to note that the problems can differ due to different severity of disasters, the time of the day, the season, the population density, the particular group affected and existing health infrastructure and whether existing local health resources are spared or these are also disrupted. No disaster management can be efficient without the help from the local population, which may be required sometime on a large scale, especially with too many people injured in a natural calamity, like an earthquake. There is a need to build on the strengths of the community. Vulnerable communities also tend to learn strategies for their survival, their own methods to cope up. These must be respected and supported. Information and training in management of the potential health transportation and first-aid methods are very important. Pan American Health Organisation in its Scientific Publication No. 575 suggests the following for health management during disasters.

1. Population Density

Closer human contact in itself increases the potential spread of airborne diseases. This accounts in part for the reported increases in acute respiratory infections following disasters. In addition, available sanitation services are often inadequate to cope with sudden increases in populations.

2. Population Displacement

The movement of disaster victims may lead to the spread of communicable diseases to which the migrant populations are susceptible.

3. Disruption and Contamination of Water Supply and Sanitation Services

Existing water supply and sewerage systems and power systems are particularly vulnerable, and may be damaged by natural disasters. In the aftermath of the 1985 earthquake in Mexico City, for example, millions of inhabitants remained without a piped water supply for as long as several weeks. Drinking water is prone to contamination caused by breaks in sewage lines and the presence of animal cadavers in water sources.

4. Disruption of Public Health Programmes

After a disaster, personnel and funds are usually diverted to relief. If public health programmes (e.g., vector control programs or vaccination programs) are not maintained or restored as soon as possible, communicable disease transmission may increase in the unprotected population.

5. Ecological Changes that Favour Breeding of Vectors

Unusual periods of rain, with or without flooding, are likely to affect the vector population density. This may involve an increase in mosquito breeding sites or the introduction of rodents to flooded areas.

6. Displacement of Domestic and Wild Animals

As with human populations, animal populations are often displaced as a result of natural disasters, carrying with them zoonoses that can be transmitted to humans as well as to other animals.

7. Provision of Emergency Food, Water, and Shelter in Disaster Situations

The basic needs of the population are often provided from new or different sources. It is important to ensure that these new methods are safe and that they are not the source of infectious disease.

Outbreaks of gastroenteritis, which are the most frequently reported diseases in the post-disaster period, are closely related to the first three factors mentioned above. Increased incidence (or at least increased reporting) of acute respiratory infections is also common in displaced populations. Vector-borne diseases will not appear immediately but may take several months to reach epidemic levels. It should be noted that humanitarian workers are at risk following sudden-impact of natural disasters as well as the disaster victims. The principles of preventing and controlling communicable diseases after a disaster are to:

- Implement as soon as possible all public health measures to reduce the risk of disease transmission;
- Organize a reliable disease reporting system to identify outbreaks and to promptly initiate control measures; and
- Investigate all reports of disease outbreaks rapidly. Early clarification of the situation may prevent unnecessary dispersion of scarce resources and disruption of normal programs.

Disaster creates stress, anxiety and depression among people affected which is very serious which require Government, NGOs and others to offer mental health services.

Selye and Levi have defined stress as a non-specific, conventional and phylogenetic-based response pattern, the primary function of which is to prepare the body or physical activity such as resistance or flight (called Eustress). If, however, the subject lacks the means of restoring either to fight or flight, i.e. of relieving the stress reaction, stress gives rise to distress which manifests itself in the form of psychosomatic symptoms or disorders.[1] Ivancevich and Matteson define stress simply as "the interaction of the individual with the environment" but then they go on to give a more detailed working definition, as follows: "an adaptive response, mediated by individual differences and/or psychological processes, that is a consequence of any external (environmental) action, situation, or event that places excessive psychological and/or physical demands upon a person." Beehr and Newman define stress as "a condition arising from the interaction of people and their jobs and characterized by changes within people that force them to deviate from their normal functioning." High levels of stress may be accompanied by anger, anxiety, depression, nervousness, irritability, tension, and boredom. One study found that stress had the strongest impact on aggressive actions, such as sabotage, interpersonal aggression, hostility, and complaints.[2]

Stress according to Yoga is imbalance. Imbalance is misery. At the mental and physical levels, it is excessive speed and thus a demanding situation which causes pain and leads to ailments and diseases. Imbalances at the emotional level manifest as upsurges which are caused by strong likes and dislikes. At the psychological level the imbalances lead to conflicts and often manifest as petty and narrow ego-centric behaviour. Lack of holistic knowledge and a balanced outlook, at the subtle levels are responsible for imbalances found at gross levels.[3]

One of the implicit functions of diasaster management team is the responsibility of overall health . . . they need to recognize the signs and proactively introduce preventative stress management to reduce or mitigate potential stressors and resultant strains.

According to researchers, Jex, Beehr and Roberts (1992), stress is an overarching umbrella concept that is comprised of stressors and strain; or the processes where a stressor leads to strain.[4] A strain, also known as distress, is the negative reaction to the stressor.

Stress is a state of mind which reflects certain biochemical reactions in the human body and is projected by a sense of anxiety, tension and depression and is caused by factors associated with disasters. The intensity of such demands that require a readjustment of resources or operational styles would determine the extent of stress. Such environmental events or conditions that have the potential to induce stress are known as "Stressors."

The stress created by desirable and successful effects is called "eustress" and the stress created by undesirable outcomes is known as "distress." It is primarily the distress form of stress which requires examination and steps to cope with it.[5] It is important to deal with stress at an early stage. Early warning signs such as headaches, back pain, irritability, insomnia, absenteeism from work or alcoholism should be taken seriously. Otherwise they could lead to serious emotional disorders as well as physiological problems such as ulcers and heart diseases. When stress is left untreated for a long time, it can develop into anxiety and depression.

"Selye" postulated a 'general adaptation syndrome' of somatic systems caused by 'non-specific stress'. It involved three stages:

(a) Alarm reaction—When an initial shock phase of lowered resistance is followed by counter-shock during which an individuals defence mechanisms are activated.
(b) Resistance—It is a stage of maximum adaptation when the individual restores the equilibrium.
(c) Exhaustion—If the stress continues or the defence mechanism falters, the individuals moves to this stage.[6]

We must provide mental health services to restore all these affected by disasters. This can be done by medical team, NGO's and society. This requires constant counselling and assurance that everything would be ok.

They need not worry. This is not an easy task. It requires constant efforts to bring them back to life. Dr. H.R. Nagendra and T. Mohan feel that Yoga, the ancient science of India, is a conscious process for gaining mastery over the mind and thereby growing faster from the animal level to become normal human beings and reach heights of greatness, and ultimately attain divinity or perfection itself. This conscious process of gaining mastery over mind helps us to manifest the innate potentialities dormant in all of us and blossom into men with the five-fold personality development mentioned above. Yoga harmonises our growth and through balance, helps in total development. Such growth brings the divine qualities like love, affection, sacrifice, service, etc., which are at the base of the four-fold consciousness. In this sense, Yoga is the science of holistic living and is synonymous with basic or real education.[7]

SETTING UP A DISEASE SURVEILLANCE SYSTEM

In emergency conditions, the routine disease surveillance system is either not up to the task, is disrupted as a direct consequence of the disaster, or cannot provide data quickly enough for timely decisions to be taken. It is recommended, therefore, that a local, syndrome-based surveillance system be prepared at the national level and temporarily instituted in the disaster aftermath. It should be a more flexible and faster reporting system than used in normal conditions. The routine surveillance system must be re-established as soon as possible. In order to collect and interpret data, it is essential that a national epidemiologist be assigned adequate epidemiologic and clerical staff who have transportation to the field and priority access to public or private laboratory facilities. In addition to the national epidemiologic staff, university departments, research centers, and bi-lateral or international agencies may provide trained epidemiologists and laboratory support nationally or regionally. The national epidemiologist should be the secretary of a disease surveillance and control sub-committee of the Health Emergency Committee. The sub-committee should provide direct feed-back to hospitals and other health facilities where surveillance data are being collected.

The epidemiologist closest to the local reporting unit should investigate suspected disease outbreaks detected by the surveillance system as soon as possible. Until epidemiological assistance arrives, initial investigation and control measures are the responsibility of the local health unit.

Background data should be collected on the geographical areas affected, the major disease risks in the affected area (e.g., whether cholera or malaria are endemic), available resources, and at-risk and affected populations.

STAGES IN HEALTH MANAGEMENT IN DISASTER AREAS

Planning for Health Services

It has been seen that there is generally chaos immediately after the disaster as individuals, non-governmental organisations, government agencies, International agencies, bi-lateral aids, start working in isolation causing confusion and unplanned action. There is less benefits as compared to the resource used. The need is to plan properly before action. Planning would promote synchronization and optimation. The planning would evolve the following steps.

Planning for health in disasters is an intellectual process of analysing and conceptualizing a system, formulating its goals and objectives, assessing its capabilities and capacities, designing alternative courses of action or plans for the purpose of achieving these goals and objectives, evaluating and initiating the necessary action for its implementation, and monitoring the system to ensure the implementation of the plan and its desired effect on the system.

Planning is one of the major functions of disaster management. In the planning stage, decisions are made about what needs to be done, how and when it has to be done by whom and with what resources. In considering these points, managers are clarifying objectives or goals and establishing policies and procedures for guiding those who will do the work. They also have to chalk out the lines of action, with proper time schedules for the execution of work. This is all part of planning.

For disaster planning is essential. 'Well begun is half-done'. This proverb means that a Job which is carefully planned is half way to being successfully completed before the actual work commences. In other words, planning saves time in the long-run because we know where we are going and how we are going to get there. Planning leads to more effective and faster achievements because everyone involved is clear about what is to be done, how, when and why. Planning ensures unity of purpose clear-cut methods of doing things, and a focus on the objectives and targets to be achieved. In short, planning is like laying the foundation for a building. Once the foundation is laid, the upper structure of the building must necessarily conform to the basic design as outlined in the foundation. The preparation or ground work, which we call planning, minimises the cost of doing a job and helps to ensure that resources are used wisely to achieve our objectives.

CHARACTERISTICS OF GOOD PLANNING FOR DISASTERS

1. Focus on Purpose

Foremost in the planning process is the need of setting goals to be reached and objectives to be achieved, e.g. control of communicable diseases, trauma control, etc. These goals and objectives are the purpose of a programme. Every programme has a purpose. Health programmes have different purposes or objectives depending upon the nature of disaster like control of communicable diseases, or improvement of sanitation, or provision of MCH care. These programmes have their objectives, both qualitative and quantitative.

In an immunization programme in a disaster affected areas, when we say that we want to 'immunise children', that is only a goal or a qualitative objective. When we specify the coverage as a percentage of the children that have to be immunised, we now have quantitative objective. Planning takes into consideration both qualitative and quantitative objectives, and formulates goals that indicate the direction in which a particular programme is to move. So the most important thing about planning is to have clear-cut objectives and goals or a purpose.

2. Continuity and Flexibility

Like learning, planning for disaster is also a continuous process as things would change during and after disaster. When objectives have been set, a plan is not in a final form. Situations change, people change and technology changes. It may be necessary, therefore to adjust the plan to changes. The plan must be flexible and the planning process must provide for adjustments. This is particularly necessary in long-term plans that cover a period of years for rehabilitation of disaster affected people. But all plans must be flexible and the updating of plans must go on continuously.

3. Harmony with Organisation and Environment

In good planning there must have been complete identification with the organisation and with the environment. In other words, the plan should not be based on high ideals and be blind to the social, economic and political conditions in the environment. Over ambitious plans should be avoided. Plans should always be realistic so that all persons affected by disasters get their normal life back.

4. Precision

Planning must be precise in its objective, scope and nature. It should be realistic in scope and pinpoint the expected results.

5. Pervasiveness

It should be pervasive activity covering the entire enterprise or organisation with all its departments, sectors and different levels of management and functioning. Planning is not the exclusive responsibility of top management only, it extends also to middle and lower managers. In lower levels individuals must know individual work assignment in keeping with the overall objectives.

6. Documentation

Planning should always be documented so that all concerned are fully committed to the implementation of the programme. The document will also serve as a blueprint for implementation.[8]

Write-up of Formulated Plan

After deciding the priorities, goals and objectives, the next major step is to prepare a write up of the plan so that this can be circulated among all persons engaged in disaster rehabilitation. This may contain a schedule (time sequence for the plan to be implemented) and procedures (a set of rules for implementing the plan) and other details so that evaluation becomes easy and meaningful.

Implementation

Plan implementation is an integral part of the planning process. It requires responsibility for translating the objectives of health plan into action. However, looking from the broader point of view, plan implementation requires cooperation, coordination and commitment at all levels of the implementing machinery starting with the Ministries of Health at the Union and State levels through to the various non-secretariat organisations in the field at the district, block or village level. It is at the implementation level that the difficulties creep in resulting in lower output. Implementation must be watched properly and timely action should be taken to improve administrative, technical, financial or personnel inadequacies.

Health Actions in Disaster Affected Areas

(i) Epidemiology of the Area

This would include the estimates of the people affected in the area and the facts of diseases in disaster affected areas so that services may be provided accordingly. In addition, the survey may be done of existing health facilities which have not been affected by disaster, and are in a position, to provide health services. In this way, we can find out the need of extra help from neighbouring districts within the state, outside the state or International level depending on the nature of disaster.

The data collected would serve as the base for planning. Health statistics provide the key to a competent, sound and efficient planning. It has been stated officially that health planning and effective operation of health services are only possible on the basis of reliable statistics.[9] Dr. Chandrasekhar, Ex-minister of Health and Family Planning (India), emphasised the importance of this subject and said:

All over the region, greater efforts were needed to have better, further, more adequate and more reliable vital and health statistics. Health statistics were extremely poor not only in India but undoubtedly in the region as a whole.[10]

(ii) Temporary Referral System

Another important area in planning during disaster is to ensure screening by general doctors and then referring to specialists to avoid unnecessary misuse of resources and providing right type of services by right experts, i.e. creating a temporary referral system in the area. In this way we can optimize the use of personnel and equipment.

(iii) Courteous Behaviour

The third important aspect of health services in a disaster affected area is the need of good and courteous behaviours of the doctors since people are in a great shock. They need both medical help and personal touch which can provide relief to them

(iv) Resource Management

Resource planning is very important so that medicines and equipment are available. We have to take care that resources should not be misused as was done in Gujarat where doctors instead of helping the disaster affected people ran away with costly equipments donated by foreign countries.

(v) Priority Setting

The medical team must also be trained to function in a disaster area as the situation is beyond normal. When available resources are insufficient to meet the needs of the disaster affected people. Therefore, there is a need to select the pressing and urgent problems. There are a number of factors (economical, technical, financial, social, political and administrative, ethical, etc.) which must be taken into consideration while laying down the priorities. This can be decided with the help of techniques like cost-benefit analysis, cost-effectiveness. Priorities have to be determined at different levels.

Pan American Health Organisation suggests the following measures for mitigation:

1. Identify areas exposed to natural hazards with the support of specialized institutions (meteorology, seismology, etc.) and determine the vulnerability of key health facilities and water systems.
2. Coordinate the work of multidisciplinary teams in developing design and building codes that will protect the health infrastructure and water distribution from damage in the event of disaster. Hospital design and building standards are more stringent than those for other buildings, since hospitals not only protect the well-being of their occupants, but must remain operational to attend to disaster victims.
3. Include disaster mitigation measures in health sector policy and in the planning and development of new facilities. Disaster reduction measures should be included when choosing the site, construction materials, equipment, and type of administration and maintenance at the facility.

4. Identify the priority hospitals and critical health facilities that will undergo progressive surveys and retrofitting to bring them into compliance with current building standards and codes. The function of a facility is an important factor in establishing its priority. For example, in earthquake zones, a hospital with emergency medical capacity will have higher priority in the post-disaster phase than a facility that treats out-patients or those who could be quickly evacuated. Create mitigation committees at the local level to identify key facilities and ensure that mitigation measures are implemented in all projects.
5. Ensure that disaster mitigation measures are taken into account in a facility's maintenance plans, structural modifications, and functional aspects. In some cases, the facility may be well designed but successive adaptations and lack of maintenance increase its vulnerability.
6. Inform, sensitize, and train those personnel who are involved in planning, administration, operation, maintenance, and use of facilities about disaster mitigation, so that these practices can be integrated into their activities.
7. Promote the inclusion of disaster mitigation in the curricula of professional training institutions related to the construction, maintenance, administration, financing, and planning of health facilities and water distribution systems.

Let us now take up separately different types of health services:

Emergency Health Operations

The casualty department provides round-the-clock, immediate diagnosis and treatment for illness of an urgent nature and injuries from accidents. Simple cases after administering preliminary treatment are discharged with instructions to attend OPD as a follow-up measure. Cases of serious nature are admitted in emergency wards to provide immediate medical care. Such patients are either discharged after 2-3 days or are transferred to permanent in-patient wards. The best services must be provided to the patients in the emergency wards as the patients and their relatives are under emotional strain and surcharged with suspense and anxiety about the consequences of the disease or calamity that has come up suddenly. Such an approach would alleviate a large part of sufferings born out of fear and suspicion of the unknown. The Public Accounts Committee (1977-78) suggested that: "In order that the emergencies are attended to quickly and effectively, it is necessary to have an efficient set-up, well-knit with other departments of the hospitals with well laid out procedure and work distributions."

Once rescued, the victims of disaster may be found injured, bleeding, in a state of shock or unconscious. A quick physical examination can largely indicate the exact cause of infirmity. Resuscitation, wherever necessary may include maintaining the potency of airways, arrestment of haemorrhage, prevention of impending shock and its management, location and immobilization of fractures using body support, splints or improvised artifacts. The collective aim of all such resuscitator measures is to enable transport of the items to nearest medical facility in as good a state of health as achievable. However, those cases who have no chance of survival may be provided medicine and treated locally. Communicable diseases caused by water and air pollution can be taken care through potable drinking water and sanitation.

Water Supply and Sanitation

Safe water and improved sanitation are a necessary condition for better health, and there can be no lasting improvement of public health without them. There is no denying the fact that inadequacy of safe drinking water, improper disposal of human excreta, solid and liquid wastes leading to unfavourable environmental condition have been the causes of many killer diseases.

Inadequacy in the availability of safe drinking water, unfavourable environmental conditions and lack of personal hygiene have been the major causes of disease and disability among people. 80 per cent of diseases caused by disaster are related to unsafe water supply and inadequate sanitation.

Sanitation has become a yardstick of socio-cultural development of a nation. It is an important health index of any developing country. Since health and sanitation has an important bearing on the productivity, sanitation also has a correlation with economic progress of a country.

In the Johannesburg Earth Summit it has been agreed to halve, by the year 2015 the proportion of people who do not have access to basic sanitation, which would include action at all levels to develop and implement efficient household sanitation systems, improve sanitation in public institutions, especially schools, promote affordable and socially and culturally acceptable technologies and practices, promote safe hygiene practices and integrate sanitation into water resources management strategies.

Sanitation is a broad term that includes disposal of human excreta, wastewater, solid wastes, domestic and personal hygiene, etc. Human excreta is the cause of many enteric diseases such as cholera, diarrhoea, dysentery, typhoid, infectious hepatitis, and those based on worm infestation, etc. Studies reveal that over 50 infections can be transmitted from diseased persons to healthy ones by various direct/indirect routes from human excreta that cause nearly 80% of sickness in developing countries.

The health implications of this state of affairs as said are appalling Improved hygiene and sanitation help reduce sickness from diarrhoea considerably. Intestinal worms infect about 10% of the population of developing countries that can be controlled through better sanitation, hygiene and water supply. As per the WHO report globally 200 million people are infected with schistosomiasis, of whom 20 million suffer seriously. Basic sanitation facilities reduce the disease by up to 77%. Sanitation facilities help check transmission of many feacal oral diseases by preventing human excreta contamination of water and soil.

Water supply and sanitation are accepted as basic needs. Urban water supply and sanitation are areas critical to the quality of life, people's health and environmental protection. They affect the productivity in the towns and cities which contribute significantly to the national development. While water supply has received greater attention, sanitation has been comparatively neglected. Inadequate sanitation leads to degradation of environment and serious health problems of waterborne and vector-borne diseases. It is, therefore, necessary that both water supply and sanitation are treated together as issues in environmental health.

Kofi Annan, United Nations Secretary-General says that "The centrality of freshwater in our lives cannot be overestimated. Water has been a major factor in the rise and fall of civilizations. It has been a source of tensions and fierce competition between nations that could become even worse if present trends continue. Lack of access of water for meeting basic needs such as health, hygiene and food security undermines development and inflicts enormous hardship on more than a billion members of the human family. And its quality reveals everything, right or wrong, that we do in safeguarding the global environment."[11]

Nikolas P. Napulbow in his editorial, "Water For All, a Human Right" has rightly said that, "water is a basic human need for health indeed, for survival and therefore it is not an exaggeration to call it one of the basic human rights. Without safe water and sanitation, there is no real development. A community ravaged by diarrhoeal diseases, dracunculiasis or schistosomiasis cannot look beyond its immediate problems towards social and economic welfare. Safe water is the doorway to health and health is the prerequisite for progress, social equity and human divinity.[12]

Infectious diseases resulting from water pollution created by disasters can be classified into four groups, depending upon the ways in which their incidence can be lessened by improvements in water supply especially during disasters.

(1) "Water-borne" diseases are those in which infectious agents remains alive in drinking water e.g., typhoid, paratyphoid, gastroenterities, etc. The incidence of these diseases can be reduced by the purification of water.

(2) "Water-washed" diseases include infection of the outer body surface, e.g., trachoma, skin ulcers scabies and typhus, bacillary and amoebic dysentery and gastro enteritis. The incidence can be reduced by augmenting water quantity.

(3) "Water-based" infections, i.e., schistosomiasis, guinea worms. The infection occurs when the skin is in contact with water or through drinking water.

(4) "Water breeding" or water proximity diseases are caused by mosquitoes, or flies living near aquatic conditions.

There is probably no single factor that has a greater effect on the health, well-being and development of a disaster affected community than the provision of ample and convenient supply of wholesome and good quality water during and after disaster. Water supply is recognised as vital for the maintenance of public health and the prevention of epidemics. Dame Barbara Ward, President of the International Institute for Environment and Development, rightly observes that, "Water is everywhere, the key to human health, clean water is a key to human comfort, health and even survival."[13] Martin Boyer, Adviser, Drinking Water Programme, UNICEF has observed that "The provision of ample supplies of safe water and the sanitary disposal of excreta have a direct and far-reaching effect upon the health and well-being of populations. Indeed, it is believed that no other single measure can make a comparable contribution to the improvement of their health and standard of living. The choice of an appropriate technology depends on local conditions."[14] To quote WHO: "One hospital bed out of four in the world is occupied by a patient who is ill because of polluted water. . . . Provisions of a safe and convenient water supply is the single most important activity that could be undertaken to improve the health of people living in rural areas of the developing world. During and after disaster this becomes a serious problem.

WHO estimates that as much as 80 percent of all diseases in the world are associated with water. Lain Guest (Geneva), a specialist in development topics submits that an astonishing number of people suffer from these water-related diseases at any time, 400 million with gastro enteritis, 160 million with malaria, 30 million with river blindness, 200 million with Schistosomiasis.[15] At the 1969 World Health Assembly, a delegate from the region (SEA) estimated that water-borne diseases accounted for 40 percent of all morality, and 60 percent of all morbidity in his country.[16] This becomes aggravated during and after disaster.

Drinking water and sanitation improvements could reduce the overall incidence of infant and child diarrhoea by one quarter and cut total infant and child mortality by more than one-half. Country programmes are increasingly taking measures to improve water supply and sanitation within their primary health care programmes. Guinea worm disease can be effectively prevented by providing safe drinking water and its global eradication is clearly possible within the next few years. As for schistosomiasis, some 60% reduction could be achieved by improving water supplies. Building latrines, giving health education and introducing selected drug therapy could reduce the prevalence even more.[17]

WATER QUALITY ASSURANCE AND PROVISION OF SAFE DRINKING WATER

As the water supply and sanitation infrastructure was damaged by the earthquake WHO recruited experts to carry out a need assessments for local water quality capacity and the capability of existing systems towards providing safe drinking water. The experts also assessed rural sanitation and health promotion needs. According to the assessments 75 to 80 percent of water supply infrastructure was damaged. Also, the sanitation situation was worse in urban areas.

Although 90 percent of the water supply was from underground sources, due to the damages in the supply network there was a high risk of contamination of drinking water during transportation. Therefore, it was decided to enhance drinking water chlorination. To this end, WHO helped, thorough provision of chlorospopes to the government for its mobile teams; primary health centres and supervisors. The water provided by tankers in the earthquake areas was also chlorinated before distribution.

In the aftermath of an earthquake, flood, or cyclone there could be a serious water crisis. It, therefore, becomes very necessary to develop contingency action plans for meeting any emergency arising due to any of the natural or man-made disasters. These contingency action plans should include:

- Coordinating measures to be taken up to ensure safe water supply.
- A communication plan to alert and inform users of the supply.
- Detailed plans to provide and distribute emergency supplies of water.

Alternative safe water supply means have to be developed in the case of water supply system becoming in operational due to any disaster or mass evacuation of people. Various practical and social considerations must be taken into account prior to assessing the emergency needs of affected community, such as:

- number of people to be served;
- quantity of water can be calculated by taking atleast 15-20 liters per person per day for needs like drinking, cooking, personal hygiene, etc.;
- quality of available water and level of contamination; and
- availability of water at the nearest source.

(a) Urban Water Supply Scheme

If the disaster has affected an urban centre and a disruption to water supply scheme has taken place, the first priority should be to put the system back into operation. Damaged portions must be replaced or repaired and the supply must be quickly restored. In the aftermath of the disaster, the water pressure and the chlorine concentration must be increased to avoid any contamination from polluted water. In case any of the portion of treatment plant gets affected by the disaster, it should be repaired and proper disinfection must be done prior to putting it back into operation.

(b) Underground Source

Underground sources are usually free from contamination and may not require any treatment. When springs are being used as a source certain changes in the water quality may take place after earthquake. Hence proper testing for water quality is required before restoration of supplies. As far as wells as the potential water sources are concerned, the location of these should be atleast 30 m away from the potential source of contamination like latrines, etc. and should be at a higher elevation. The wells must be properly covered. For additional precaution, the drinking water from these sources must be boiled or disinfected prior to use.

(c) Surface Water

The usage of surface water as a water supply source should be the last option. Muddy, coloured, polluted water should not be consumed. The water from the surface sources should be treated to remove turbidity, colour and other impurities and should be disinfected. For this purpose mobile water treatment plants as an *ad hoc* measure could be pressed into service. Mobile plants need be made available mounted on a truck alongwith all accessories which include a centrifugal pump run by an engine, a rapid sand filter unit, chemical solution tank, chlorine solution tank and other necessary accessories.

Water Storage in Emergency

Emergency storage of water can be done in canvas, rubber coated nylons and plastic containers. Polyethylene containers erected in pits dug to size can also be used as storage. The total storage capacity for water distribution should be equal to the amount required for 24 hrs. Elevated water tanks must be erected using drums, iron sheeting and wooden poles, etc. For long-term emergency camps, all the storage tanks must be covered to protect from dust, and other contaminations. Proper arrangements for proper water discharge and water outlet, etc. must be provided in the storage tanks. Special attention must be paid for proper sanitation near these tanks.

Distribution of Water

In emergency situations water is usually distributed through tankers. The individual's families and local groups must be provided with water containers to store water. Special care has to be taken in checking the quality of water prior to transporting the water for distributions.

SANITATION

The damage and destruction of amenities included revamping sanitation infrastructure in the urban areas in Gujarat disaster. Here WHO assisted through building toilets and garbage bins in the temporary camps housing the victims. Also WHO supported the development of a solid waste collection programmes to supplement existing municipal services, and the spraying of disinfectants and insecticides in the camps. Support to train workers to carry out various sanitation-related activities, providing required equipment and supplies and supervision to support the relief work was also given by WHO.

In rural areas the thrust was on the construction of sanitation facilities at health centres, training health staff as sanitation promoters and educators and promoting sanitation services and healthy sanitation behaviour in the villages.

The success of the collaboration in the health sector is visible from the lack of epidemics in Katch district, the most badly affected area, after the earthquake. This was made possible through a coordinated response to disease and water quality surveillance, and the provision of basic water, sanitation and health amenities. Apart from the rehabilitation of systems, the surveillance system's prompt response also helped preventing epidemics. The coordinated system was also useful in reducing an overlap of activities between the various agencies working in the area.[18]

Potable Drinking Water

If water is the mirror of health, as an old proverb says, it can also become a source of disease when sanitation breaks down. Water is a basic human need for health—indeed, for survival—and therefore it is not an exaggeration to call it one of the basic human rights.

Without safe water and sanitation, there is no real development. A community ravaged by diarrhoeal diseases, dracunculiasis or schistosomiasis cannot look beyond its immediate problems towards social and economic welfare. Safe water is the doorway to health and health is the prerequisite for progress, social equity and human dignity.

An adequate quantity of water, by itself, is not enough to safeguard health. Unsafe water supplies lead directly to diseases that affect hundreds of millions of people, mainly living in the tropics.

An accessible and safe water supply, improved personal and domestic hygiene, and stronger community participation are the main ways to avoid water-borne diseases. But to be really effective they must be accompanied by other measures such as pollution control and proper drainage of surface water. Since environmental protection of fresh water sources is the basic step to ensure a sustainable clean water supply, this must always be an integral component of both environment and health programmes.

Drinking water and sanitation improvements could reduce the overall incidence of infant and child diarrhoea by one quarter and cut total infant and child mortality by more than one-half. Country programmes are increasingly taking measures to improve water supply and sanitation within their primary health care programmes. Guineaworm disease can be effectively prevented by providing safe drinking water and its global eradication is clearly possible within the next few years. As for schistosomiasis, some 60% reduction could be achieved by improving water supplies. Building latrines, giving health education and introducing selected drug therapy could reduce the prevalence even more.

Our studies on cost reduction through optimization of water supply and wastewater systems suggested that any integrated solution to the problem of water supply in the big cities should include:

- Integration of water and wastewater management, coupled with health education for cost-effectiveness and promotion of preventive measures for health;
- Prospecting for water resources through state-of-the-art techniques of remote sensing and geophysical surveys;
- Protection of water sources against pollution;
- Decentralization of water supply, matching the required quality and quantity with the supply through waste recycle and reuse;
- Maintenance of the water distribution system, which can prevent up to 50% of the purified water from being lost; and
- Application of mathematical programming techniques with exact fluid flow relationships in the design of water and wastewater systems, so as to ensure functionality and to conserve material and financial resources.

In the aftermath of any disaster, the immediate need of the situation is to provide sufficient portable water to the affected population. By providing the potable water various problems like spread of epidemics can be avoided.

So, in a disaster affected area water gets polluted because of collapse of buildings and large number dead bodies scattered all around. There is a need of ensuring potable water supply. Immediately, if the existing water supply is in operation, disinfecting the sources and taking other measures to provide safe drinking water to avoid the attack of communicable diseases which would be fatal.

FOOD AND NUTRITION

So, food has to be procured from neighbouring areas to feed the disaster affected people. There is a need of ensuring safety of food otherwise it can cause a number of diseases. Therefore, pure food may be procured and kept safely to feed the affected people.

Food and nutrition assumes an important role, when an emergency situation is created by strike of any disaster. While performing the exercise of food collection and distribution, the basic tenet of nutrition and balanced diet is to be kept in mind. Also, hygiene and sanitation measures have to be taken and duly maintained, which otherwise may worsen the already demolished and deteriorating conditions in a disaster. Food security becomes important. Food distribution has to be very quick and this can be ensured by the most feasible and available mode of transport such as road, rail or air. Likewise a fair distribution practice has to be adopted for the vulnerable population through the system of ration and adequate sanitary measures should be ensured and adopted during the mass feeding programmes.

HYGIENE AND SANITATION

Disaster affected areas must be made hygienic or where people are temporarily transferred in camps, there must be hygienic conditions and sanitation so that communicable and water borne diseases may not spread.

Hygiene and sanitation assume great importance in health management in disaster situations. Sanitation can be described as the means of collecting and disposing of excreta and community liquid wastes in a hygienic way. Keeping in mind the different areas, their water supply levels, solid conditions and population density, a proper planning of sanitary system should be done. Adopting any sanitation option should be guided by these conditions, as this will greatly minimise the problem of excreta disposal during disaster. However, when the existing sanitation system gets disrupted, rapid repair should be done and temporary arrangements for discharging sewage should be made. Adequate precaution and sanitary measures should be taken in the temporary shelters and camps.

Smita Mishra and Ragnhild Lund in their working paper, "Environmental Hazards, Women's Work and Health in Rural Kutch, Gujarat" (Institute of Rural Management, Anand, March 2003), stated that there was considerable damage to the health-related infrastructure in Kutch. The only hospital with all facilities in Bhuj town collapsed. Of the others, 21 Community Health Centres, 227 Sub-Centres, 800 Anganwadi Centres (Child and Maternal Care Centres), 6 Integrated Child Development Services Storehouses were all either entirely or partially damaged or the structures were weakened and were unfit for operation.

Impact on Health Facilities by Super Cyclone in 1999 in Orissa

The devastating super cyclone had caused enormous damage to infrastructure facilities at all levels of the health care delivery system. Around 1,485 peripheral health institutions were damaged, either partially or completely. Around 80% of the quarters of the medical and para-medical staff were damaged in this cyclone. Electricity failure caused difficulties in providing emergency medical services at health Institutions. It also caused total breakdown of the cold chain system meant to preserve costly vaccines and life saving drugs. Lack of mobility due to inadequate availability of vehicles and roadblocks restricted the out-reach of health services to people affected by the cyclone.

Out of the three medical colleges and hospitals of the state, the MGCG Hospital and Medical College has been severely affected in the cyclone of 17.10.99, and the October 29-30 super cyclone has caused damage to the buildings and equipment of the SCB Medical College and Hospital, SVPOGIP and AHRCC, Cuttack. The SCB Medical College and Hospital, which is an old and premier institutions of the country, has sustained irreparable loss to its buildings and equipment.

Social Security: Health

Large-scale damage to health infrastructure has led to disruption of health services in the cyclone affected areas. The following areas have been decided to be taken up for assistance:

Repair and reconstruction of health infrastructure is being carried out at PHC (Primary Health Care) level by the government as well as UNICEF. Additional support for strengthening of laboratories both in terms of providing the medicine supplies and manpower, as well as adequate hospital waste management in the CHC (Community Health Centre) is being provided by WHO.

This is accompanied by community involvement in various PHC services and training for doctors in disaster preparedness. Measure to achieve the positive health status in the affected areas: provision of continued support for diseases surveillance, establishment of communication network for various health institutions is being provided. WHO is financing projects on Community Health Care through participation of the Community.

The Action Aid as well as UNICEF are taking up Psycho-social counselling initiatives for the victims.[19]

Most of the damage due to the quake occurred in Kutch district. The service deliveries (Immunization, pre- and ante-natal care and other reproductive health-related services) particularly those relating to maternal care and child care were severely disrupted. The private medical facilities were also damaged in Bhuj town. All operational medical services were deployed for people with injuries. However, attention to promote full health care was not paid especially on women who are the major sufferers in terms of shelter, work, health, spouse, children. The gender differences need to be incorporated in any post-disaster relief operations especially to those living in vulnerable environment.

All hospitals and health facilities were made functional within a short time after the earthquake with temporary and alternative structures. The Bhuj civil hospital that had collapsed has been reconstructed, with the assistance of the Prime Minister's Relief Fund, at a cost of over Rs. 100 crores. The new building for the Bhuj hospital adopted the base isolation technology that was developed in New Zealand. Engineers from the New Zealand were also involved in the installation of isolators. It is a huge building with state-of-the-art equipment. It was inaugurated by the Prime Minister of India on 14th January 2004. Now this huge building has remained a structure only and has failed to become an institutions, as the state government has been unable to get it running. To have it working on the scale it has been designed, there is a need of sufficient funds. These funds are far in excess of the current outlay needed to run a district hospital. Besides the existing district hospital staff is also incapable of running it. This building, which is easily the most imposing and magnificent structure in Bhuj is the center of a huge debate. And the reconstruction effort draws a lot of criticism because of its being non-functional.

As regards other facilities, 6 community health centers, 24 primary health centers, 184 sub-centres, 9 dispensaries and 183 Anganwadis have been constructed. A number of other buildings are under construction. 1976 anganwads have been repaired. In the health sector, the reconstruction work is funded mainly by the European Union and NGOs. Most of the works funded by NGOs have made good progress whereas those funds by the European Union have been delayed because of elaborate procedure laid down.[20]

The progress of Health structures in the Rural areas of Kutch is as follows:

As stated in a Pan American Health Organisation document, the following areas are also important:

Priority Environmental Health Services

Primary consideration should be given to services essential for protecting and ensuring the well-being of the people in high risk areas, with emphasis on prevention and control of communicable diseases as there is danger of infections taking a massive scale.

Communications and Transport

Effective management of health relief requires access to and control of adequate transport and communication. Because the health sector's resources are usually insufficient to meet those needs, advance planning is particularly important to ensure that other institutions and sectors provide sufficient support in the event of a disaster. As part of pre-disaster planning, the Health Disaster Coordinator should make arrangements with entities such as the ministries of transport, public works, and communications; the armed forces; non-governmental organisations; private passenger and freight transport companies; private and state telecommunications companies; and ham radio operator clubs.

Responsibility and coordination for emergency government transport and communications should be centralized in a single office of the National Emergency Committee, which can coordinate their use for defined relief needs. The importance of developing a good working relationship with national telecommunications agencies and/or private sector telecommunications service providers cannot be overemphasized.

Health Measures

Due to shortage of water and food, people in drought-affected areas were likely to suffer from the following diseases:

1. Water borne diseases (Diarrhoea, dysentery, etc.),
2. Common type of diseases (Anemia, Malnutrition, etc.), and
3. Skin diseases (Scabies, etc.).

In order to tackle these problems, both curative and preventive health measures were to be taken in the following manner:

- The Control Room of State headquarters as well as the control rooms at the District and Sub-divisional headquarters to function round the clock.
- Supply of adequate medicine, disinfectants, Halazone tablets, ORS packets, etc. and other life saving medicines to drought prone areas of the districts.
- Chlorination of drinking water sources.
- Formation of minimum of two mobile health units in each district.
- Opening of Medical Relief Centre at vulnerable areas.
- Detection of Grade-III and Grade-IV Malnutrition amongst children and aged persons.
- Close liaisoning with District Administration Authority, ICDS personnel at the Block level.
- Weekly Diseases Surveillance Reports are to be submitted by Districts to the State Headquarters for monitoring the situations.

Availability of Drinking Water

Rural Water Supply

- During 2002-03 there was acute drinking water problem in all the districts due to depletion of ground water level. However, the following contingent plan had been prepared to tackle the situation.
- In order to overcome the likely distress situation in drinking water in some rural areas, where the surface water was normally deficient, water had to be transported by tankers. It was estimated that 10 such tankers will be required for about 10 months. Hydro-fracturing of about 1,000 existing bore wells was

required to improve their yield, for which Rural Development Department was pressed into service.

- It was assessed that about 9,000 tube wells have become defunct either because they have outlived their utility or ground water is not accessible. Apart from that, a number of new habitations have also come up. In order to provide the minimum required tube wells in replacement of the defunct ones and to cover new habitations with focus on SC/ST habitations having a population of 100 or more about 6,000 new bore wells will be immediately required. The cost estimate on this cost was estimated to Rs. 3000 lakh @ Rs. 0.50 lakh per bore well.
- In the western part of the State, about 8,000 tube wells had the problem of depletion of water level for which extension of riser pipe was apprehended for which approximately a sum of Rs. 200 lakh would be required.

Urban Water Supply

Scanty rainfall had adversely affected the urban water supply in most of the Urban Local bodies in general and those in the drought-affected and distress pockets in particular. The surface sources of water had been drying up. The ground water situation had also deteriorated. Source improvement measures like construction of cross-bundh, etc. for storage of water, sinking large production well, laying of connecting pipe, renovation of infiltration gallery, intake well had been planned.

Water Resources Management

Water Resources Management mainly demands conservation of water, reduction of wastage of surplus water, improvement of canal systems, creation of new MIPs and renovation of completely derelict MIPs to combat drought situations. Accordingly the action plan for specific actions depending on the resources was planned.[21]

CONCLUSION

Most of the people in disaster affected area become horrified and are afraid of drastic consequences. For them, the life becomes standstill. What is needed to bring them to normal life is counselling which need to assure them of good days ahead and bright future life. Pan American Health Organisation stresses the need of Training. To quote:

Training in all components of the disaster management program is necessary if activities are to be properly implemented. The failures in disaster mitigation, preparedness, and response are largely due to the gaps that exist between different professions and a lack of specific training for health care and public health personnel. Many health professionals have never received training, experienced a disaster situation, or participated in disaster management activities. Professionals employed in other sectors such as public works, financing (involved in construction of health facilities), foreign affairs, or the national disaster management agency (humanitarian assistance) should be aware of disaster preparedness and mitigation issues as they relate to the health sector.

Pan American Health Organisation suggests the Structural Health Disaster Management as given below.

The National Health Disaster Management Programme

The program's areas of responsibility are promotion, establishment of standards, training, and coordination with other institutions and sectors, as outlined on next page.

Promotion

- Health and social aspects and benefits of disaster management with other sectors, including the private sector;
- Inclusion of disaster reduction into development activities of other programmes and divisions of the ministry of health and other health sector institutions; and
- Public education through mass media and health educators.

Establishment of Standards

- Building and maintenance standards for health facilities in disaster prone areas, taking into consideration mitigation and preparedness measures;
- Norms for contingency planning, simulation exercises, and other preparedness activities in the health sector;
- Lists of essential drugs and supplies for emergencies; and
- Standardized telecommunication protocols.

Training

- In-service training of health personnel (from disaster prevention to response);
- Promotion of disaster management in the curricula of undergraduate and graduate schools in health sciences (such as schools of medicine, nursing, and environmental health); and
- Inclusion of health-related topics in disaster management training for other sectors (e.g., planning and foreign affairs).

Liaison with other Institutions and Sectors

- The national disaster management agency or other agencies with multisectoral responsibility;
- Disaster focal point or commission in other sectors (e.g., national disaster management agency, legislature, foreign affairs division, public works departments, NGOs);

- Disaster programs in the health sector in and outside the country particularly in neighbouring countries or territories; and
- Relief organisations at the national or international level (bilateral and UN agencies, NGOs).

In the event of disaster, the programme is responsible for: Mobilization of the health response; and providing advice and coordinating operations on behalf of the head of the health sector (minister of health), and supporting the health response in case of large-scale emergencies resulting from natural, technological, or man-made disasters.

Notes and References

1. Dr. H.R. Nagendra, New Perspectives in Stress Mangement, Swami Vivekanand Yoga Prakashan, Bangalore, 2003, p. 9
2. Peter Y. Chen and Paul E. Spector, "Relationship of Work Stressors with Aggression, Withdrawal, thief and substance use: An exploratory Sudy, *Journal of Occupational and Organisational Psychology,* Rand MC Nolly, Chicago, 1976.
3. Dr. H.R. Nagendra and R.P. Nagarthma, *op. cit.*, p. 41.
4. Ritu Kappula, Under the Influence of Stress, in *Human Capital*, Vol. 7, No. 10, March 2004, pp. 36-37.
5. Jito Chandan, Organisational Behaviour, Vikas, New Delhi, 1994, pp. 182, 192.
6. H. Seyle, The General Adaptation Syndrome and the Disease of Adoptation, *Journal of Clinical Endrocology,* 1946, p. 117.
7. H.R. Nagendra and Shri T. Mohan, "Yoga in Education", Swami Vivekananda, Yoga Prakashna, 1986, p. (iii)
8. 'Management Training Modules for Medical Officer', *Primary Health Care,* National Institute of Health and Family Welfare, pp. 97-98.
9. WHO, *WHO Chronicle,* 1966, No. 20, pp. 301-9.
10. WHO, SEARO: 20th Session of the WHO Regional Committee for South-East Asia, New Delhi, October 1970, p. 101.
11. "Water and Sanitation for Cities", *Building Materials News,* World Habitat Day, Oct. 6, 2003.
12. Nikolas P. Napulbow, Water for All: A Human Right, in *World Health,* July-Aug., 1992, p. 3.
13. Barbara Ward, "The Key to Health", in *World Health,* January 1977, p. 3, UNICEF, Assignment Children, 34, April-June, 1976, p. 11.
14. UN, 1970, Report on the World Social Situation, New York, 1971, pp. 167-68.
15. M.C. Gupta and Vinod K. Sharma, "Orissa Super Cyclone, 1999", National Centre for Disaster Management, IIPA, New Delhi, pp. 68-69.
16. Reading and Case Studies on Disaster Management, Centre for Disaster Management, Vol. II, p. 45-46.
17. *World Health,* July-August, 1992, p. 7.
18. *Sangam,* Newsletter of UN Inter-Agency, Vol. I, June 2004.
19. *World Health,* July-August, 1992.
20. GOI, Department of Agriculture and Co-operation, Ministry of Agriculture, States Report, Orissa, pp. 188-89.
21. Centre for Disaster Management, LBSAA, Mussorie Readings and Case Studies on Disaster Management, 2006, pp. 45-46.

12

CHAPTER

Health and Stress/Strain

INTRODUCTION

Inspite of the proliferation of health institutions both in public and private sector, health problems are on the increase. An interesting phenomenon of health problems is rising cases of diseases caused by stresses and tensions for which medical treatment is inadequate as the medical science deals mostly on physical plane. This has also led to the consumption of medicines on a large scale causing side-effects. It is being realized that the existing health system has failed to provide quality health services and that is why new institutions dealing in the science of Yoga, medication, are coming up in a big way to strike at the root causes of ill health. We may keep in mind that these institutions also failed in treating patients suffering from diseases arising from stress as the first requirement of such institutions is to change the mind set of the people under stress from the present values borne out of affluence to mental equaminity which is a Herculean task. It has been rightly said that it is easy to destroy the mountains than to change the minds of the people. These institutions appear from outside attractive but a depth analysis of these institutes would reveal that these institutes are also charging huge money and are simply engaged on physical aspects of Yoga.

Selye and Levi have defined stress as a non-specific, conventional and phylogenetic-based response pattern, the primary function of which is to prepare the body or physical activity such as resistance or flight (called Eustress). If, however, the subject lacks the means of restoring either to fight or flight, i.e. of relieving the stress reaction, stress gives rise to distress which manifests itself in the form of psychosomatic symptoms or disorders.[1] Ivancevich and Matteson define stress simply as "the interaction of the individual with the environment" but then they go on to give a more detailed working definition, as follows: 'an adaptive response, mediated by

CHART 12.1

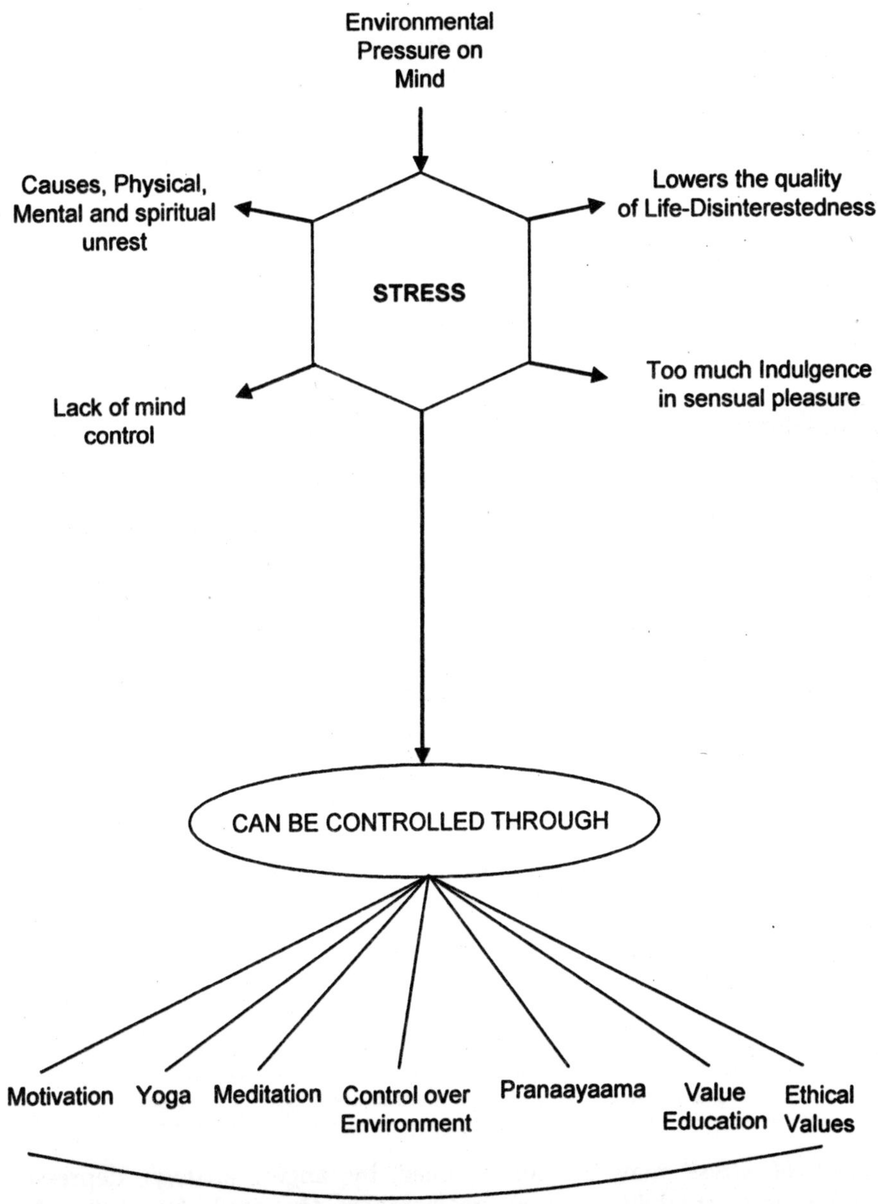

individual differences and/or psychological processes, that is a consequence of any external (environmental) action, situation, or event that places excessive psychological and/or physical demands upon a person," Beehr and Newman define stress as "a condition arising from the interaction of people and their jobs and characterized by changes within people that force them to deviate from their normal functioning." High

CHART 12.2

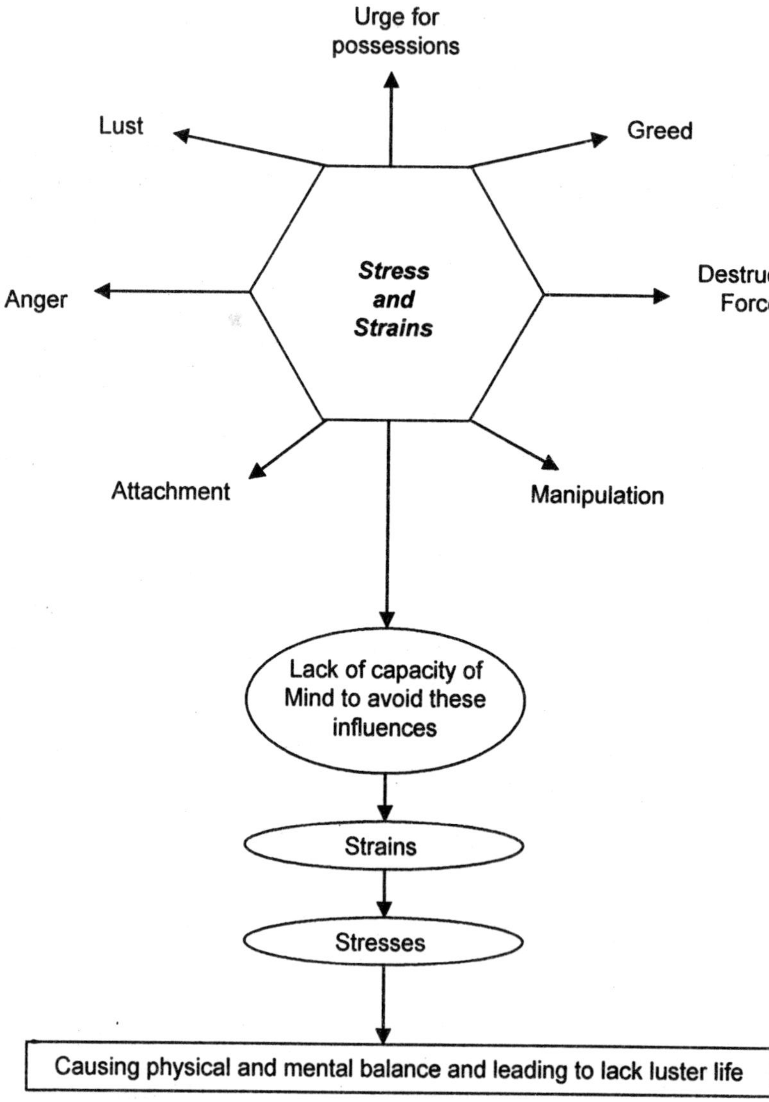

levels of stress may be accompanied by anger, anxiety, depression, nervousness, irritability, tension, and boredom. One study found that stress had the strongest impact on aggressive actions, such as sabotage, interpersonal aggression, hostility, and complaints.[2]

Stress according to Yoga is imbalance. Imbalance is misery. At the mental and physical levels, it is excessive speed and thus a demanding situation which causes pain and leads to ailments and diseases. Imbalances at the emotional level manifest as upsurges which are caused by strong likes and dislikes. At the psychological level the imbalances lead to conflicts and often manifest as petty and narrow ego-centric behaviour. Lack of holistic knowledge and a balanced outlook, at the subtle levels are responsible for imbalances found at gross levels.[3]

One of the implicit functions of HR is the responsibility of overall organisational health. . . they need to step up to the plate, recognize the signs and proactively introduce preventative stress management to reduce or mitigate potential stressors and resultant strains.

According to researchers, Jex, Beehr and Roberts (1992), stress is an overarching umbrella concept that is comprised of stressors and strain; or the processes where a stressor leads to strain. In other words, a stressor is the physical or psychological stimulus present in the environment (e.g. work overload due to shortage of staff, poor lighting on the shop-floor, unclear job expectations or role ambiguity). A strain, also known as distress, is the negative reaction to the stressor (i.e. job burnout, substance abuse, violence, depression, anxiety). Not all stressors produce strain. An individual may also have a positive response to a stressor, and this is known as eustress. Eustress, or good stress, occurs when the individual constructively manages their response to a stressor.[4]

Stress is a state of mind which reflects certain biochemical reactions in the human body and is projected by a sense of anxiety, tension and depression and is caused by such demands by the environmental forces or internal forces that cannot be met by the resources available to the person. The intensity of such demands that require a readjustment of resources or operational styles would determine the extent of stress. Such environmental events or conditions that have the potential to induce stress are known as "Stressors"

The stress created by desirable and successful effects is called "eustress" and the stress created by undesirable outcomesis known as "distress." It is primarily the distress form of stress which requires examination and steps to cope with it.[5] It is important to deal with stress at an early stage. Early warning signs such as headaches, back pain, irritability, insomnia, absenteeism from work or alcoholism should be taken seriously. Otherwise they could lead to serious emotional disorders as well as physiological problems such as ulcers and heart diseases. When stress is left untreated for a long time, it can develop into anxiety and depression.

"Selye" postulated a 'general adaptation syndrome' of somatic systems caused by 'non-specific stress'. It involved three stages:

(a) Alarm reaction—When an initial shock phase of lowered resistance is followed by counter-shock during which an individuals defence mechanisms are activated.
(b) Resistance—It is a stage of maximum adaptation when the individual restores the equilibrium.
(c) Exhaustion—If the stress continues or the defence mechanism falters, the individuals moves to this stage.[6]

Feeling stressed is a danger signal: a sign that you are reaching the limits of your resources. Stress is bad for health as well as a cause of increasing inefficiency and worsening relationships. The danger is that when under stress we ignore our health, and put our relationships under increasing strain. This sets up a vicious cycle because poor health and poor relationships then add to the stress. It is important, therefore, to focus not only directly on the stresses but also to look after one's health and relationships.

This idea is clearly enunciated in the Katha Upanishad where the God of Death tells Nachiketa that human beings have been created in such a way that they cannot but want to enjoy the outside world. Only in rare moments of inner awareness we are conscious of a divine spark in us. Even then our biological urges pull us down towards the mundane things of the physical plane. This results in a situation where a person is aware of the presence of perfection within and is eager to reach it but is hindered by powerful urges. Obviously, the result of this conflicting pull is tension.[7]

In modern society there are different kinds of diseases and nervous tension which can also be counted as one of them. But it is different from most other diseases because there is no germ or virus causing it. It is the result of the malfunctioning of the body-mind interaction. In other words, we can say that nervous tension is a psychosomatic disease in the true sense of the term. The word "psyche" means the mind and "soma" means the body. Nervous tension is the result of the way we have consciously or unconsciously chosen to live. When we speak of tension we should understand that the primary need of the mind and the body is that the mental and physical functioning be regulated. [8]

Nervous tension is a kind of recurring imbalance resulting in the daily wear and tear of the body. The two aspects of it which we need to understand are how it occurs and how we give expression to it. It comes in different guises, so to say. It may take the form of emotional or mental stress which is generated by our personality as it interacts with the environment everyday. This can also be called "social stress." In addition, there is another form of stress called the "digestive stress." It is the tension which results due to our poor eating habits. Therefore, it would be a mistake to think that the causes of stress are merely external: at home or in the place of work, that overwork alone causes stress. There are many other causes, such as poor eating habits.

Apart from these we have another common form of stress called environmental stress in the present times. It may be the result of many factors such as smog, noise and air pollution.

Each of us thus has a psychophysical system in the body which reflects our state of mind through physical diseases. If we suffer from nervous tension, fatigue or tremendous strain at the mental level, it is sure to come out in the form of aches and pains or more serious diseases such as hypertension, ulcer, stroke, cancer, heart attack and others. In fact, the doctors and psychologists are strongly of the opinion that most diseases are closely linked with a state of sustained nervous tension which has become an invariable component of our daily routine.

Sustained nervous tension is therefore a common phenomenon today. It stems directly from different kinds of frustration, worry and despondency. Each day we have to meet various forms of challenges at home, in our place of work or even at play. These are in addition to the ordinary demands imposed on our mind and body by he process of living. The result of this is acute nervous tension which shows itself in the form of impatience, anger, anxiety or fear. If we take an unhealthy diet, or if we have the habit of smoking, drinking or an addiction to drugs, they too result in different kinds of tension. In short, we can say that we are living in a world of tensions.[9]

Janina Gomes in his Article, "Still the Chattering of the Mind states."[10]

> All of us in life experience moments of disharmony. We find we are often at cross purposes with life, with events, with daily happenings, with others. Out of all this disorder and disharmony, if we can build lives of harmony and orderliness, we will succeed if not at all times, at least in the most crucial moments in stilling the chattering of our minds.

Ever since the dawn of civilization, man has been constantly engaged in the pursuit of unraveling mystery of nature with a view to arriving at the fundamental values of life. Today, the world is in a state of turmoil, the causes of which seem to be beyond man's comprehension and capabilities. Paradoxically enough, man seems to be lost in the world of plentitude. It's soul is starved in the midst of unbounded materialistic pleasures and comforts that science and technology of today have placed at his disposal. The harder he strives to extricate himself out of the web of these problems, the more he is caught and involved in it. Underneath the morass of conflicting values lies man's quest for the real meaning of life and the destiny to which it leads. Science does not help us to find answers to the fundamental moral and spiritual values of life or "how to live" and here we see that the advancement of science has led to mankind, is lopsided growth and development. Sanskrit Literature is full of details as to how to lead our lives decently without causing tensions, stresses and depression. Since we have forgotten our ancient literature and its value, such problems are on the rise.

Human being is the best creation of God and is endowed with logic, perception and capacity to verbalize his experiences. He can make his life pleasurable depending upon how does he use his own resources and experiences. He can induce tension and stress in others by imparting wrong information and can also lesson his worries by imparting correct information.

Present day society is highly competitive. Every one strives for power, prestige and possession to excel over one's own fellow being. This competitive process obviously poses many challenges for the society and the susceptible individuals and may cause anxiety, stress and tension. These are the related terms having almost similar genesis and outcome and are often used to denote hardship of life. Scientifically, however, they are different.

Anxiety refers to a fear reaction in which the cause of the fear is not a specific object. Stress refers to a condition resulting from disturbances to physical or psychological well-being. Tension is readiness for action generally with no action possible and often refers to the strain resulting from stress. Under these situations, logical process is constricted, slowed down and emotional process took up the individual's control.

D.R. Kaarthikeyan suggests the need of harmony to avoid problems—Physical, mental, social, spiritual. To quote him:

> Revered Shri Vethathiri Maharishi says, 'Harmony is a precious treasure of human life'. Real success and satisfaction, happiness are the different facets of harmony. If one is to enjoy the benefits of life to the fullest, it is necessary to develop and maintain harmony; and for this understanding the philosophy of nature is required.
>
> Harmony should be maintained in all spheres of life, and these are:
>
> Between body and life;
> Between wisdom and habits;
> Between self and society;
> Between the purpose of life and the method of living; and
> Between will and nature.
>
> The more one understands life, the more one will achieve harmony; and success will be proportionate to that. No doubt harmonizing life is a difficult task, but it is worth all the striving, for it is the only way to equip oneself to enjoy life to the fullest extent and to reach the goal of life, which is the perfection of consciousness. By the development of knowledge man comes to understand the Cause-and-Effect system, which is a Law of Nature.

The greatest wealth is to live content with life for there is never want where the mind is satisfied and save oneself from stress and mental tensions. Richard Howell in his article, "The importance of spirituality in our lives" in *Hindustan Times* (Aug. 13, 2002) rightly emphasizes that Medical Profession paid a great price when it detached itself from all religious and philosophical references in order to obey only laws of science. There are so many human problems created by technical progress that in great industrial firms, psychologists and moralists occupy prominent places alongside technical experts and economists.

We should clearly understand that the problems is rooted in the minds and therefore stress management is to be managed at mental level though we may take physical help as a sound mind is in a sound body. Swami Chaitanya Keerti in his Article, "In Search of Eternal India" (*Hindustan Times*, Aug. 14, 2002)" rightly feels: The rise of consciousness, the light of enlightenment, the blossoming of flowers of meditations and their fragrance in the form of love and compassion that has blessed this part of the earth has never been experienced so much anywhere else.

For almost ten thousand years, thousands of people have reached the ultimate explosion of consciousness. Their vibration is still alive, their impact is in the very air, you just need a certain receptivity, a certain capacity to receive the invisible that surrounds this strange land, says the Master in Osho Upanishad.

The Upanishads declared: "Amritasya Putrah! O Sons of the Eternal and Immortal! Wake Up:" Osho says that only those who have heard this clarion call and are on this amrit path—the eternal path, are the real citizens of India. People accidentally born here are not the real citizens.

Physical ailments form but one tribe of hordes that barbarously attack us; even more relentless and cruel are our mental sufferings. As we progress in our knowledge of the curative processes for ameliorating the physical sufferings, we observe that the mind's ill-health affects the body much more than what one could imagine; and this kind of suffering proves all the more difficult to deal with. Mental disintegration is more dangerous, for, it brings about not only misery to the sufferer but a kind of dangerous disharmony in and excruciating intolerance with the surroundings of such an individual.

On the whole it means each one of us who is suffering (and is there anyone who is not?) from this inner malady is an unhappy centre spreading all around him unhappiness and restlessness. A solution to these problems, very complicated and extremely confusing to the average mind, is what we seek individually and collectively. The results of such investigations conducted by the ancient enquiries and the data collected from their personal experiences constitute the bulk of our scriptures.

Today instead of searching for any radical solution and specific cure for this problematic disease and consequent suffering in life, what man actually does in society is to collect around him various kinds of "escape-distractions" and compromise-dopes, through all kinds of foul methods. He vainly hopes to drown his sorrows in ever so many unhealthy indulgences. By these methods at best man succeeds in turning his mind away from the actual facts of life as they are. To analyse scientifically and to observe closely the nature and behaviour of our outer world-of-objects and the inner instruments-of-experience in us, are the methods employed in the Upanisads, by which the Seers have discovered a happy solution for the great problems of man and his life.

Vedanta is the Science of life. It explains the art of living.[11] People, who thus follow religion as an escape from themselves, ultimately come to gain nothing except perhaps a lingering sorrow, dulled by a blind faith that benumbs the very capacity to perceive their own tragedies of life ! Scientific detachment, honest observation, logical conclusions and heroic decisions alone can help an individual to come away from his own life's fallacies.[12]

Thus, stress management is a very complex problem as it involves mind whose control is very difficult. Until and unless, we learn to control the mind, stress would continue. Stress management requires change of existing value system based on materialism to spiritualism. There is a rat race for material comforts and possessions of material resources resulting into recoiling on such persons in the form of stresses, tensions, depression and many other ailments. From those material possesions, they wanted to lead a life of quality and peace but what has been the result? They spend the physical resources in getting treatments in nursing homes without getting peace. Thus, the stress requires overhauling our existing value system and change it with our old value system enshrined in our sacred literature—Shrimad Bhagvad Geeta, Vedas, Mahabharta, etc. if we follow the values as given in our ancient wisdom we would be getting many benefits like.

(1) Mental peace, which every body requires but does not work for it in practice.

(2) Enjoying a life of quality with vigour and vitality.

(3) Creating more centres of Yoga as there would be no need of such a big health infrastructure causing more problems than solutions.

(4) Less expenditure on health services and thus less material requirements.

(5) Creating a stimulating physical, social and spiritual environment radiating peace.

(6) Avoiding tensions among nations as stated in UNESCO preamble that war begins in the minds of men, it is he minds of men that are to be reformed."

(7) Creating harmonious interpersonal relationships.

(8) At home, society, Nations and international level, there will be peace and spiritual prosperity.

Classification

Many scholars are writing and producing literature on stress management for special categories of individuals like stress management for executives, stress management among police personnel, political elite, Bureaucracy, students, women, etc. However such classification is of no use as stress is the same in all. Stress does not differ in different categories of personnel. Stress may however differ in severity and to deal with people in stress, we have to understand the level and severity of stress. It may be stressed that stress management in this book is for all without any distinction in status.

Approach

Approach to stress is understood wrongly. We are seeing today that every third shop is of a chemist as we think that medication can cure stress which is totally fallacious. We also find the opening of many gyms, religious institutes, training institutions for stress management which is also not a right approach. Stress is mental and need be dealt on mental level. Until and unless we do not purify our minds, there can be no mental peace. We shall discuss various approaches to control stress.

Causes

There are many causes responsible for stress:

(1) Wrong use of mind for greed, lust, manipulation causing turbulence in mind and disturbing the mental equanimity.
(2) Filling the mind with impurities responsible for stress like hatred, lack of service to humanity, self centred.
(3) Always planning harassing other people and disturbing the pece and tranquility of mind.
(4) Lack of right thinking causing destructions of mind causing mental turbulations.
(5) Lack of practices leading to mental purity like yoga, meditation, etc.

Effect of Stress

1. Poor health leading to many health problems—depression.
2. Low productivity/efficiency at work.
3. Lack of interest in life and work.
4. Absence of harmony in social life.
5. Absence of right thinking.
6. Degenerated mental environment.

Today, man is subjected to a large number of stress situations in the modern fast way of life and his balance is frequently disturbed. The system is constantly kept under sympathetic stimulations without enough time for the parasympathetic to do its job. This repeated sympathetic stimulations lead to intermittent upsurges of heart rate, blood pressure, poor digestion, elevated blood glucose, etc. when this happens over a number of years it becomes a habit for the heart and the blood vessels to remain in a stimulated state and they lose the capacity to come back to the resting levels. This is the main cause for the increasing incidence of high blood pressure and diabetes among people today.[13]

Mental Health

There is very close relationship between mental equanimity, peace and happiness of an individual and his physical health and efficiency. A mentally tense, anxious and sick person has a tendency to develop various symptoms of organic disorders. Thus, other conditions remaining equal a normally serene and cheerful person may be expected to have various pathological symptoms in his body.

Consciousness shrinks in a mentally abnormal person, and his shrunken consciousness finds expression through his pathological organic disorders. The consciousness of a diseased person has a trend towards continuous contraction. The domain of consciousness of a mentally and organically sick person becomes narrow, clouded and depressed. The ancient Indian seers used the conception of 'mental equanimity' instead of the concept of 'mental health'. Sri. Aurobindo used the concept of mental serenity in the same sense as the concept of 'mental equanimity' of ancient Indian seers. The concept of 'mental equanimity' is more satisfactory than the concept of mental health because the former alone can produce spiritual development in an individual.[14] Swami Vishnu Devananda states:

तदेवार्थमात्रनिर्भासं स्वरूपशून्यमिव समाधिः
Tad everthamatra-nirbhasam svarupa-sunyam iva samadhih

When consciousness of subject and object disappears and only the meaning remains, it is called samadhi.

Samadhi is a merging of the mind into the essence of the object of meditation. Nothing exists but that pure awareness.[15]

Let us take the role of mental health in Government. Mind is the most powerful part of the human system. It is a Super Computer. We don't realize its potential or devise ways and means to harness this most important source. We can achieve excellence, provided we know the secret of tapping human mind. We generally notice that most of us are not mentally positive as one or the other problem concerning us continuously bogs us down. Many of us become mental wrecks and a liability. The health institution, instead of solving their problems, cause further deterioration. 25 percent of people in every organisation are a liability and the other 75 percent are not contributing as per their potential. We should try to create positive mental attitudes among them. Positive mental attitude is a state of mind that reflects among the people. Positive mental attitude is a state of mind that reflects the strength of ones belief in what we do. It generates inner and voluntary emotions, which enhances motivation, resulting in positive thoughts. Positive thinking is the key to development and is result-oriented.

Ethical behaviour is considered as a blend of moral qualities and mental attitudes. The requisite moral qualities include not only the willingness to serve the public but also the willingness to behave competently, efficiently, honestly, responsibly, objectively, fairly, and accountably. Mental attitudes include awareness of moral dilemmas inherent in policies and conflicting claims on the substantive and procedural aspects of policy, an empathy for divergent views held not only by some members of the public but also by professional colleagues, and a sensitivity to paradoxes of rules that may lead to frustrating and unkind actions. Thus, an appropriate blend of moral qualities and mental attitudes become an essential ingredient for moral government and administration. Such a mixture strengthens the basis of legitimate and effective government, which is founded on public trust and confidence.

We get a moral government by creating those conditions within which a moral government can operate. This is done by making it possible for officials to acquire the necessary traits and by practicing the same. An exemplary public servant is not simply the one who obeys and behaves within the confines of law but is also one who strives for a moral government. Such is the duty of those who wish to be involved in the difficult and complex world of government. This is the essence and basis of a moral state.[16]

Public life is in a desperate state today, with vice regal regalia dominating it with its fierce ferocity and crushing criminality, sounding the death knell of ethics, morality, and value system. There is dire need to save it. Public men, at whatever station of life they function—must be 'men' for the public; leaders must lead; and most importantly, politicians must stop 'politicking'. Public opinion which is often branded as meaning neither public nor opinion—must be built up against acceptance and tolerance of unethical behaviour and action by anybody, howsoever high and mighty he may be. Crisis of confidence—which admittedly is a function of culture—must be restored in public life; otherwise, the ancient civilization that we boast of, will be no more; there will remain no public, no life, worth living, without ethics.[17]

The ancient Indian philosophers laid stress on mental equanimity for the general well being of individuals. The mind of an ordinary person is usually very restless. Myraids of desire produce upheavals in the mind of an individual. Over and above this, the mind of an ordinary person is affilicated by several tensions.

The ancient Indian philosophers maintained that if the mind of an individual usually remains in a disturbed state, he is very likely to develop pathological symptoms. An individual with pathological mental symptoms quite often develop certain pathological organic symptoms because there is very close relationship between the body and the mind of an individual. The mind of an individual becomes free from anxiety and miseries, if there is peace in his mind.[18]

The mind is a reservoir for numerous powers. By utilizing the resources which are hidden within it, one can attain any height of success in the world. If the mind is trained, made one-pointed and inward, it also has power to penetrate into the deeper levels of our being. It is the finest instrument that a human being can ever have.[19]

Spiritual Health

Individuals can have perfect health only when they are able to ascend from the lower to the higher states of consciousness, and remain perfectly poised in the higher plane of consciousness for a considerable duration of time. Perfect health is a comprehensive concept which includes mental equanimity, physical fitness and spiritual development of an individual.

The most crucial problem with which mankind is faced at present is the problem of health in its comprehensive sense. Health in its comprehensive sense means perfect physical fitness, mental serenity and vivid comprehension of the higher planes of consciousness in an individual. Healing means restoration of an individual to his normal state of physical efficiency, mental equanimity and clear comprehension of the higher planes of consciousness.

Health has its base in spiritual powers. We can arrange different lectures on spiritually which can keep the health of the people in good shape as well move them to positive action. J.L. Gupta in his article, "Power of Prayer" in the *Daily Tribune*, dated August 31, 2000 stated that, "Today, we care for what we eat, but not for what is eating us. We worry about what we wear, not what is wearing us out. We build houses and furnish them at considerable cost to make them comfortable. Then we look for the fastest cars to get away from our homes. We get every place air conditioned so that we do not sweat at work or on the road of life. Then we spend more—we buy a treadmill or join a gym, even to go to a health-club all to be able to sweat out."

Such indeed is the dichotomy in our lifestyle. In the new millennium we are moving fast, at a rather rapid pace, but we are not aware of the direction. We are rudderless. No, wonder, we have problems—of body and mind—All tension and lot of stress. There is not a moment of peace and rest. No time to stand and stare. Resultantly, the medicos claim a substantial share of our earnings, regularly.

Shirish Joshi rightly stresses the need of spiritual health. To quote him: that the notion that religious faith can promote physical well being is not new. Most of us have heard of cases in which someone, by sheer faith and will have, miraculously recovered from a terminal illness or survived far longer than doctors thought possible. What is new that such rewards of religion are becoming the subject of study by scientists.[20] A study found that religious folks had lower blood pressure, less depression and anxiety, stronger immune system and generally spent less money on medicines than people who did not believe in the existence of God and were less involved in religious activities in temples.

Scientists cannot prove that God heals, but they can now prove that belief in God has a beneficial effect. There is little doubt that healthy religious faith and practices can help people get better.

As a result of many studies, which say that prayer can help people feel better and live longer, many medical schools in the USA are offering courses in spirituality, religion and health.

Man without divine knowledge wanders in darkness. He is like a tree without fruit, flower without fragrance, a stream without water. Such a life is absolutely barren and worthless.

S.K. Kiran Kumar and K.A. Geetha have rightly summed up: Holistic approach to health represents a revisioning of the human endeavour to restore order in the organismic functioning, that has occurred in the past several centuries within the medical profession. The holistic health movement is the reflection of the growing dissatisfaction among the professional as well as lay people about the capacity of modern medicine in delivering the health care. A shortcoming of modern medicine is its failure to recognize the interactive nature of the different aspects of human existence viz., physical psychological, social and spiritual in the etiology of illnesses and in the maintenance of health and well-being.

Since modern medicine is itself a development within the framework of science, many have argued that the change needs to be brought about in the very framework. Thus, holistic movement is viewed as a by product and manifestation of the contemporary thrust on the revision of the scientific framework. One can find this trend in the works of behavioural, natural and social scientists which are contributing for major change in the world view. It involves a fundamental shift in cognition leading to radical alternations in the belief and assumptions about the nature of the universe, about the human nature, about organism environment interaction, and about the nature of consciousness. The newly emerging worldview is described as holistic paradigm (Krippner, 1991).

In the final analysis, the physical, social, mental and spiritual balance is the most desirable for holistic health. Unless a person is physically fit and active; he cannot perform at his best level. On the other hand, it is the mind, which accounts for 80 percent of physical and social problems. These are called psychosomatic diseases. Lastly, it is the spirit which ultimately directs the mind and through it to the body. We should devise ways and means to ensure synergy of the physical, social, mental and spiritual capabilities, which would release the infinite potential powers and generate efficiency and happiness in the the society.

The secret of right action in reality is not a secret. It does not lie in any formula that we repeat. There is no magic by means of which we can follow the path of idleness and yet make our life productive. No! The secret lies in our own motives, in our power of application. It is not the strong physical vehicle which makes the productive human being; it is skillfulness in action, knowing how to adjust ourselves quickly, how to perform a task with the least expenditure of energy. This is what gives immediate success. We should take action in time to solve problems before they become violent and result in destruction and unpleasant atmosphere.

Gita has given us some thoughts which if followed can remove tensions and stresses.

कर्मण्येवाधिकारस्ते मा फलेषु कदाचन ।
मा कर्मफलहेतुर्भूमा ते सङ्गोऽस्त्वकर्मणि ॥ 247 ॥ Bhagavad Gita

Man has a right to action alone, not to the renunciation of action. If out of egoism he forcibly tries to renounce all action, he will not succeed in the attempt (III.5); for his nature will compel him to act (III.33; XVIII.59, 60). In this way he will be abusing his authority, and by refusing to perform an obligatory duty he will also have to bear the evil consequences of violating the commands of the scriptures.

योगस्थ: कुरु कर्माणि सङ्ग त्यक्त्वाधनंजय ।
सिद्धयसिद्धयो: समो भूत्वा समत्वं योग उच्यते ।। 2/48 ।। Bhagavad Gita

Arjuna, perform your duties established in Yoga, renouncing attachment, and even-tempered in success and failure; evenness of temper is called Yoga (48).

The word 'Yoga' bears a peculiar meaning in the Gita and the Lord conveys that peculiar meaning by defining it as equanimity. The Lord thus establishes identity between Yoga and equanimity, and shows that one can become a Yogi by attaining equanimity through any discipline whatsoever.

दूरेण ह्यवंर कर्म बुद्धियोगाद्धनंजय ।
बुद्धौ शरणमन्विच्छ कृपणा: फलहेतव: ।। 2/49 ।। Bhagvad Gita

By declaring action with a selfish motive as far inferior to the Yoga of equanimity, the Lord has shown that the fruit of actions prompted by desire is the attainment of fleeting and momentary pleasure whereas the fruit of Karmayoga is realization of God. Thus, there is no comparison whatsoever between the two. The word 'Karma' in this verse cannot be interpreted in the sense of prohibited action, for such action is altogether worth renouncing and its fruit is nothing but untold misery and suffering. Therefore, it cannot be cited as a fit subject of comparison to bring out the glory of the Yoga of Equanimity.

बुद्धियुक्तो जहातीह उभे सुकृतदुष्कृते ।
तस्माद्योगाय युज्यस्व योग: कर्मसु कौशलम् ।। 2/50 ।। Bhagavad Gita

Endowed with equanimity, one sheds in this life both good and evil. Therefore, strive for the practice of this Yoga of equanimity. Skill in action lies in (the practice of this) Yoga.

We should avoid favouring some at the cost of others. Our actions should be fair and impartial.

"Many people confuse attachment with love. But in attachment you become selfish, interested in your own pleasure, and you misuse love. You become possessive and try to gain the objects of your desires. Attachment creates bondage, while love bestows freedom. When yogis speak of non-attachment they are not teaching indifference, but are teaching how to genuinely and selflessly love others. Non-attachment, properly understood, means love. Non-attachment or love can be practiced by those who live in the world as well as those who are renunciates."[21]

Kaibara Ekken, the Japanese sage has nicely put it as: If by study, enquiry or thought, we have learned the truth, we should then put it into practice in both our speech and action. Let what we say be true and what we do discreet. Regulate the emotions, and suppress anger and selfish desires. Shake off evil and cling to good. Discovering our faults, let us not hesitate to correct them. Towards others let us be considerate. All this is the way of true action. . . Without putting what we have learned into practice, it bears no fruit.

All these would divert the energy in positive channels and thus reduce stress or lead stress free life.

A few remedies for overcoming fatigue are to increase our interest in whatever work we undertake and to perform it joyfully. Often our daily duties become monotonous resulting in boredom and fatigue. This can be relieved if we make the atmosphere of our place pleasant.

Monotony can be cured by genuine love for our work.

Of the innumerable techniques prescribed by he rishis for self-development, the most popular ones are the path of selfless dedicated service (karma yoga), the path of discriminative knowledge (jnana yoga), and the mystic path of self-development through disciplined contemplation (raja yoga).

According to Sage narada, true devotion for the Lord is superior and nobler to all these, because devotion is the final outcome of all other methods of self-development.

This supreme devotionis indeed, as a technique, even superior to the path of action, the path of knowledge, and the path of disciplined contemplation. (Narada Bakti Sutra II:I; 25).

All the other paths are the means that take the seekers to the final goal of spiritual experience, but in devotion there is very little difference in essence between the means and the end, between way and the goal. Love alone is love's own end and fulfilment. Devotion is both the means and the end. As long as residual vasanas (inherent tendencies) are still lingering in the devotee's personality, so long is devotion only the path. But when, as a result of his love for the Lord, his vasanas disappear totally, a stage comes when his supreme love itself becomes the Lord of love Supreme.

Than all other paths, devotion is the one most readily available and most easily attainable. (Narada Bhakti Sutra VI:1:58)

Having dedicated all activities unto Him, the devotee should turn all desire, anger, pride and so forth toward him alone. (Narada Bhakti Sutra VI: 2:65).

Having gained this supreme devotion, the devotee attains perfection and immortality and becomes extremely satisfied. (Narada Bhakti Sutra I:1:4)

Because Love is of the nature of peace; it is of the nature of supreme Bliss. (Narada Bhakti Sutra VI: 1:60)[22]

CONCLUSION

Techniques of Stress Management

Uma Arulnidhi stated, Meanwhile, over all his years in his pursuit of spiritual truth, he had found that certain techniques of physical exercise and meditation were useful, even necessary, tools- in that exercises served to keep the body sufficiently healthy so that one could pursue one's spiritual search without the worry, loss of energy and suffering of disease; and meditation served to quiet the mind to enhance insight, sharpen awareness and enable deeper, subtler spiritual enlightened persons of the past and present, when he wanted to convey his philosophy to the world he felt that it must be conveyed along with such practices as he had personally found efficacious and felt confident of transmitting to others so as to be useful and practical for them. He realized that there are books full of eternal Truth always available for anyone to open and read: the problem is that we cannot seem to fully grasp those truths through books, no matter how well written they may be, or how many times we read them! A personal dedication and systematic, persistent practices of body and mind should be the best way to fully realize and integrate spiritual knowledge in one's life.[23]

When we face life's problems and are confronted with turbulent or worrying events, we often get so obsessed with the problem that our minds chatter and weave round and round the problem to no avail. This chattering of the mind disturb our mental poise and ease and makes us compulsively obsessed with the happenings. The result—a loss of equilibrium and balance.

Deep down inside us is a felt need for a still mind. In fact, there are ways to experience this stillness in the thick of the battles of our lives. In the midst of confusion and conflict, we can retain a stillness that quietens us and creates a certain distance between us as experiencing selves and our circumstances. [24]

To maintain calm in situations of threat, hazards, disorder and conflict is not easy. It is a life-long lesson we have to learn. It comes through practice, through trial and error, through many failed efforts, through the process of human growth and evolution.

Stillness is a divine gift. The human heart has divine treasures which unfold through patient effort and calm. Stillness is not passivity but experiencing calm in the midst of trials. It is the ability to respond to life with courage and the ability to stand the test without turbulence.

But to be still is not to be frozen in one's mindset or state of mind. Those who are frozen in a certain state do not move and are not evolving or growing. Those who move and flow with life are, however, those who like the ripples in a still pond, experience movement but maintain an underlying stillness that makes life a movement of grace and harmony.[25]

All of us in life experience moments of disharmony. We find we are often at cross purposes with life, with events, with daily happening, with others. Out of all this disorder and disharmony, if we can build lives of harmony and orderliness, we will succeed if not at all times at least in the most crucial moments in stilling the chattering of our minds.

Follow the heart. A pure heart sees beyond the intellect; it gets inspired; it knows things that reason can never know, and whenever there is conflict between the pure heart and the intellect, always side with the pure heart, even if you think what your heart is doing is unreasonable.

When it is desirous of doing good to others, your brain may tell you that it is not expedient to do so, but follow your heart, and you will find that you make less mistakes than by following your intellect.

The pure heart is the best mirror for the reflection of truth, so all these disciplines are for the purification of the heart. And as soon as it is pure, the truth will flash upon it in a minute; all truth in the universe will manifest in your heart, if you are sufficiently pure.

Louis Lavelle states that the meaning of holiness. Love transports us beyond ourselves; it is like an inspiration that is constantly being renewed, a power that is always present, sustaining us. Louis Lavelle the meaning of holiness.

Rediscovering ourselves and trying to build a new life from the wreckage of the earlier one which has been causing depression and despair are effective strategies to overcome the problem of tension. With strong determination we can resolve the trouble which may at first sight seem insurmountable. Bringing about effective changes is totally up to us as long as we are prepared to accept the responsibility for our behaviour, actions and attitudes. As a good General can inspire his soldiers to move forward fearlessly, fight boldly and win glorious victories against the most invincible enemies so also is an answering determination able to inspire an individual to achieve remarkable feats of courage in the battle of life.

Individuals can thus determine the course of their own lives if they have sufficient confidence and unshakeable faith in themselves. It is not right to just sit back and wait for fortune or luck. One should depend rather on one's own acts, thoughts, efforts, skills and values. These induce positive thought currents that we have to make our own life significant. Nothing else or no one else can do this for us. It is for us to formulate a workable strategy of meaningful existence and carry it throughout life. Then we should have no time to indulge in our predilection for being depressed.[26]

Stress as the author feels is caused by lack of control over mind which becomes susceptible to senses and impulses. Mind is quickly influenced by selfish motives and lust for worldly pleasures. When there is no control over mind, the individual is engulfed by lust, greed, anger, attachments and manipulations (see Chart 12.1) The result of all these is stress and strains which cannot be cured simply by medicines and physical exercises. For this we have to control our mind.

When non-acquisitiveness is established, an understanding of the purpose of birth is gained. When the yogi no longer desires to have possessions he frees himself from the material world. This gives him a perspective of the purpose of his birth, both in this life and in past one's. He gains comprehension of the law of Karma and understands what lessons remain to be learned before attaining Realization.[27]

Let us have a great ideal, an ideal that will startle us with its greatness. That is the only kind of an ideal to hold before our mind's eye and to work for. Little by little our imperfections and difficulties will vanish and instead of regarding life as a drudgery, instead of shirking from it, we shall bless this life which offers so many opportunities. We shall find joy even in the little daily tasks and wherever we are placed we shall know happiness.

पात्राकलित वेदानां शास्त्रमार्गानुसारिणां
तदेतु अरिकालस्य करिकालस्य शासननम् ।। Karikala Chola.

This inscription means that the order of Karikala, who is the kaala (death) of enemies, is that those who follow the vedic path should be protected and those who pursue evil paths should be punished.

There are many diseases for which modern medical science has not discovered a remedy, but these mountaineers do not even suffer from these, Perhaps fresh food, fresh air, and, above all, free thinking with no anxiety is responsible for their health. Millions of patients all over the world who suffer from psychosomatic diseases can be helped through right diet, juices, relaxation, breathing, and meditation. Preventive and alternative medicine should not be ignored.[28]

Notes and References

1. Dr. H.R. Nagendra, New Perspectives in Stress Mangement, Swami Vivekanand Yoga Prakashan, Bangalore, 2003, p. 9.
2. Peter Y. Chen and Paul E. Spector, "Relationship of Work Stressors with Aggression, Withdrawal, thief and substance use: An exploratory Sudy, *Journal of Occupational and Organisational Psychology*, Rand MC Nolly, Chicago, 1976.
3. Dr. H.R. Nagendra and R.P. Nagarthma, *op. cit.*, p. 41.
4. Ritu Kappula, Under the Influence of Stress, in *Human Capital*, Vol. 7, No. 10, March 2004, pp. 36-37.
5. Jito Chandan, Organisational Behaviour, Vikas, New Delhi, 1994, pp. 182, 192.
6. H. Seyle, The General Adaptation Syndrome and the Disease of Adoptation, *Journal of Clinical Endrocology*, 1946, p. 117.
7. Swami Gokulnanada, How to Overcome Mental Tension, Ramakrishna Mission Institute of Culture, Calcutta, 1997, pp. 20-21.
8. *Ibid.*, p. 1.
9. Swami Gokulananda, How to overcome Mental Tension, Ramakrishna Mission, Institute of Culture, 2000, pp. 1-3.
10. *The Daily Tribune*, Sept. 12, 2002.
11. Swami Chinmayananda, Atma Bodha, Central Chinmaya Mission Trust, Mumbai, 2001, pp. (ii) and (iii).
12. *Ibid.*, p. 2.

13. Dr. H.R. Nagendra and R. Nagarantha, New Perspectives in Stress Management, Swami Vivekananda Yoga Prakashnana, 2002, p. 27.
14. A.K. Sinha, Science and Tantra Yoga, 1993, p. 9.
15. Swami Vishnu Devananda, *op. cit.*, p. 185.
16. O.P. Dwivedi, "Reflections on Moral Government and Public Services as a Vocation, in *IJPA*, July to Sept. 1995, p. 297.
17. O.P. Dwivedi, "Conclusion: A comparative Analysis of Ethics, Public and Public Service", James, S. Bowman and F.A. Elliston (eds.) Ethics, Government and Public Policy, New York, Greenwood Press, 1988, p. 318.
18. Bata K. Dey, Ethics, Maladies and Remedies, in *IJPA*, July-Sept. 1995, p. 461.
19. Swami Rama, Living with Himalayan Masters, the Himalayan Institue Press, Pennsylvania, 1999, p. 313.
20. *The Sunday Tribune*, Sirish Joshi, August, 19,2000.
21. Swami Rama, Living with Himalayan Masters, The Himalayan Institute Press, Pennsylavania, 1999, p. 58.
22. *The Tribune*, Nov. 24, 1980.
23. *Aliyar*, 2000, *op. cit.*, p. 128.
24. *Aliyar*, 2002.
25. R.H. Singh, "Yoga and Heath", Science and Philosophy of Indian Medicine, Baidyanath Bhawan, Pvt. Ltd. Nagpur, 1978.
26. Swami Gokulnanda, How to overcome Mental Tension, Ramakrishna Mission Institute of Culture, 2002, pp. 224-25.
27. Swami Vishnu Devananda, Meditation and Mantras, Delhi, Motilal Banarsi Das, 1978, p. 179.
28. Swami Rama, *op. cit.*, p. 348.

13
CHAPTER

Health and Housing

HOUSING is a State subject. The Union Government is, however, responsible for the formulation of policy with regard to programme and approaches for effective implementation of social housing schemes, particularly those pertaining to weaker sections of the society. A comprehensive Housing and Habitat Policy, 1998 had been formulated to address the issues of sustainable development, infrastructure and for strong public-private partnership for shelter delivery. The objectives of the policy are to create surpluses in housing stock by creating an enabling environment and facilitate construction of 20 lakh additional dwelling units each year in pursuance of National Agenda for Governance. It also seeks to ensure that housing alongwith supporting services is treated as priority sector at par with infrastructure. The Central theme of the policy is strong public-private partnerships for tackling housing and infrastructure problems. The Government would provide fiscal concessions, carry out legal and regulatory reforms and create an enabling environment. The problem of housing shortage compounded with the population explosion has also been addressed by this policy. This document clearly identifies the respective roles of the Central Government, the State Government, local authorities, financial institutions, research standardisation and technical institutions. However, since housing is state subject, State Governments have to play the primary role in formulating specific action plans and programmes suited to local needs and conditions duly involving local bodies and citizen groups.

The National Agenda for Governance has identified 'Housing for All' as a priority area, with particular emphasis on the needs of the vulnerable groups. As per this programme, it is proposed to facilitate construction of 20 lakh additional units every year, with emphasis on Economically Weaker Section (EWS) and Lower Income Group (LIG) sections of the population as also the needs of SC/ST and other vulnerable groups. Out of

20 lakh additional houses, 7 lakh houses are to be constructed in urban areas and remaining 13 lakh in rural areas. This would require an additional investment of around Rs. 4,000 crore per year.[1]

The 'Working Group on Housing' for the preparation of the 'Tenth Plan Approach Paper' has observed that 90 percent of the housing shortage relates to the poor and that there is need to increase the supply of affordable housing to low income groups through a proper process of allocation of land, extension of funding assistance and provision of support services. All the issues identified by the Working Group relates to the sphere of activity and responsibility of state governments and local bodies, and therefore, the success of the National Housing Policy depends largely on the efforts of state governments.

Providing better living conditions for people is now a global concern. The Millennium Development Goals envisage achieving significant improvements in the lives of at least 100 million slum dwellers by the year 2020. In this context, urban planning and governance structures have to be made more effective, and incorporate an explicitly pro-poor focus on land rights and affordable low-cost housing to meet the burgeoning demand for shelter in urban areas.[2]

Dr. Roderick J. Larence in his article, "Housing and Health" in the *World Health*, March-April 1991 clearly stated that the meaning of housing, like the meaning of home, varies from person to person, between social groups and across cultures. Houses are commonly accorded an economic value, an exchange value, an aesthetic value, an exchange value, and a use value—whereas, in addition to these, a home is usually given a sentimental and a symbolic value. All these values, as well as domestic roles, routines and rituals, are not simply expressed by individuals; they are acquired, nurtured, transmitted, reinforced, or modified by interpersonal communication (for instance, between parents and children, or between members of the same social or professional group).

From this perspective, the interrelations between housing and health are very different when viewed from the resident's point of view. Trying to understand those viewpoints requires an approach that may be in conflict with arbitrarily defined solutions drawn up and applied by national governments or by international agencies. During this century, the practice of prescribing minimum standards for the quality of a wide range of environmental entities—air, water supply, and building materials, for variance—has led to a significant improvement in site planning, building construction and housing design in both industrialized and developing countries. Yet when these standards are examined in terms of their rationale and objectives, it becomes clear that they have commonly been drawn up with economic, opinions and well-being of local populations have been largely undervalued or else ignored.

Studies of the housing conditions in large cities of both industralized and developing countries today show that those people who do not have regular employment, who cannot afford to pay high rents or mortgage payments, and who need to live in urban neighbourhoods readily accessible to the job market, have the most unfavourable housing conditions. Although slum clearance has meant that vast numbers of unfavourable dwellings have been demolished, overcrowding has often increased, not by choice as some claim, but through economic necessity. These processes and their consequences are the crux of housing and health problems in many cities. In essence, the presence of substandard housing is not merely an architectural or technical planning problem but also, basically, an economic and political one explicitly related to the equitable and ecological use of natural resources.

Few public or private institutions today bother to identify and monitor the costs and benefits of development policies, or the specific changes that may be brought about the products for housing sites, communities or larger ecosystems, so that informed decisions can be made, costs and benefits correctly assigned, and negative impacts reduced or overcome. Most housing built during this century, and especially since the Second World War, did not benefit from this kind of approach, and the legacy for current and future generations is a grim one. For example, many housing units have been found to contain toxic building materials. Outside walls have inadequate thermal insulation, so they are hard to heat, and condensation and dampness favour the growth of mould or fungus. The indoor air quality often cannot be adequately regulated by cross-ventilation, and sound insulation may be lacking altogether.

Is it any wonder that respiratory illness and allergies have become a primary cause of morbidity and mortality in some European countries? Furthermore, new (or formerly unknown) diseases such as Legionnaires' diseases such as Legionnaires' disease have been identified. Room humidifiers, air ventilation systems and cooling towers, as well as hot and cold water supply ducts, have been found to nurture *Legionella* bacteria and transmit them throughout the indoor environment, or discharge them into the immediate vicinity of the building. An ecological perspective raises some fundamental issues. We could begin by asking why the water supply has become prone to bacteria; or ask whether it is necessary to install mechanical ventilation and air-conditioning systems in high-rise housing when it might be simpler to avoid constructing internal rooms that are devoid of both daylight and natural ventilation? Are there not alternative principles and practices for building construction and housing design even when high density housing is unavoidable.[3]

Housing is directly connected with health as people living in Delhi in crowded areas of old Delhi fall ill because of poor, congested, unventilated, polluted water, etc. The people in crowded cities are not living in a house but huddled together in a common place. Some of the houses are only one room where all the activities are done. Most of the illness are associated with poor housing. A personal visit of the author found that a room has been made three tyred sleeper at night. The condition of housing is miserable. The recent trend in high-rise of real estate prices has made it impossible either to purchase or get on rent a good accommodation. The Government of India and State Government have failed to solve the housing problem causing innumerable problems to economically backward population. The Government has been proposing to construct big hospitals like All India Institute of Medical Sciences and expansion of secondary and Primary Health Care? There is no need of spending on these hospitals. People would not get total treatment here? Why? Government must read about health and its essentials. One of these is good housing. People living in so-called houses would be regular visitor to hospitals as they have not the basic means to keep healthy. Politicians and administrators have no time to provide health care to the people, i.e. food, clothing and shelter. In addition, pure air and potable water are the life of the people which they do not get. The Government is busy in signing agreements with World Bank, USA, etc. for big project loosing sight of the people living under the Nose of the Government

The situation of Housing is very serious as one in five families live in slums. Even those who are living in urban areas are without good facilities, half of the urban population is without sanitation facilities. The Government is making efforts but without positive results.

According to the above definition, very few people live in houses. The definition pin points the essentials of housing:

1. Living space according to the number of members in the family. 80 percent of the population in India have no living place but a so-called house where people are living together. It must have some open space which can be used for expanding family.
2. The house must have the facilities of pure air, potable water, energy, light, sewerage disposable otherwise house would be stinking.
3. It must have adequate security and privacy.
4. There must be some park and other entertainment facilities nearby.
5. Cost of the house must be affordable to lower strata of society.
6. Educational and health facilities must be near the house.
7. The government must subsidise the housing for the poor.
8. The neighbourhood must also be clean so that children can play and do not catch any infection.

Hippocrates' approach is appropriate for an understanding of the interrelations between housing and health. It can be complemented and enriched if the architect, the housing administrator or the public health officer ceases to be a passive observer and assumes the active role of an "enabler" who, in contrast to an "expert", is willing to integrate his or her explicit professional knowledge with the tacit know-how and experiences of lay people.

Public participation in the definition and management of housing is important for at least two reasons. Firstly, only by involving the community is it possible to establish a real understanding of the customs and values of people in their domestic setting. Where participation has been adopted, it often happens that certain basic institutional assumptions about housing and health have been proved incorrect. Secondly, public participation can be a useful form of public health education by increasing the awareness of lay people about the complex range of social, economic and political factors that are involved if we want to improve unhealthy housing and reduce homelessness.

According to Mrs. Christiane Vedma, Former Deputy Editor, *World Health*, Housing policies and public health rarely figure today in the manifestos of governments or political parties. It is not surprising, therefore, that we see many indications that all is not well, such as new human illness, increasing homelessness, and a declining quality of housing and human settlements in many countries. A fundamental change in human values and behaviour is necessary. This change can be promoted by a much better dissemination of knowledge, know-how and experience between professionals and lay people, and between the public and private sectors. The current worsening situation in the largest cities of both industrialized and developing countries must be seen as a challenge to the planners, because housing and health are fundamental anthropological concepts as well as basic human rights.[4]

This strong feeling was shared by Christopher Alexander, an American architect with a difference. He is a caring architect—one who believes that his role does not end with the completion of a drawing because, as he says, life does not come out of a drawing; life can only come out of a process, the process of building, in which everybody must participate and most particularly those who are going to use the building and to live in it.

Beauty and harmony play an important role in giving people a sense of belonging, just as old buildings did, whether they were vast cathedrals and palaces or a simple shack. And beauty and harmony can only be obtained with what Christopher Alexander calls "Wholeness"; each part—even the smallest—of the whole is expressly designed and made to serve the same purpose as the whole itself.

In "Places for the Soul", a film produced and directed by Ruth Landy, a public information officer with WHO in Geneva, Christopher Alexander expresses forcefully that the only long-term chance for survival of man and his planet depends on his building harmonious relationships with his environment. There is still a long way to go before we can achieve this, and those who are trying to express this view in "concrete" terms are still only pioneers. Their voice needs to be heard at the highest political levels so that future policies are inspired by their achievements.

Christopher Alexander, Centre for Environment Structure, Berkeley, CA, USA clearly defines that "In all countries of the world, people are suffering from modern forms of housing. These have, unnecessarily, gone in a direction which is inhumane, inefficient, expensive and unpleasant.

"It has happened because they have assumed, wrongly, that there is no alternative. Imagination on the part of the architects, and the will to take into account people's expressed needs, can provide alternatives. These needs are enough space, beautiful rooms, beautiful light, outdoor space of one's own, a sense of private uniqueness, communal quality in the public land, convenience of parking. The Shirotori Housing Project that I hope to be able to build in Nagoya, Japan, will provide just that. Every inhabitant of the 500 apartments in a low-rise high-density building will have a garden of their own. They will have a beautiful common space for children to play, for community links to be formed, and for contact with nature. They also will have the opportunity to determine their own physical layout, and thus create for themselves a real home."

An article "Cities of tomorrow" by Dr. Layi Egunjobi, in the *World Health*, 1991 " Less than ten years from now, no fewer than 24 of the world's great cities will have more than ten million inhabitants each. Five of these—and four of them are in developing countries—will have passed the 15 million mark. Even the cities that will not reach these staggering dimensions are undergoing such rapid growth that they seem to be heading for catastrophe. Hasty efforts are under way to provide for the needs of city-dwellers, whether in matters of housing, job opportunities or social and health services. Yet once again we have a situation where only a minority of the inhabitants are able to enjoy an acceptable standard of living. It follows that every effort at health promotion must be aimed at narrowing the gulf between rich and poor."

The primary health care approach and inter-sectoral cooperation combine to form the strategy of choice. As in the rural areas (which we have to safeguard from the threat of galloping urbanization), it is local action, situated firmly in a national, regional and even worldwide context, that has the best chance of succeeding in the great cities of tomorrow. Now more than ever, we have to "think globally and act locally."

The health authorities must convince the local powers-that-be of the important role of health in development matters, and must promote the right kind of leadership in the heart of the urban community to ensure the participation of everyone in health activities.

Health for All is our common objective, shared by us all. Not only can it lead us to greater equity and justice: it can also give the cities that human dimension on which their very survival depends.

Prof. Chen Changhui and D.R. Solving Ekbald in their article, "High-density life in China, in the *World Health*, 1991 clearly observe that what causes stress in cities is a subject of keen debate among psychologists, psychiatrists, sociologists, architects and city planners. These problems vary from country to country. The People's Republic China, which accounts for one-fifth of the world's population, is at present undergoing urbanization and rapid social and economic development. How do people cope with life in the great cities of China?

Health care has made significant progress, increasing average life expectancy (at present 70 years) and reducing infant mortality, both of which trends tend to augment the population. At the same time, the family structure is changing as extended families give way to nuclear families. In addition, an enormous rural labour force is being transferred to the cities.

As a result, the urban housing shortage is now a serious problem. City planners and architects are under great pressure urgently to provide more housing. Two demographic factors are particularly relevant to the housing shortage. One is the large youthful population, and the other is the more housing. Two demographic factors are particularly relevant to the housing shortage. One is the large youthful population, and the other is the move away from agricultural occupations as part of the new economic strategy. China's emphasis on urban-based industrial development, on the one hand, and its efforts to restrict urban growth by controlling rural-to-urban migration, on the other, have made the Chinese experience of urban development unique.

These changes have profound effects on the people, especially on such vulnerable groups as children, the elderly and the disabled. But it is becoming clear that people reared in the traditional Chinese culture are likely to be more tolerant of high-density living and have lower levels of stress than people educated with Western traditions. The Chinese people have developed cultural norms and values which encourage the maintenance of harmonious relationships between man and nature, and which use various coping mechanisms involving space, time status and emotional management.

The National Plan of Action, prepared by the Government of India for the Habitat Conference defined adequate shelter, in the Indian context as the one "which would include adequate living space with provision for incremental development and proper access to physical and social infrastructure and services including energy, fuel, potable water, waste disposal and sanitation services, and education, health and recreational facilities. It must have adequate privacy and security, as also lighting and ventilation. The location of the shelter must be suitable with reference turk place markets, communication services, and social and cultural amenities. . . . The endeavour of the government and the people of India would be to maintain the cost of such adequate shelter at an affordable level. . . The critical task is to ensure that access to adequate and affordable shelter is available to all, including people living in poverty, the vulnerable and the disadvantaged, either through the market or through well targetted and transparent subsidies." (pp. 99-100, India Country Report). There is a need to take rational decisions to ensure what is contemplated. Worlds written or spoken are of no use unless put to action.

GENESIS OF SLUMS AND MAGNITUDE OF THE PROBLEM

"Slum" is defined as that area where the buildings are in any respect unfit for human habitation; or by reason of dilapidation, overcrowding, faulty arrangement of buildings, streets, lack of ventilation, light or sanitation facilities or combination of these factors, are detrimental to safety, health or morals (Slums Improvement and Clearance Act, 1956).

Approximately, 68.8% of the country's slums population 'was concentrated in the 300 Class I cities and less than 1/3rd of this population resides in the remaining 3300 urban centers'.[5] (Slums are not fit for settlement and are a danger both for residents and the urban population living nearby. Roosevelt has rightly said that poverty anywhere is a danger to prosperity.

Sh. Aditya Prakash, retired Principal of the College of Architecture, Chandigarh, has termed the growth of slums in the City Beautiful of Chandigarh, as a "planning failure." He says, "The slums should not have been allowed to sprout in the first place. The need of the hour is to solve poverty and shelter problems and it can be done through proper planning."

Evolution of Slums

Urbanization has been considered as an index of development but in case of developing countries like India, urbanization is not the outcome of merely the growth potential generated by urban settlements. It has been largely due to people work relationship in rural areas, in which land is the essential medium and which is right now so critically balanced that even small addition to population is pushing people out of agriculture to non-agricultural occupations. Thus, by and large, in India, urbanization is emerging as merely a process of transfer of rural poverty to urban environment, which only results in concentration of misery. This has resulted in the malfunctioning of most of the urban settlements leading to emergence of number of imbalances and problems. Thus, most of these settlements suffer from improper and haphazard development, absence of basic infrastructure and services, uncontrolled and unchecked growth of slums, lack of housing, high degree of visual and environmental degradation and uncontrolled traffic. The cumulative effect of these factors is the degradation of quality of life in urban settlements and huge amount of subsidies is required to maintain them. These facts are more evident in case of larger cities especially sector and super-metros.

Problems of Urban Areas Especially Human Settlements

Urban areas have not received much attention in terms of the planning, development and management despite the fact that cities and economic development are inextricably linked. Because of high productivity of urban areas, economic development activities get located in cities. Accordingly, it is desirable that human settlements are provided with necessary planning and development inputs so that the orderly growth and development is ensured. This would also be necessary for ensuring efficient functioning of human settlements for improving their productivity and for providing desirable quality of life to its residents in order to cater to their both economic and physical and metaphysical needs. The urban development strategy for any state thus assumes importance of not only its economic emancipation but also its physical well being.

Concept of Slums[6]

The concept of slums and its definition vary from country to country depending upon the socio-economic conditions of each society. Irrespective of location, whether in the core of the city, in the form of old dilapidated structures or in the outskirts, in the form of squatting, slums have often been characterised:

(a) Physically, an area of the city with inadequate housing, deficient facilities, overcrowding and congestion.
(b) Socially, slum is a way of life, a special character which has its own set of norms and values reflected in poor sanitation, health values, health practices, deviant behaviour and social isolation.
(c) Legally speaking, section 3 of the Slums Areas (Improvement and Clearance) Act, 1956 defines slums as areas where buildings:
   (i) are in any respect unfit for human habitation; and
   (ii) are by reason of dilapidation, over-crowding, faulty arrangements of streets, lack of ventilation, light or sanitation facilities or any combination of these factors which are detrimental to safety, health and morals.

Section 3 of Slum Areas Act, 1956 defines slum areas by Notification in the official Gazette. The slum areas are declared, which require:

(a) repair,
(b) stability,
(c) natural light and air,
(d) system of dump,
(e) water supply,
(f) drainage and sanitary conveniences, and
(g) facilities for storage, preparation of cooking of food and disposal of waste water, the buildings deemed to be unfit if it is so for effective in one or more of the said matter and not found reasonably suitable for occupation in that condition.

Slums a Great Danger to the Populations

S. Saksena and P.N. Govindarajuler in their article, "Health Care For Urban Slums with special reference to Bangalore City" have rightly sensed the problem. To quote them:

"Slum-dwellers have the worst of both the worlds—urban and rural. On one side they suffer from economic hardships, lack of education and absence of health infrastructure like the rural population. On the other hand, they also suffer the ill-effects of over-crowding, pollution and rootlessness characteristic of large metropolitan cities."

They further add that, "Most comforts and conveniences of the cities are sustained by the work done by slum-dwellers. As such, the affluent and the privileged have the moral responsibility to try to mitigate and alleviate their suffering. Rural population may be ignorant of the "goodies" they are missing, but a slum-dweller is painfully aware of the privations suffered by him due to his constantly rubbing shoulders with urban effluence and conspicuous consumption with resultant and resentment."[7]

A Survey on the health status of adolescent girls in Patiala, carried out by a team of expert lady doctors, has revealed that 92.5 per cent of girls in urban slums are anemic while the percentage of such girls in urban areas is 88.6 and 86% in rural areas. It was further found that 38.7 percent girls in urban slums were severely anemic.

Not only mental disorders but problems relating to physical abuse (15.2%), domestic violence (30.2%) and sexual abuse (10.2'%) were seen in urban slums indicating poverty, illiteracy and low status of women in this category. (*The Hindustan Times*, 24 Dec., 1999)

It is paradoxical situation that on the one hand they provide all services to urban population on the other, they cannot meet their needs. Over a period of time, slum-dwellers are beginning to see themselves as citizens contributing to the economy and, therefore, deserving their own place in the sun. It is the slum and pavement dweller, who provides the vast network of services that the middle and upper classes enjoy at cheap rates. These services include the entire food supply network (vegetables, milk, eggs, butter, bread, meat, poultry as well as restaurant services), clothing, laundry, vending and sales, transport, conservancy, communication, construction and domestic services for homes, offices. The slum-dwellers, if united, have the power to bring to a halt the entire urban system, so powerful is their role in urban economy.[8] Most of the slum-dwellers are immigrants of villages or towns and then migrate to slums or another form of low-income urban housing. They move to the place after the migrant has established himself in the city with a job, a network of friends and some sort of understanding of the political and bureaucratic structure of the municipality. However, this pattern of movement from rural to slum is a very common one. Some move permanently. This usually happens when a migrant already has a well-establishment network of relatives and friends living there. Some of migrants come not only from rural areas but also from other urban centres of the country. Others never settle permanently in the city but stay only long enough to take advantage of the economic opportunities available there before returning to their place of origin.[9]

Within the existing broad loose definition, following housing areas can be categorized as "slum":

(i) Inner city blighted areas;
(ii) Squatter settlements on both private and public land;
(iii) Illegal land sub-divisions (unauthorized colonies);
(iv) Urban villages;
(v) Resettlement colonies (like those in Delhi); and
(vi) A squatter settlement improved under the environmental improvement scheme.[10]

Despite all the efforts being taken by the departments. In providing housing and basic civic amenities to the urban poor living in the slum areas, the population in these areas has increased. As is evident from a census report for the town of Bombay. The report says:

"Preliminary findings of the state government's ongoing census on slums in Mumbai suggest that the city's slum population has doubled over the last five years. Officials concerned with the census say that over 60 lakh slum-dwellers have been enumerated against the 40 lakh recorded when the census was last updated in 1995."[11]

Housing Questions

Our sample consisted of 125 three-generation households in the Western District of Beijing, and the interview questionnaires dealt with dwellings as well as social, sanitary and health conditions. Among the results were the following:

— Existing multiple dwelling units are usually designed for nuclear family requirements, and the educational level among the high–rise inhabitants seems to be above that of persons in other types of dwellings;
— People are more crowded than in developed countries, but the traditional living courtyard has less private space than multi-storey dwellings; and
— Multi-storey homes are better equipped for cooking and personal hygiene, and have better access to public and social services, the high-rise blocks being closest to most of the city facilities:

Stress levels are not correlated with age, sex or life satisfaction but with the type of dwelling. The elderly in traditional houses report least satisfaction with living in the present outmoded, crowded dwelling, but are most satisfied with life. Coping with traditional Chinese life seems to be more difficult for those who live in modern apartments and results in a decreased social network and social exchange;

— Indirect signs of psychosomatic symptoms are an inability to sleep because of the noise, and concern about lack of privacy among young mid-rise dwellers;

— Adverse behaviours (such as excessive alcohol consumption) are quite rare; and
— Children rarely show somatic and mental symptoms, but those who live in high-rise apartments spend significantly fewer hours outdoors in winter as well as summer, by contrast with children in multi-storey homes.

Recent Developments[12]

The Valmiki Ambedkar Awas Yojana (VAMBAY) was launched on 2 December 2001 to ameliorate the conditions of the urban slum dwellers living below poverty line who do not possess adequate shelter. The primary objective of VAMBAY is to facilitate construction and up-gradation of dwelling units for the Slum dwellers and providing a healthy and enabling urban environment through community toilets. Since its inception GOI subsidy of Rs. 928.09 crore has been released for construction of 4,41,204 dwelling units and 65,286 toilet seats The GOI subsidy for construction of toilet seats was released under 'Nirmal Bharat Abhiyan', a sub-component of VAMBAY. Under this programme, the sanitation units, with a 10 seat or a 20 seat toilet block meant for men, women and children with separate compartments for each group and special design features are maintained with the help of contribution from those who uses them.

VAMBAY was the first scheme of its kind meant exclusively for slum dwellers with a Government of India subsidy of 50 per cent, the balance 50 per cent arranged by the State Government. VAMBAY, along with National Slum Development Programme (NSDP), has been subsumed in Integrated Housing and Slum Development Programme launched on 3 December 2005 along with Jawaharlal Nehru National Urban Renewal Mission (JNNURM).

BASIC SERVICES TO THE URBAN POOR

For integrated development of slums through projects for providing shelter, Basis services and other civic amenities with a view to provide utilities to the Urban poor in select 63 cities Sub-Mission on Basic Services to the Urban Poor (BSUP) has been launched on 3 December 2005 by the Hon'ble Prime Minister. The sub-Mission on BSUP is implemented on a demand-driven basis for which State Governments are required to prepare and submit City Development Plans (CDPs); Detailed Project Reports (DPRs) and also to sign Memorandum of Agreement (MoA) making a commitment to undertake urban reforms. Salient features of BSUP are as follows:

- The Sub-Mission is to be implemented in 63 select JNNRUM cities.
- To be implemented over 7 years beginning with the year 2005-06.

- Central share in the form of Additional Central Assistance as full grant
- 50 per cent of the project cost in respect of cities having million plus population or above to be borne by the Central Government
- 90 per cent of the project cost borne by the Central Government for projects from cities/towns in North Eastern States and Jammu and Kashmir.
- 80 per cent of the project cost borne by the Central Government for projects from the remaining cities
- A minimum of 12 per cent beneficiary contribution for houses. For SC/ST/BC/OBC/PH and other weaker sections, 10 per cent beneficiary contribution.
- Access of Central assistance predicated upon the State/Urban Local Bodies/Parastatals agreeing to the reforms.
- Reforms to ensure improvement in urban governance.

Since the launch of BSUP, an amount of Rs. 87.33 crore has been released as on 31 May, 2006.

INTEGRATED HOUSING AND SLUM DEVELOPMENT PROGRAMME (IHSOP)

In cities/towns not covered under BSUP an Integrated Housing and Slum Development Programme is implemented. The IHSOP has subsumed Valmiki Ambedkar Awas Yojana (VAMBAY) and National Slum Development Programme (NSOP). For IHSOP, COPs are not required. Salient features of IHSOP are as follows:

- Central share in the form of Additional Central Assistance as full grant.
- Per cent of the project cost borne by the Central Government.
- 90 per cent of the project cost borne by the Central Government for projects from cities/towns in special category States.
- A minimum of 12 per cent beneficiary contribution for houses. For SC/ST/BC/OBC/PH and other weaker sections, 10 per cent beneficiary contribution.
- Access of Central assistance predicated upon the State/Urban Local bodies/Parastatals agreeing to the reforms.
- Reforms to ensure improvement in urban Governance.
- Cities/towns to prepare and submit Detailed Project Reports.

We concluded that both positive and negative effects arise from the three types of dwelling. The traditional courtyard home satisfies psychological needs (for instance, privacy, child-rearing and welfare of the elderly), while its structural conditions, the lack of modern facilities and safety features are disadvantages. Modern homes, on the other hand, seem to have a negative influence on psychological comfort. Can the experiences of Western industralized countries help to open up a new approach to city planning in China that fits in with the Chinese cultural background? We believe this is possible. Ideally the dwelling environment should provide opportunities for establishing and sustaining constructive social relations. Those who plan and build homes must start from a holistic approach, by which we mean that people's symptoms and illness, with their causes and consequences, have to be appraised in both a medical and a psychological and social perspective. This approach suggests that the link between housing and health may be quite indirect, and that unless the intervening processes are understood, changes in the physical structure of the housing alone may have no beneficial effect on health if they do not simultaneously have a beneficial effect on intervening factors.

CONCLUSION

As a matter of fact, inadequacy of housing for the vast majority of the urban poor with its attendant evils is the single most important factor for the fast degradation of the urban environment in India. Improvement in some of the basic management, as discussed earlier, cannot be implemented effectively unless the problem of settlements and human habitations for the vast majority of urban poor is taken care of clustered houses are also a cause of communicable diseases. Housing is most essential for healthy life.

Population Explosion I

1947	—	342 million
1991	—	846 million
2001	—	1003 million
2015	—	1250 million

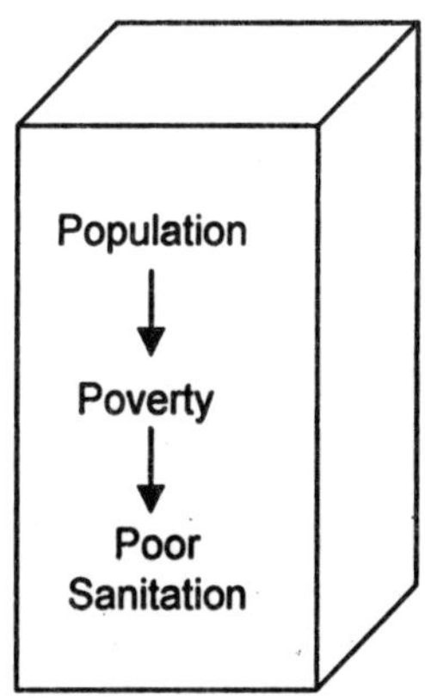

Notes and References

1. India, A Reference Manual, Ministry of Information and Broadcasting, New Delhi, 2007, p. 385
2. Karnataka Human Development Report, 2005, p. 155.
3. Roderick J. Lawrence, Housing and Health, in *World Health*, March-April, 1991, p. 21.
4. Rodericks J. Lawrence, *op. cit.*, p. 22.
5. Sanganal, Ashok, "Participation of Slum Dwellers in Urban Governance" Shelter, Vol. III, No. 1, p. 35.

6. Gurumukhi, K.T., 'Slum Related Policies and Programmes', *Shelter*, Vol. 3, No. 2, April 2000, pp. 57-58.
7. Goel, S.L., "Planning and Administration of Urban Basic Services: A Case Study of Una (H.P.) in 'Development Planning and Administration", Ed. S. Bhatnagar and S.L. Goel, pp. 167-68.
8. *Shelter*, Vol. III, No. 1, p. 35.
9. *Ibid.*, p. 42.
10. Risbud, Neelima, "Slum Improvement in India—Some Issues", Delhi Vikas Patra, p. 27.
11. *Indian Express*, Chandigarh, Dated 7, Nov., 2000.
12. India-2007, A Reference Annual, Ministry of Information and Broadcasting, GOI, 2007.

APPENDIX 13.1

INTRODUCTION

Shelter is a basic need for human existence—for protection from the elements as well as to raise families. And. just as provision of shelter facilitates human existence, access to drinking water, sanitation and hygiene rank foremost among the basic services that affect human development. Access to safe drinking water and basic sanitation impacts not only poverty and health indicator but also has critical gender implications in terms of women's work and women's health. This chapter deals with these three facets of human development in Karnataka.

I. HOUSING

While all human beings need shelter, for the poor, even the most basic shelter may be beyond reach because they do not own land or because the cost of building materials and construction is too high. Shelter is a basic human need. The National Housing and Habitat Policy, 1998 provides the framework for the implementation of shelter programmes in the country. The national agenda on housing envisages the creation of 2 million houses every year. The Habitat policy and the national agenda recognise housing activity as an engine for substantial employment generation in the country. The Working Group on Housing for the preparation of the 'Tenth Plan Approach Paper' has observed that 90 per cent of the housing shortage relates to the poor and that there is need to increase the supply of affordable housing to low income groups through a proper process of allocation of land, extension of funding assistance and provision of support services. All the issues identified by the Working Group relate to the sphere of activity and responsibility of state governments and local bodies, and therefore, the success of the National Housing Policy depends largely on the efforts of state governments.

Providing better living conditions for people is now a global concern. The Millennium Development Goals envisage achieving significant improvements in the lives of at least 100 million slum-dwellers by the year 2020. In this context, urban planning and governance structures have to be made more effective, and incorporate an explicitly pro-poor focus on land rights and affordable low-cost housing to meet the burgeoning demand for shelter in urban areas.

The housing scenario

In Karnataka, 54.9 per cent of households live in permanent houses, as compared with Kerala, which has the highest percentage of households (68.1 per cent) living in permanent houses among the southern states. This is above the national average of 51.8 percent. A high 35.6 percent of households in Karnataka have semi-permanent houses, a high proportion among southern states, and above the national average of 30 per cent. Urban households perform better, with 77.9 per cent households living in permanent houses, as compared with only 42.6 per cent in rural areas. The scenario is reversed with regard to temporary houses. (Table 13.1)

Karnataka (78.5 per cent) stands fourth among the southern states with regard to the number of households living in houses that they own. This is less than the national average of 86.66 per cent. Karnataka, with 18.7 per cent households living in rented houses, ranks just after Tamil Nadu (19.9 per cent) among the southern states. However, the proportion of households owning houses in rural areas is quite high at 91.2 per cent (Table 13.2).

Across districts, only 24 per cent households in Raichur district live in permanent houses and 44.3 per cent are in semi-permanent houses, as compared with Bangalore Urban district, where 89.7 per cent households live in permanent houses. The proportion of temporary houses is the highest in Koppal district (33.8 per cent) followed by Raichur (31.7 per cent), Gadag (28.1 per cent) and Bellary (24.5 per cent), all of which are in north Karnataka.

Bangalore Urban district tops the state in respect of households living in permanent houses in urban areas (92.1 per cent) while Bidar (a low HDI district) tops the state in respect rural households living in permanent houses (74.5 per cent). Raichur has the lowest percentage of rural households living in permanent houses (13.7 per cent) and Gadag has the lowest percentage of urban households (41.3 per cent) living in permanent houses. Data indicates that Bangalore Urban has the least percentage of semi-permanent houses (6.4) in respect of urban areas.

Data on the tenure of households indicates that the lowest percentage of families (45.69) that own houses are to be found in Bangalore Urban, which is below the state average of 78.46 per cent. The highest percentage of households in Bangalore Urban lived in rented houses (0.73). The highest percentage (90.94) of households that own houses is in Chamarajnagar (a low HDI district) followed by Udupi (90.42) and Bidar (90.19). In Udupi, a high HDI district, we find only 7.37 per cent of households in rented houses. A low 68.3 per cent of rural households in Kodagu district own their houses, followed by Bangalore Urban (69.0 per cent) while 95.7 per cent of rural households who own houses are situated in a relatives underdeveloped district like Bidar. The urban scenario shows that in Bangalore Urban, only 43 per cent households own houses while 54 per cent live in rented houses.

There appears to be little correlation between the economic development of a district and house ownership patterns. House ownership is high in the predominantly agrarian north Karnataka districts where land values are less likely to be affected by speculation consequent on urbanisation as in Bangalore Urban. Migration to cities is a factor that pushes up the percentage of persons living in rented houses.

Policy interventions

Given the relatively low percentage of house ownership in the state, Karnataka has long recognised the significance of housing as an important component of the Minimum Needs Programme. Indeed, Karnataka had launched a state-funded housing programme for the poor through the Ashraya and Ambedkar housing programmes in 1993-94, long before the National Habitat Policy was formulated. The state has one of the best housing programmes in the country.

Housing schemes

The Ashraya programme provides assistance of Rs. 20,000 of which Rs. 10,000 is a subsidy and the remaining Rs. 10,000 is a loan. For SC/ST beneficiaries in both Ashraya and Ambedkar programmes, the entire provision of Rs. 20,000 is a subsidy. In the urban Ashraya programme, the assistance is Rs. 25,000 with a beneficiary contribution of at least Rs. 5,000. The state launched the ambitious 'One Million Housing Programme' in October 2000, which envisaged the construction of one million dwelling units in rural and urban areas during the period 2000-05, i.e. 2,00,000 houses each year. Rural housing has been given primacy with an annual target of about 1,70,000-2,20,000 houses. The annual target for the urban programme is 30,000. The cost of urban projects is usually very high.

A village-wise demand survey was conducted by gram panchayats during May-June 2003 and it has been estimated that there are 12.26 lakh houseless people and 10.43 lakh people without house sites who have asked for assistance under the programme. Since 2001-02, a large number of new village settlements known as Navagramas has been created adjoining, and preferably abutting existing village settlements to decongest villages. So far 2,399 Navagrama have been created to provide better amenities. Table 13.2 gives details of houses constructed under the state and Central government sponsored housing programmes during 1999-2004. State sponsored schemes constitute 80 per cent of the rural housing programmes and 87.5 per cent of the urban housing programmes implemented in Karnataka. The state had invested over Rs. 18,912 million till March 2004 to create 8.96.269 dwelling units.

Recommendations

It would be no exaggeration to state that the poor find it difficult to borrow for housing Commercial banks are unwilling to lend to the poor, and even if they are willing to do so, lending norms guidelines and collateral security requirements mean that the most needy get excluded. Hence, in Karnataka, institutional lending is channeled through the state government. The concerns of banks can be met by organising an institutional partnership with local bodies and microfinance structures that would ensure loan recoveries cost-effectively and also facilitate savings for home loans to meet credibility requirements. There is definitely a need for banks to have a fresh look at the lending norms for the poor to enable them to access funds for housing.

Currently, provision of infrastructure facilities like water, electricity, sanitation, internal roads and drains is not being financed under any housing programme. This has resulted in poor occupancy and a poor quality of life for occupants in the settlements. Infrastructure provision is extremely resource intensive and should not be left to cash-starved local bodies to provide; it should be funded by the state since the ability of the poor to contribute is meager.

In Karnataka the state survey reveals that 14.31 lakh families are houseless and 15.08 lakh families do not own house sites. The number of houseless families is the highest in Belgaum (1.07 lakh) followed by Gulbarga (1.02 lakh), Kolar (0.99 lakh), Mysore (0.96 lakh) and Tumkur (0.94). Public policy must focus on targeting resources to districts where the problem of houselessness is most acute.

An evaluation-*cum*-audit of the gender sensitive initiative that mandates that house, title deeds shall be in women's names must be taken up to assess the impact of this step in changing gender relations and empowering women.

The National Urban Renewal Mission (NURM) is expected to be the major vehicle for urban renewal in the country, providing substantial financial assistance for urban infrastructure and provision of basic services for the urban poor. Accordingly, the city development plans and strategies must focus on enabling the poor to better access services. Those working in the urban informal especially women, must be included in the agenda for urban regeneration.

Karnataka Habitat Policy

The state's millennium policy envisages:

1. Construction of 2,00,000 houses each year and 10,00,000 houses during the period 2000-05 through state government sponsored Ashraya and Ambedkar the latter scheme is for Scheduled Castes and Scheduled Tribes housing programmes as well as Centrally sponsored housing programmes for the poor;
2. Preparation of a reliable database for implementing housing programmes for the poor in rural and urban areas;
3. Ownership of the dwelling units shall be in the name of women except in the case of widowers, ex-servicemen, and the physically disabled;
4. Quotas for the Scheduled Castes/Scheduled Tribes in allocation in 2002-03, the Quotas increased to 40 per cent for SCs from 30 per cent and for STs to 10 per cent from three per cent;
5. Quotas for the physically disabled were enhanced from three per cent to five per cent in 2003 and for senior citizens without any income, it is two per cent;
6. Establishing a Special Purpose Vehicle (SPV), the Rajiv Gandhi Rural Housing Corporation as the nodal agency to implement the housing programmes;

7. Providing a subsidy at Rs. 10,000 per unit to all (poor) beneficiaries and an additional subsidy of Rs 10.000 for SCs/STs for houses constructed in rural areas;
8. Procuring, preferably by direct purchase from landowners lands required for housing in rural and urban areas;
9. Providing house sites free of cost to eligible beneficiaries in both rural and urban areas;
10. Encouraging beneficiary participation in construction;
11. Providing guarantee for funds borrowed from HUDCO and other financial institutions;
12. Facilitating housing for certain socio-economic groups such as beedi workers, porters in agricultural market yards, weavers, artisans. leather artisans, *safai karamcharis,* fisher people; and
13. Beneficiary selection through gram sabhas.

Some Innovative Strategies

Beneficiary participation

Local bodies and SPVs have traditionally constructed housing projects with little input from beneficiaries. Over the last five yeas however, beneficiary instruction has become the preferred mode of implementation, particularly in the districts of south Kamataka. This mode of construction is facilitated by the presence of reasonably skilled construction labour such as masons and underemployed farm labour, which doubles as semi-skilled or unskilled construction labour. At present. about 80 per cent of the construction of houses for the economically weaker sections (EWS) in rural area is constructed by beneficiaries. This has the advantage of ensuring that dwelling units address the social, cultural and occupational needs of the beneficiaries far more effectively than agencies constructed core housing could hope to achieve. Beneficiary participation takes the form of direct participation in construction, supervision of work, attending to simple, yet significant, tasks such as curing cement blocks or masonry to provide additional funds for construction of the dwellinq unit. The generation of local employment and use of locally available building materials is a crucial economic outcome of this approach. There is better accountability for the funds since these are made available to the beneficiaries only when they attain the prescribed benchmarks. 'Self-help' housing does not, however, mean that beneficiaries are deprived of technical inputs. Taluk panchayat engineering staff, Nirmithi Kendras and the Karnataka Land Army Corporation (KLAQ) provide construction support to beneficiaries who are unable to construct their own houses. In urban areas, 'core' housing is provided by agencies as a matter of policy to prevent speculation in land, since land markets are poorly organised and there is heavy demand for house sites, even by the non-poor and there is every likelihood that sites may be sold to speculators, thus defeating the purpose of the programme.

Women's empowerment

The decision of the state to select only women beneficiaries for assistance under the housing programmes (barring some exceptions) and give hakku patras (title deeds) for house sites and houses only in the names of the women of the household, has had a critical impact on ownership patterns in a society where land, houses and assets traditionally belong to men. It is a significant step towards promoting gender equity.

Community participation

The selection of beneficiaries was initially entrusted to the Ashraya Committee. Now gram panchayats identify and select beneficiaries, and the very poor will hopefully now be in a position to articulate their demands. This is a significant step towards governance through community participation.

Social equity

There is specific targeting of Scheduled Caste and Scheduled Tribe people through the Ambedkar (100.0 per cent) and Ashraya programmes (50.0 per cent).

Source: Government of Karnataka: Karnataka Human Development Report, 2003, Planning and Statistical Department of Karnataka, Bangalore, pp. 155-60.

TABLE 13.1

Distribution of households by tenure and type: Karnataka and selected states: 2001

State	*Area*	*Tenure Status*				*Type*		
		Total	*Own*	*Rented*	*Any other*	*Perma-nent*	*Semi-Perma-nent*	*Tempo-rary*
India	Total	191964	166353	20230	5380	99432	576.64	34816
	%	100.0	86.66	10.53	2.80	51.8	30.0	18.1
	Rural	138272	130491	49.13	28.67	56829	494.02	32010
	%	72.03	94.37	3.55	2.04	41.1	35.7	23.1
	Urban	53692	358.62	153.17	2513	426.0	83.62	2809
	%	27.97	66.79	28.53	4.68	79.3	15.4	5.2
Karnataka	Total	10232	80.28	1909	295	5616	3645	971
	%	100.0	78.5	18.7	2.8	54.9	35.6	9.5
	Rural	66.75	6085	416	174	28.43	3009	821
	%	65.24	91.2	6.2	2.6	42.6	45.1	12.3
	Urban	3557	1943	1493	121	2770	636	150
	%	34.76	54.6	42.0	3.4	77.9	17.9	4.2
Kerala	Total	65.95	61.10	332	154	44.94	1424	673
	%	100.0	92.6	5.0	2.3	68.1	21.6	10.2
	Rural	49.43	4663	163	116	31.91	1185	564
	%	74.95	94.3	3.3	2.4	64.6	24.0	11.4
	Urban	1653	1447	196	37	1302	239	109
	%	25.05	87.5	10.2	2.3	78.8	14.5	6.6
Tamil Nadu	Total	14174	11007	28.22	345	8295	2572	3304
	%	100.0	77.7	19.9	2.4	58.5	18.1	23.3
	Rural	8275	75.54	556	165	3914	1672	2688
	%	58.38	91.3	6.7	2.0	47.3	20.2	32.5
	Urban	5899	3452	22.66	180	4381	900	616
	%	41.62	58.5	38.4	3.0	74.3	15.3	104
Andhra Pradesh	Total	168.50	137.95	2715	340	9221	3589	4034
	%	100.0	81.9	16.1	2.0	54.7	21.3	23.9
	Rural	12676	114.57	1001	218	69.62	3077	3633
	%	75.23	90.4	7.9	107	47.0	24.3	28.7
	Urban	41.74	2337	17.13	123	32.59	512	401
	%	24.77	56.0	41.1	2.9	78.0	12.3	9.6

Maharashtra	Total	19063	15311	30.20	732	11021	6553	1475
	%	100.0	80.3	150.8	3.8	57.8	34.4	7.7
	Rural	10994	9891	724	378	4434	52.74	1281
	%	57.67	90.0	6.6	3.4	40.3	48.0	11.7
	Urban	80.70	5419	2296	354	65.87	1289	194
	%	42.33	67.2	28.5	4.4	81.6	15.9	2.4
Gujarat	Total	96.44	82.07	1181	255	6300	2849	492
	%	100.0	85.1	12.2	2.7	65.3	29.5	5.1
	Rural	5886	5458	324	1.4	3000	2453	431
	%	61.03	92.7	5.5	1.8	51.0	41.7	7.3
	Urban	37.58	2749	857	151	3300	395	62
	%	38.97	73.2	22.8	4.1	87.8	10.5	1.6

Source: Registrar General of India, Census of India, 2001, Housing Profile Table H-4, H-5 and H-6.

TABLE 13.2

Houses constructed under State and Central Schemes: 1999-2004

Sector	*Area*	*Scheme*	*Years*					*Total*
			1999-00	*2000-01*	*2001-02*	*2002-03*	*2003-04*	
STATE	Rural	Ashraya	53630	71794	136889	11527	108747	486324
		Matsya Ashraya		1598	1851	1066	264	4779
		Ambedkar	22712	17619	26489	18417	16247	101509
		Ambedkar						
	Urban	Ashraya	7746	28702	34274	20020	17966	108708
		KSCB (Hudco)	1000	1080	1000		8356	
		KSCB (SC/ST)		1000	1080	1000		3080
		Total	86088	125697	205929	159575	14432	721662
CENTRAL	Urban	KSCB (Vambay)				10312	7985	18280
	Rural	Indira Awas Yojana	36636	27785	29069	28910	24222	146639
		PMGY			2217	3360	4112	9686
		Total	36626	27785	31313	42582	36302	174608
		G. Total	122714	153482	237242	202157	180674	893189

Source: Rajiv Gandhi Rural Housing Corporation Limited, Progress reports of various years.

TABLE 13.3

Distribution of households by location of drinking water: Karnataka, 2001

Location	*Total*	*Percent*	*Rural*	*Percent*	*Urban*	*Percent*
Access within the premises	3248	31.7	1236	18.5	2011	56.5
Access outside the premises	4749	46.4	3696	55.4	1054	29.6
Access away from the premises	2235	21.8	1734	26.1	492	13.8
Total no. of households	10322	100.0	6675	65.2	3557	34.8

Source: Registrar General of India, Census, 2001, House Profile, Kartanaka.

14
CHAPTER

Health and Violence

At least three and a half million people on our planet die every year as a result of injuries caused by accidental or intentional violence. Whether on the roads, at home, at work or at play, the risks of injury to individuals have been neglected for too long, and the need to prevent and reduce them has so far received little public attention.

Today, public health is improving in many countries, and life expectancy at birth is increasing everywhere. It is therefore less acceptable than ever before that so many peoples should meet a violent and premature death, or that millions of others should become permanently handicapped. More than half the deaths of young people are due to injuries, and injuries represent the main cause of potential years of life lost.

As a result of negligence, indifference or foul play, millions of people each year require medical care after accidents or acts of physical violence. At a time when economic crises are jeopardizing efforts to improve the health of mankind, injuries of all kinds cost the world community almost US$ 500 thousand million a year in medical care and lost productivity.[1]

In devoting World Health Day 1993 to the prevention of accidents and injuries, the World Health Organisation wishes to draw attention to the sometimes disastrous consequences for individuals and society of accidents and acts of physical violence, which very often can be prevented.[2]

Safety must have priority

The fact is that, where road traffic is concerned, economic interest take priority over those of public health. It is not pure chance that the countries which build particularly fast cars only "recommend" maximum speeds on their motorways. While airliners and trains have devices—the black box—that record all the circumstances whenever can accident occurs, there is nothing comparable for private vehicles, yet they cause far more deaths than air or rail travel.

Furthermore, there are not yet any devices to limit motor vehicle speeds (within approved limits) in towns or on motorways. For the sake of economic gain-even though there is no proof that profits suffer from such measures—we decline to tackle the problem of road safety at the most basic level.

International organisations have little influence on road safety. The European Economic Community, for instance, harmonizes regulations governing automobile production and their free circulation within the Community, for instance, harmonizes regulations governing automobile production and their free circulation within the Community; but it does nothing about limiting their speed at the point of construction, except in the case of heavy lorries.

WHO itself interferes very little in this field, yet it ought to be drawing up a charter for road safety. Is it really acceptable to export to the developing world heavy trucks that were designed for the roads of the industrialized countries? The power and speed of these vehicles make no economic sense, because on inadequate roads they consume more fuel and wear out more rapidly; besides this, they are particularly dangerous in regions where road traffic is poorly regulated and where the local residents have no experience of heavy traffic. Contrary to present policy, it would be better to promote vehicles which have low fuel-consumption and are hardy and well adapted to the road conditions of the developing world.

The love of speed, the appetite for alcohol-and the fear of upsetting those who profit from both-conspire to leave road safety dependent on each individual's decision to respect other people's lives—or not, as the case may be. We refuse to separate road safety from private behaviour and, in the name of individual freedom or the freedom to manufacture and sell, we produce only disablement and death. Doesn't this amount to an attack on freedom in much more important areas? So long as we go on producing vehicles that do not match the traffic rules and refuse to equip them with well-tested regulatory systems, we are encouraging death and disablement on the road.[3]

Road Traffic Hazards: Hidden Epidemics

More than 20 million people are severely injured or killed on the world's roads each year. The burden falls most heavily on developing countries, where it will grow heavier still because of the rapid increase in the number of vehicles.

In addition to the direct costs of road injuries and deaths, the increase in the number of vehicles and reliance on certain transport policies have other serious health implications as well as wider social, economic and environmental impacts.[4] In some countries, air pollution from road transport causes even more deaths than those resulting from traffic accidents.[5] Besides the direct impacts on respiratory and heart disease, Motorized transport produces around a quarter of the anthropogenic emissions of gases leading to climate change.[6] These "hidden epidemics"

CHART 14.1

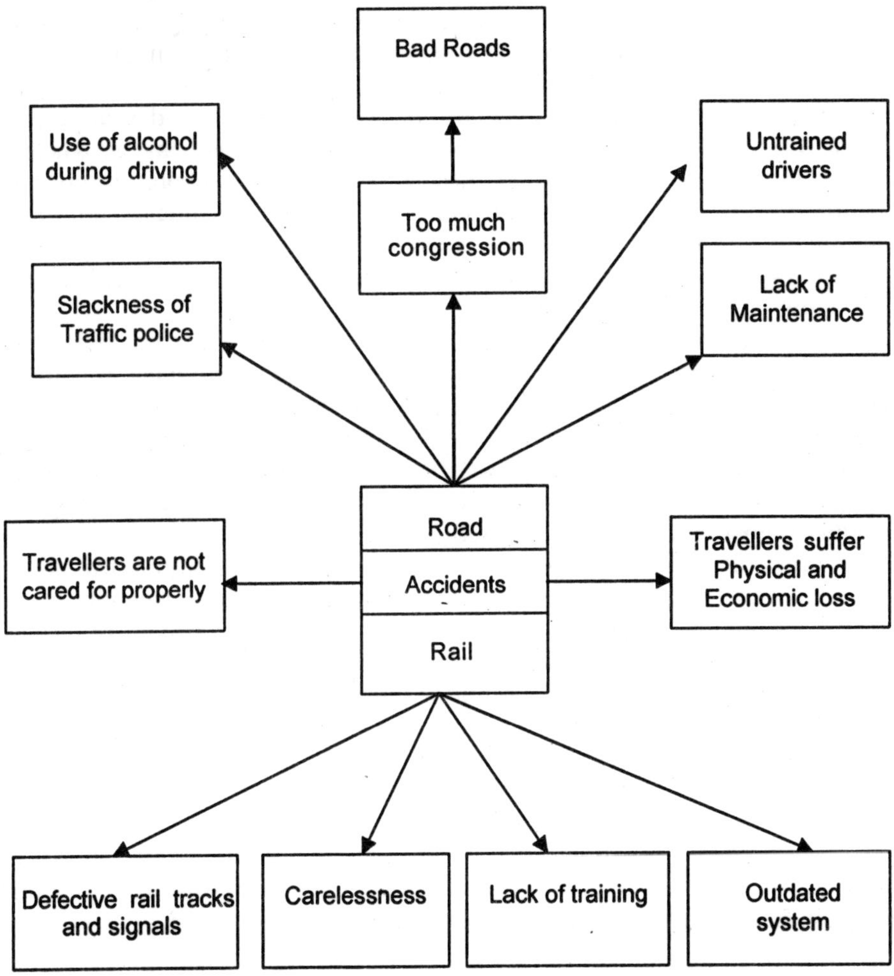

receive relatively little national or international attention compared with the focus on major communicable and non-communicable diseases.

To a large extent, road injuries are preventable. There are available and affordable interventions that can prevent injuries and save lives: to date, most of the evaluation of these interventions has been carried out in developed countries, and more research is needed on their effectiveness in developing countries. Renewed efforts are under way to increase world-wide awareness of the problem and its solutions and to encourage the introduction of road safety policies and practices. Several countries are using integrated strategies to deal with traffic risks and enhance the benefits of transport and land-use policies to promote physical activity and cohesive projects for community development[7].

Emergency Medical Services for Road Accident

In the more developed countries the response of ambulances and the like to reach the scene of an accident are short and many lives are saved as a result. In India, the average response time is much longer with the consequence that some lives are lost that with a quicker response time might have been saved. However, response time is not the only important factor. The quality of post-accident treatment also has a bearing on whether or not an accident victim lives or dies. In some areas, Highway Patrol and Traffic Aid Posts have been introduced to improve response time and quality of treatment. To achieve quick response time and prompt high quality medical attention requires a higher degree of co-ordination between the many agencies involved.[8]

A large proportion of the world's population live in rural areas and a majority of these people are involved in agricultural activities. In spite of their numbers, people living in rural areas do not have access to adequate health care, and in most countries we do not have detailed epidemiological information about their health problems. This is partly because information on details of illness and injury do not get recorded in city hospitals, which is where most research is conducted.

Agriculture related injuries in our study villages amounted to about 20 minor and three moderate-to-serious injuries per thousand people every year. This obviously means that in a country life India agriculture-related serious injury and deaths would be in the region of 5 million and half-a-million respectively. Most of the minor injuries are due to hand tools.

In consultation with farmers, artisans, engineers and product designers we were able to make fodder-cutting machines much safer without increasing the cost significantly. This has been done by incorporating a warning roller before the crushing mechanisms and attaching a blade guard which pushes children's hands away before the blade can touch the fingers. Over a hundred farmers in this area have not fitted these devices to their machines.

Similar improvements to equipment such as threshers, tillers and harrows can make farming a much safer occupation. But many more professionals will have to be involved and many more people will have to take up such work seriously. Otherwise the unnecessary maiming and killing of millions of farmers and their families will continue around the world.[9]

As for occupational accidents, it is recognized that 70% of them are due to human error, which can be avoided by training and constantly drawing attention to the risks. An unsafe work environment accounts for 30% of cases; it is essential to introduce safe equipment and non-hazardous chemicals, and to improve work conditions. The best precaution would be to use only technologies with built-in safety measures.[10]

One of the tragedies of modern-day society is the extent to which we are confronted with violence. Violence exists throughout the world and takes many form, but one of the most shocking and insidious forms of violence is that which affects girls and women.[11]

CHART 14.2

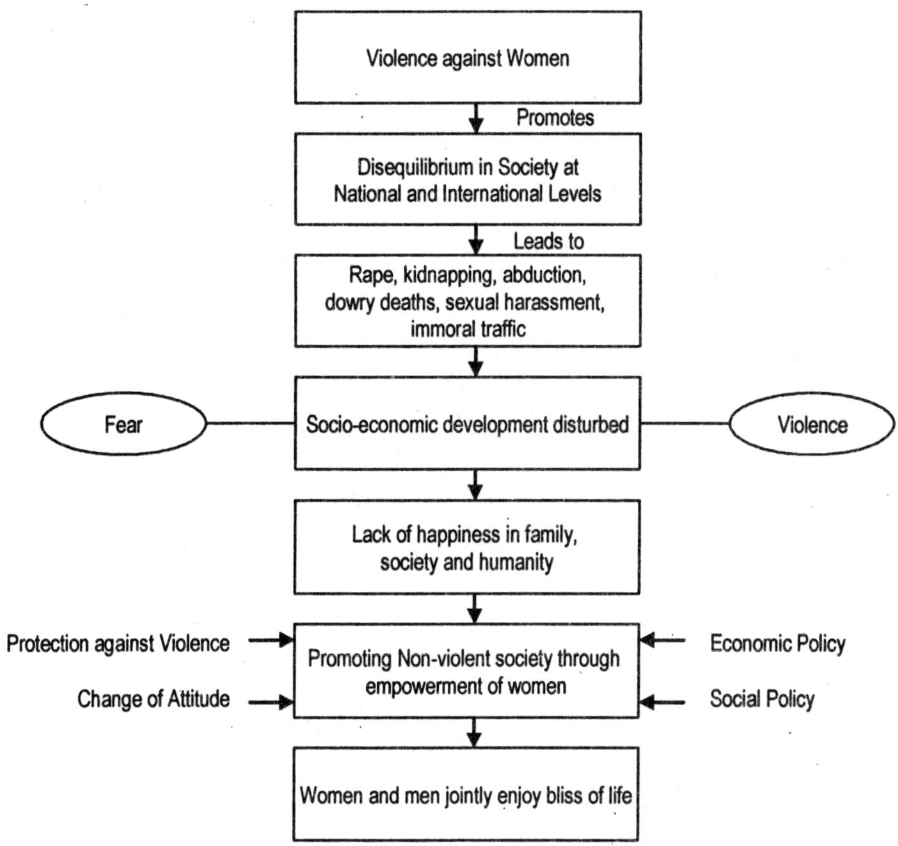

According to the United Nations, violence against women consists of "any act of gender-based violence that results in, or is likely to result in, physical, sexual or psychological harm or suffering to women, including threats of such acts, coercion or arbitrary deprivation of liberty, whether occurring in public or private life. Violence against women shall be understood to encompass but not be limited to: physical, sexual and psychological violence occurring in the family and in the community, including battering, sexual abuse of female children, dowry-related violence, marital rape, female genital mutilation and other traditional practices harmful to women, non-spousal violence, violence-related to exploitation, sexual harassment and intimidation at work, in educational institutions and elsewhere, trafficking in women, forced prostitution, and violence perpetrated or condoned by the State."

Violence against women is viewed as one of the most crucial societal mechanism by which women are forced into a subordinate position. It is a manifestation of unequal power relation, which has led to man's domination over and discrimination against woman.

Violence is defined as a physical act of aggression of one individual or group against another or others. Violence results in or is likely to result in physical, sexual, psychological harm or suffering. This also includes the threat of such act; coercion or arbitrary deprivation of liberty in public or private life and violation of human rights of women in situation of armed conflicts.

While the basic reason for violence against women is their inferior status in a male dominated society educationally, economically, politically and socially, there are other factors too. The increasing criminalization of society, media images of violence, poor enforcement of legal provision, unabashed consumerism and erosion of traditional values have all added to it.

The issue of violence against women has been the most pervasive themes of the new women's liberation movement in India since its rise in 1974-75. First it was the horrifying rising toll of fire in the growing number of dowry deaths, then from 1980 with the cases of Mathura, Maya Tayagi and Rameeza Bi, the problem of rape burst out of the shadows to stand as and Rameeza Bi, the problem of rape burst out of the shadows to stand as the symbol of women's oppression. Finally, the last few years have seen dramatic revivals of the ancient customs of Sati as well as female infanticide and female foeticide.[12]

Violence against women is an important force that helps to keep the structure of patriarchy intact. It makes gender discrimination a live and terrifying experience for women, and ensures their subjugation. We have used the term gender-based violence to describe acts that cause physical, sexual or psychological harm to women. Such acts are based in the unequals relations that exist between men and women in society. The most important thing to remember about gender-based violence is that, it is all pervasive—it can occur in all kinds of situations (within the family, at the workplace, in public places, in the community, and even when in the custody of the state) and at all stages of a woman's life.[13]

Violence against women means any act of gender-based violence that results in, or is likely to result in, physical, sexual or psychological harm or suffering to women, including threats of such acts, coercion or arbitrary deprivation of liberty, whether occurring in public or private life. Violence against women, including threats or fear of violence is a permanent constraint on the mobility of women and limits their access to resources and basic activities. Such violence are impediments to the achievement of the objectives of equality, development and peace. It violates and impairs or nullifies the enjoyment by women of their human rights and fundamental freedoms.

The term "violence against women" following the declaration of UN Commission on the Status of Women (1993), is usually defined as "any act of gender-based violence that results in or is likely to result in, physical, sexual or psychological harm or suffering to women, including threats, such as acts, coercion or arbitrary deprivations of liberty, whether occurring in public or private life."[14]

Broadly, violence against women can be divided in two categories:

(a) Physical, sexual and psychological violence occurring within the community, including rape, sexual abuse, sexual harassment and intimidation at work, in educational institutions and elsewhere, trafficking in women and forced prostitution; and
(b) Physical, sexual and psychological violence occurring in the family, including bettering, sexual abuse of female children in the household, dowry-related violence and other traditional practices harmful to women, non-spousal violence and violence related to exploitation.

The nature and forms of violence is intertwined within physical, mental and psychological levels. Prevailing forms of violence are wife beating and cruelty at home, molestation, rape, sexual harassment at workplace, etc. It occurs regardless of age, marital status, caste, relation. Violence includes physical, sexual emotional, psychological, social and economic abuse by one member of a family/society to control or dominate women in the family/society.

Physical violence includes slapping, punching, beating, shoving with or without weapons.

Sexual violence includes rape, molestations, harassment. Rape is forcing a woman to have sex against her will. It is a violation of an individual's rights over here body.

Emotional violence can include all intentional attempts to minimize the victim's concern and to make them feel bad. Humiliating the victim in public and private places.

Psychological violence is any threats that are made or carried out with the intent of financial or emotional injury, blackmail or humiliation.

Economic violence creates financial dependence.

Intimidation as a form of violence can include making women afraid by using looks, action and gestures: by destroying their property or by displaying weapons.

Isolation can be used to control and limit what woman does, whom they see and where they go.

Using privilege to control is also a form of violence. By treating a woman or child like a servant and having the last world about everything, the abuser is acting like a master. He is defining and rigidly abiding by the traditional roles of men and women.[15]

Violence against women must be seen in its broadest sense. Violence not only refers to the physical and mental abuse to which women are subjected. It also refers to the hidden violence that women face when they are discriminated against or denied basic human rights such as education, food, medical care, and a safe environment in which to live.

Violence affects women throughout their entire life span from the in utero period right through to old age. In some instances, the capacity to determine the sex of a child before it is born has been used to prevent the birth of girl children. In other cases, girls have been subjected to differential feeding practices, which may affect their physical and mental well being for the rest of their lives. Discriminatory practices in childrearing, such as keeping girl children away from school to work in the home, can be seen as a from of violence which may be detrimental to the girls' own health and that of their future children.

Within the family structure many women across societies suffer various types of abuse at the hands of their partners. Elderly women, too, are often the victims of mental and physical abuse within the confines of their family, or through the neglect and disinterest shown to them by society as a whole.

When a woman works outside her home she may encounter different forms of violence, from the lack of security on the streets to the overt or hidden violence and discrimination she faces in her place or work. Too often women are afraid to speak out against violence or abuse in the workplace for fear of losing their position.

These are but a few examples of the daily violence women and girls experience, and which result from the status they are accorded in society. All forms of violence against women represent an abuse of human rights.

We must not allow these violations of human rights to go unrecognized and unchallenged. We must open our eyes to all forms of violence against women and combat them on all fronts: behind the doors of family homes; in the community; on the streets of our villages and towns; at work and in the political and economic institutions that govern our societies. Let us use the occasion of World Health Day, 1993 to speak out strongly against this abuse of human rights and take strong measures to put an end to all forms of violence against women.[16]

In the ultimate analysis, there can be no two opinions about the need for stringent laws, sensitive judiciary, effective law and enforcement machinery and vigilant women's groups to deal with such atrocious crimes against women. But what is needed more than anything else is a total revolution in the thinking of our society that always blames the woman for the crime of which she is the victim, not the perpetrator.

Mahatma Gandhi strongly feels that, "If only the women of the world would come together they could display such heroic non-violence as to kick away the atom bomb like a mere ball. Women have been so gifted by God. If an ancestral treasure, lying buried in a corner of the house unknown to the members of the family were suddenly discovered, what a celebration if would occasion. Similarly, women's marvelous power is lying dormant. If the women of Asia wake up, this will dazzle the world. My experiment in non-violence would be instantly successful if I could secure women's help."

Major Health Problem

In today's world, violence against women constitutes a major public health problem. In the US, nearly two million women a year are beaten in their homes and it is a fair assumption that many more such cases go unreported. Cases of rape are even more numerous and even less frequently reported; it has been estimated that only one rape is reported to the US authorities for every ten actually committed. Many other countries do not even have data on these crimes, since frequently it is not socially or culturally acceptable for women to reveal that they have been beaten or raped, nor are such revelations recognized.

Seldom seen as a public health issue, violence against women is a significant cause of female morbidity and mortality around the globe. In the USA, for example, wife abuse is the leading cause of injury among women of reproductive age. Between 22% and 35% of women who visit United States emergency clinics are there for symptoms related to on-going abuse.

But women in the USA share the reality of violence with women in virtually every other culture in the world. Data from developing countries reveal that one-third to over half of women surveyed report being beaten by their partner. Not uncommonly, beatings are part of a pattern of emotional and physical abuse that escalates over time. In Papua New Guinea, 18% of all urban wives surveyed had sought hospital treatment for injuries inflicted by their husbands. A survey of one Caribbean island revealed that one in three women had been sexually abused as a child.

Wife abuse also provides the primary context for many other health problems. Again, research from the USA indicates that bettered women are four to five times more likely to require psychiatric treatment and five times more likely to attempt suicide than non-battered women. And they are at increased risk of alcohol abuse, drug dependence, chronic pain, and depression. In one US study of the use made of health care, a history of rape and/or assault was a stronger predictor of physician visits and outpatient costs than were a woman's age or other health risks such as smoking. Along with physical injury and emotional trauma, rape survivors run the risk of becoming pregnant or contracting sexually transmitted diseases, including AIDS.

Violence poses a powerful obstacle to achieving other goals that are high on the development agenda. During pregnancy, for example, it threatens the goal of "Safe motherhood" for all women. Battered women run twice the risk of miscarriage and four times the risk of having a low-birth-weight infant.[17]

Abuse and neglect of children is an emotional crippler and disabler of both children and adults. The cost of inaction far exceeds any potential cost of prevention.

As we approach the 21st century, the numbers of maltreated children continue to increase. It is clear that by paying more attention to this problem, on prevention just as in recent decades we have eradicated smallpox and are eliminating poliomyelitis and other scourges of childhood. Abuse and neglect of children is an emotional crippler and disabler of both children and adults. The cost to society of not dealing directly with the problem far exceeds any potential cost of the prevention efforts.[18]

Daily observation and statistics confirm that any other age group, are both the instigators of violent behaviour and its victims.

What is sure is that aggression and violence intrude more and more into our daily lives; the instantaneous and worldwide coverage by the media makes sure of that. Another certainty, which daily observation and statistics confirm, is that adolescents and young adults more than any other age group are at one and the same time the instigators of violent behaviour and its victims. In the industrialized world, and in many Third World countries, violent death—which includes suicide, murder and accidental death—heads the list of causes of death among those aged 15 to 24, especially young men.

For if young people are often violent in their individual and collective behaviour, isn't this because in many ways our societies do violence to them? In other words, even though there are many palliatives for violence in young people in the form of education, regulations or even repression, the true remedy lies somewhere else. At the end of an article about violence in young people and the possible solutions, the executive director of the American Council for Crime Prevention concluded: "The burden is on us. Unless we help our young people develop a sense of stake in their communities and their futures, there may be neither communities nor future."[19]

In the aftermath of war, health workers must recognize that they have a key social role to play in reconstructing services, and that battle-related injuries and deaths are just the tip of the iceberg.

The post-war situation might, on the other hand, offer some opportunities for influencing change and ensuring that the new health sector operates equitably and efficiently. Priority issues will need to include rehabilitation services for the disabled, reconstitution of the community structures and family and other networks, and maternal and child health care programmes.

Health workers must recognize that—although conflict is political—they, like other development workers, have a significant social role to play, and that direct battle-related injuries and deaths are just the tip of the iceberg.[20]

The consequences of armed conflict on a population's health are so drastic that the international community must look beyond the effects of war and examine its root causes. This will call for simultaneous action at several levels:

- Doing everything possible to settle political and economic differences by means other than violence.
- Insisting on respect for the Geneva Convention's rules governing the protection of non-combatants, which 174 signatory governments have accepted.
- Training the civilian and military health services to cope with a sudden influx of injured and to ensure their speedy transport to first aid stations.

- Teaching as widely as possible the principles of first and wartime surgery.
- Rehabilitating those very seriously injured in war so as to reintegrate them into society and restore their dignity and self-reliance.

Only by taking this global approach to the problem shall we be able to combat that most murderous of human scourges—collective violence and war[21].

Unacceptable Epidemic

The Coalition was brought together by a mutual belief that the current level of violence and the resulting injuries are unacceptable. Violence can no longer be treated as merely a law enforcement issue but must be addressed as an epidemic affecting each one of us. The Coalition members are in agreement that violence and violence prevention are the concern and responsibility of all segments of the public and private sectors. Moreover, a multi-disciplinary approach utilizing the specific talents and expertise of the various disciplines can call attention to the problem, promote and implement prevention and intervention programmes, and evaluate programme effectiveness in order to significantly reduce violence and the resultant injuries. In addition, the Coalition provides a forum for influencing public policy regarding public health violence prevention in Los Angeles.[22]

The need is curb all sorts of Violence, which causes many health problems. We should cultivate love for peace and harmony through education and training of mends violence in any form is a grave danger making the lives of people miserable and worse. In 21st century, we must curb it at all levels from all causes and eliminate from this globe.

Notes and References

1. Hiroshi Nakajima, M.D., Ph.D, World Health Day, 1993, Handle life with care; prevent violence and negligence, *World Health*, 46th Year, No. 1, January-February 1993, p. 3.
2. *Ibid.*, p. 3.
3. Claude Got, Too to pay for freedom, *World Health*, 46th Year, No. 1, January-February 1993, p. 8.
4. Dora, C., Phillips, M., Transport, environment and health. Copenhagen, World Health Organisation Regional Office for Europe, 2000 (WHO Regional Publications, European Series, No. 89; http://www.euro.who.int/transport/Publications_1, accessed 23 September, 2003).
5. Kunzli, N., *et al.*, Public health impacts of outdoor and traffic-related air pollution; a European assessment, Lancet, 2000, 356:795-801 (http://www.euro.who.int/transport/HIA/20021107_3, accessed 23 September 2003).
6. Metz, B., *et al.*, eds. Climate Change, 2001, Mitigation, Cambridge, Cambridge University Press for the Inter-governmental Panel on Climate Change (IPCC), 2001.

7. Dora, C., Racioppi, F., Including health in transport policy agendas: the role of health impact assessment analyses and procedures in the European experience. *Bulletin of the World Health Organisation*, 2003, 81:399-403.
8. Dr. S.L. Goel, Man-made Disasters, Accidents: Road and Railway Accident, p. 141.
9. Dinesh Mohan, Avoidable dangers on the farm, *World Health*, 46th Year, No. 1, January-February 1993, pp. 12-13.
10. I.G. Badran, Accidents in the developing world, *World Health*, 46th Year, No. 1, January-February 1993, p. 15.
11. Mrs. Suzanne Mubarak, First Lady of Egypt: *World Health*, 46th Year, No. 1, January-February 1993, p. 16.
12. UNIFEM and Marry, Support Services to Counter Violence Against Women in Haryana, A Resource Directory, New Delhi, 2003.
13. UNIFEM and Sanhito, Support Services to Counter Violence Against Women in West Bengal, Kolkata, 2002, p. 13.
14. UNIFEM and Sakhi, Support Services to Counter Violence Against Women in Kerala, A Resource Directory, 2002, p. 15.
15. *Ibid.*, pp. 15-16.
16. Mrs Suzanne Mubarak, Spokes women against violence and injury, *World Health*, 46th Year, No. 1, January-February 1993, pp. 16-17.
17. Lori L. Heise, Violence against women, *World Health*, 46th Year, January-February 1993, p. 21.
18. Richard Krugman, Child abuse and neglect, *World Health*, 46th Year, January-February 1993, pp. 22-23.
19. Michel Manciaux, Violent youth, *World Health*, 46th Year, January-February 1993, pp. 24-25.
20. Anthony Zwi and Antonio Ugalde, Victims of war, *World Health*, 46th Year, January-February 1993, pp. 26-27.
21. Remi Russbach, Warfare and health, *World Health*, 46th Year, January-February 1993, p. 28.
22. Billie Weiss, Violence Prevention Coalition, *World Health*, 46th Year, January-February 1993, p. 30.

15

CHAPTER

Health and Sports

Sports are an integral part of education system since sports promote health, discipline and alertness in life. Today, only few students who take part in competition of games enjoy all the facilities. The purpose of sports should be to involve each and every student in one sport or the other. In addition, sports must be played by all people even after the school and college life. Sports provide relaxation and dynamism since sports rejuvenate the body and mind. Sport can:

(i) Protect people from all diseases which are the product of sedatic life and causing cardio-vascular diseases, diabetes called life time or lifestyle diseases
(ii) Encourage people to enjoy life by remaining active as sports are activities of body and mind.
(iii) Sports avoids people from lethargy which is slow poisoning
(iv) Sports promote discipline, good will and enthusiasm
(v) Sports indirectly keep away persons from wasting time in bad company.
(vi) Sports are sure way to good health.

F.J. Tomiche in his article, "Sports and Health" has beautifully said: There can be no doubt about it: sport offers the best antidote to the tensions and stress that are everyday hazards as our lives become increasingly competitive:

> "There can be no doubt about it: sport offers the best antidote to the tensions and stress that are everyday hazards as our lives become ever more competitive. It offers a respite from our daily cares and contributes a vital element of balance and relaxation. Individual sports, such as swimming, athletics or gymnastics, offer a school for

CHART 15.1

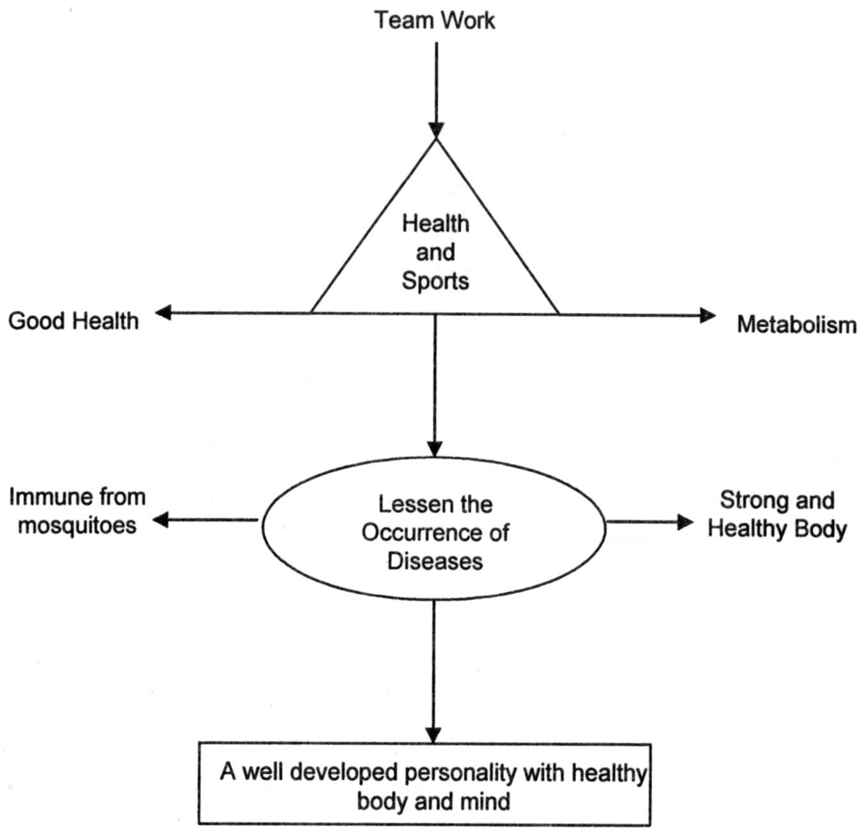

character formation, where self-discipline and stamina can be developed. Individuals exert themselves to improve their own performances. However modest these may be, and to set themselves new goals. Team games like foot-hall, rugby, hockey or water-polo, on the other hand, encourage another set of qualities, among them coordination with colleagues, the team spirit and a sense of belonging. What we call the sporting spirit combines fair play, dexterity, self-control and good manners. It was in this context that Baron Pierre de Coubertin, re-founder of the modern Olympic Games, commented: "The essential thing in life is not so much to win as to fight fair."

On the physiological level the benefits of sport are too well-known to need repeating here. All the same it is worth recalling that sport has a beneficial effect on general hygiene. There is nothing better than a good shower after the sweat of physical effort, and it is just what tired muscles cry out for.

Besides all this, athletes noticeably smoke and drink less than those who take no regular physical exercise, and the roles played by alcohol and tobacco in respiratory diseases, lung cancer and cirrhosis of the liver have today been clearly established. It follows that a healthy sporting life is in itself an excellent way of preventing quite a number of killer diseases. It has even proved effective in curbing accidents at work; workers in Soviet factories are called upon to do five or ten minutes of exercise every day and this, according to the specialists, has both reduced the number of accidents and increased productivity.

In addition, sports keep and maintain health lifestyles:

In the space of a few decades, there have been remarkable reductions in morbidity and mortality due to infectious and parasitic diseases in most developing country in all regions of the world. However, other threats of health in the form of the so-called "Western degenerative" or "lifestyle" diseases are emerging at rates that far outstrip what would be expected from the fact that people are living longer.

In many developing nations, already beset with economic, social and other health problems, the rates of heart disease, diabetes and hypertension are as high as or even higher than in major developed nations. These chronic diseases impose a destructive drain on communities through their association with sickness and premature death.[1]

Beneficial at any age

At whatever age a person starts, sport has a health-giving effect, although obviously the intensity and the nature of the effort involved varies with age. The consumption of oxygen determines the intensity of effort in the human body; that consumption reaches its maximum around 20 years of age, and then progressively decreases as the years pass by. Women in general absorb 25 to 30 per cent less oxygen than men do. But regular training can increase the absorption of oxygen in both women and men by as much as 20 to 30 per cent compared with a person who is not in training.

Around the age of 35, the heart rate decreases in men and this in turn reduces the maximum consumption of oxygen. People at this age should ease up their efforts, resist the temptation to go flat out in competitive sports, and stop racing against the clock.

Beyond the age of 45, sport is the best antidote to a sedentary life and over-indulgence in food—two leading characteristics of the affluent society. And in the "Third Age", physical exercises help to keep limbs supple and to avoid such accidents as fractured hips to which the elderly are particularly prone. At all ages, countless invalids, heart cases and disabled persons have managed to restore themselves to normal activity, thanks to having embarked on the right sort of physical activity.

There are some detractors of physical exercise who claim that the benefits which may be derived from sport fall very far short of compensating for the risks entailed. No human activity, whether it is merely boiling an egg or mending an item of clothing, is totally free from potential danger. Even walking on a lonely path, with no likelihood of ice about. can carry certain risks; you could be stung by a wasp or you could twist an ankle. But to set the benefits of sport on the same level as the dangers that can quite easily be avoided is to deny all the evidence—or merely to put up a lame excuse for not doing any physical exercise.

In fact the number of professional sportsmen and women is tiny today if compared with the total of amateur athletes. Those few thousands of footballers who are paid fabulous sums, or the hundred or so tennis players whose game merges into "show-business", represent a negligible total of individuals compared with the millions of teenagers who express their joy of living by kicking a ball about. The big difference between these two categories of athletes is that the first mentioned lay claim to newspaper headlines and television interviews, while the others play their games in simple anonymity.[2]

We can thus plead that sports should not be restricted to only those who are to play national and International games but should be expanded in schools, colleges, so that people at all ages play games to remain active and avoid lifestyle diseases sports are essential from children to old people. In this way sports can keep us all healthy and active. We have to propogate the need of playing sports to keep fit and healthy. People must be educated to find time for sports inspite of their being too busy. After some time, they would not be able to do much work as they would catch some lifestyle diseases. Being busy only in work and neglected sports would lead them nearer to some diseases and lack of enjoyment of life.

By sport we do not mean solely competitive games. The term also includes the normal physical exercise that is indispensable for everyone who wants to enjoy a balanced and healthy life. Sport is not the preserve of the few who are particularly gifted or who happen to be offered the chance of special training. It is a need of every individual, of whatever age and physical condition, and is an essential factor in a balanced existence.

So when we speak of food for athletes, we are really talking about the sort of simple rules that everyone can apply. Sport is not something additional to or outside of normal life, and similarly food for sportsmen and sportswomen is not some inaccessible ideal that may only be contemplated from afar with envy and frustration. Every individual should be able to find through sport the total fulfilment of his or her capability; all we need to know is the kind of food that will be most conducive to that full realisation of self.

It would be quite wrong to think of food for athletes as if it were somehow magical, as if certain ingredients offered an instant formula for record-breaking performances. There is no miracle food. What really matters is to maintain the right balance, or to recover it once it has been lost.[3]

Sports and Health and well being: In a feature in Hindustan Times dated October 9, 2007 on "Anti-Lifestyle, Your Health is in your hand", the Hindustan Times has brought the views of different persons. Dr. S.K.

Aggarwal from Amritsar observes that we come across a number of youngsters suffering from heart diseases or other lifestyle ailments like diabetes and hypertension. But they can't blame it on modern day pressures alone. They also owe their sufferings to lack of knowledge on health issues and a casual attitude towards health. Most of them believe in the statement. I'd rather die young than live on a diet of lettuce and boiled fish'. With such an attitude they are only inviting trouble.

Simple lifestyle modifications like changes in dietary habits and regular exercise can lower blood pressure and also improve a person's response to blood pressure medications. Obesity is common among hypersensitive patients and its prevalence increases with age. Some very obese people have a syndrome called sleep apnea. This syndrome is characterized by periodic interruption of normal breathing during sleep and may contribute to hypertension. A regular exercise schedule may help lower blood pressure over a period of time. It is equally important to keep a healthy attitude.

Dr. Gurkirpal Singh Sidhu from Barnala observes that people themselves are to blame for their messed up lives. They seem to be too busy or rather lost in the mad rush. The IT boom has led to more complex round-the-clock jobs, addicting to health and social problems. Irregular lifestyles are leading to ailments like high blood pressure, diabetes and stiff joints. If we regularly ignore or suppress the symptoms, the ailment will come to stay at a later stage, which may lead to irreversible changes in the body. Beware! Sometimes it gives no signal. That's why such ailments are referred to as silent killers. Fortunately, we can prevent them, and at no extra cost. This can be done at an early stage if we are alert and responsive to the abnormal functioning of our body. Healthy lifestyles do not mean swanky outings or mouth-watering dishes. A balanced diet, plenty of water and regular exercise can work wonders. If it is difficult to maintain an exercise schedule, simply applying dietary restrictions and adopting correct postures and sleeping patterns will go.

It is not the responsibility of the government or some NGO to regulate our lifestyle. The choice is with us. Nothing should outweigh our concern for health. Why wait for a symptoms to occur when we can take preventive measures beforehand. A stitch in time saves nine.

Dr. Amita Dadwal SAS Nagar observes, that earlier, cardiac diseases, hypertension and diabetes were linked with old age. But of late, these diseases, aptly called 'lifestyle diseases', are on the rise in youngsters even in their early 20s. Youngsters resort to smoking and alcohol very early in life. They subsist on junk food, aerated drinks and processed foods, which can make them sluggish and weak, You are what you eat.

Obesity is common due to the sedentary life we lead. Despite being busy, our bodies do not get the exercise we need to burn the extra calories, which go on pilling. Most of the foods and snacks contain transfat, which is harmful to the heart. But it is as if we can't do without them. We have become so lazy that we prefer to use cars or two-wheelers even for short distances. Walking is a wonderful way of keeping healthy. To start with, a 20 minute brisk walk can do wonders. Climbing stairs is another way of keeping the heart fit. Not finding time for exercise is a lame excuse. If we can find the time to eat, drink and make merry, we can certainly take out time to look after ourselves. Stress, another silent killer, can be controlled through various ways. Meditation, pranayam, yoga and regular walks are real stress-busters. A periodic visit to the doctor can help. We should be prosperous, but not at the cost of our health. If we can work hard for monetary gains, why not enjoy the fruit of labour as well with good health and longevity. Try and overcome your weaknesses. Don't let them overcome you.[4]

Although there is no clear-cut proof that physical activity prevents cardiovascular disease and prolongs life, regular physical exertion of a certain intensity is needed for the human body to function at its best. This conclusion emerged from the International Conference on Sports Cardiology held earlier this year in Rome.

The 300 participants from nearly 40 countries also agreed that physical activity ought to be considered within the framework of healthy life habits. It should not be aimed only at, or restricted to, improving cardiovascular health, but should envisage better health in general. It is very likely that, in so doing, life expectancy too will be increased while the risk of developing myocardial infraction (heart attack) will decrease.

Organised by the Giovanni Lorenzini Foundation, in collaboration with the Italian National Olympic Committee and the Italian Federation of Sports Medicine, the Conference had two aims. It sought to assess the present state of knowledge on work physiology in athletic performances, and at the same time to study the role of physical activity maintaining cardiovascular health. Delegates agreed that physical activity should be carried out within the limits of good common sense, otherwise it might even prove dangerous. Depending on a person's age, health status and training status, it might be advisable for someone planning to undertake fairly strenuous physical exercise—particularly if it is competitive in nature—to undergo a medical examination.

Exercise should be of such a kind that it can be practised throughout a lifetime, the Conference suggested. The beneficial effects that physical training can have on cardiovascular and other functions do not persist for a long time. Thus it is not enough to have been an athlete in youth; much more valuable is to remain physically active at a later age.

There was general agreement that the actual mechanism whereby exercise improves health is not fully understood. However, physical activity ought to be maintained above a certain threshold, for instance, about 2,000 calories (8.4 megajoules) per week should be expended in strenuous exercise, during which the heart rate should reach 130-150 beats per minute. Physical activity has been found to increase HDL (high-density lipoproteins), although it takes several months to do so. These lipoproteins are beneficially involved in the transport and elimination of blood cholesterol.[5]

For professional sports players, a special branch of medicine has developed by the name of sports medicine, Jack Refshuage in his article, "Sports Medicine" in the *World Health,* 1978 clearly says that sports medicine is not a new or modern practice. Ever since mankind has existed the human body has been submitted to study. Early man, in order to survive, found he must employ only the required energy and technique needed to overcome his difficult moments in hunting. Equally basically, it is probable that supreme or maximum performance was required only for survival in attack or defence, or in competition with his fellows.

Nowadays, sport is an effective means of obtaining measures of work capacity, speed and execution of manoeuvres, power potential and physical endurance. In fact, these studies have made us aware that we must not only evaluate the relative degrees of excellence that the body can obtain, but we must also define the limits that effort and performance must not exceed.

The conviction that health is linked with physical and mental activities goes back to antiquity. Greek literature of the sixth century B.C. indicates these benefits, and in the virile and well-recorded Greco-Roman era remedial therapy was practised and extolled.

In modern times, it is only during the last two to three decades that the worth and role of sports medicine have been recognised, and even now in some of the more developed countries the academic establishments still ignore its value and its inevitable development as a discipline.

Jack Refshuage in his article, "Sports Medicine" in the *World Health,* 1978 clearly says that it has been said that it is easier to describe the discipline of sports medicine than to definite it. In some countries it is confined to medical graduates only, while in others it is composed of a single professional specialty. Some see it as a combination of both medical and paramedical professionals. There is increasing acceptance around the world that suitable and regular physical activities are generally beneficial, but it must also be appreciated that programmes for elite competitors and programmes for "fun sport" participants must be individually designed, while the inherent risks in any such programmes must be calculated and covered to the best of the organisers' ability.

The "descriptive definition" I propose is that put forward by the Australian Sports Medicine Federation. This Federation in its present form is 16 years old and rapidly expanding in numbers and activities. It is a multi-disciplinary organisation with representation from many different specialties, including general and specialist medical practitioners (team physicians), psychiatrists, psychologists, exercise physiologists, physiotherapists, physical educators, podiatrists (specialists in the care of the foot), nurses sociologists and coaches.

This varied membership offers a team approach to sports medicine, and enables us more adequately to practice our aims and principles. These are:

- to supervise the medical care of organisations which promote and conduct physical activities in sport and recreation. Such medical care should help to safeguard and improve the physical and mental health of the community;
- to foster the scientific study of both the normal and harmful aspects of physical activity and to encourage research into such matters;
- to promulgate information of use to sporting bodies;
- to co-operate with kindred national and international bodies such as the International Federation of Sports Medicine (FIMS);
- to act in liaison with the Australian Olympic Federation and similar national sporting bodies;
- To act as an advisory body in matters pertaining to sports medicine and in matters relating to national health and fitness;
- To act as a co-ordinating body for all the Australian State groups, to promote policy and undertake such tasks and responsibilities as may be incidental to the Federation's aims. The Federation also produces the Australian Journal of Sports Medicine and the Australian Sports Medicine Newsletter.

So far, only few formal post-graduate courses in sports medicine have been recognised by national governments and national medical associations. The most outstanding of such courses is the six-year sports medicine study held in East Germany. The United Kingdom and the United States hold various courses and FIMS has basic programmes available. These are probably suitable for any countries that may wish to initiate studies of this kind.

There is growing determination in many developed and developing countries to establish such courses, and undoubtedly this has in part been stimulated by increased media coverage of international and national sporting events, where naturally the greatest emphasis is accorded to the successful countries.

Governments too are anxious to promote health orientation by physical activity, and in affluent countries where health insurance covers medical costs, the health percentage of the gross national income has escalated to such a degree that governments are being forced to take measures to contain this expenditure. One aspect of this escalation has been the growth of numerous "Sports Medical Clinics", in many cases staffed by medical and paramedical graduates without any sports medicine experience.

If governments are to control such clinics they must have some means of introducing an accreditation system, and it would be natural for them to turn to their sports medicine association for guidance. It seems logical that the most acceptable form of accreditation would be the completion of an appropriate course in sports medicine which would meet the requirements of the National Medical Association.

In Australia, the Australian Sports Medicine Federation proposes to initiate such a course next year, in conjunction with the Royal Australian College of General Practitioners. It will initially be developed for medical practitioners, but the Federation hopes later to establish such courses for physical educationalists and physiotherapists in consultation with and under the auspices of their own educational authorities. Courses for coaches are already in action and are being upgraded.

A further stimulus to the initiative of the Australian Sports Medicine Federation has come from our Asian neighbours, who would like to see such a course made available for their graduates, which they could adapt to their own needs as their sports medicine associations develop and consolidate.

The proposed course to be set-up for general practitioners in Australia would incorporate such topics as basic sports anatomy and kinesiology, exercise physiology and biochemistry, fitness tests, including methods and interpretation for athletes and non-athletes, training and conditioning for sport, exercise and disease—the preventive and therapeutic effects of exercise as well as medical contra-indication to sports, nutrition and drugs in sport, and the effects of environment on sport performance. The course will also deal with paediatrics and adolescent sports medicine, the effects of age on sports and recreation, the prevention and treatment of injury in sport, the psychology and sociology of sport and recreation and the role of the team medical officer.

Jangveer Singh in his article, "Price of Success" in *The Tribune* dated 14th Oct., 2007 observes that ten years back Information Technology and IT Enables Services was a sunrise industry in India. The government wisely gave the industry a free hand to frame employee policies which it did with aplomb. Today, the industry is entrenched in the metros and fast moving to tier-three cities with demand outstripping supply. IT and BPO jobs are the new panacea for a man on the move to build a bright future for himself.

However, the progress achieved in this sector in the last 10 years has come at a price. Workers, especially in the Business Process Outsourcing (BPO) sector, are complaining of mental and physical problems due to the nature of their work. Tight deadlines and ambitious targets cause similar problems in the IT sector with "burnout" becoming commonly used word and heart attacks striking down youngsters, a thing never heard in the decade earlier nine-to-five jobs available in India.

Even as the country copes with the new jobs and the new cultures it brings in its fold, things appear to be coming to a head. There is a rising concern among researchers, health workers, psychologists and now even the Union Health Ministry that there is a disconnect somewhere and some corrective action is needed to protect "young lives."

Eantosh Sharma in his article "Sports, Society and the Women", in *University News*, August 16, 2004 observes that sport is as old as human society itself. It is an institution which has its own traditions and values. Being an institutionalized and competitive activity, it involves vigorous physical exertion or the use of relatively complex physical skills by individuals whose participation is motivated by a combination of intrinsic satisfaction association with the activity, itself and external rewards earned through participation.

Society as an activity offers an opportunity of self-knowledge, self-expression and self-fulfilment; personal achievement, skills acquisition and demonstration of ability; social interaction, enjoyment, good health and well-being. It promotes involvement, integration and responsibility in society and contributes to the development of society, especially when sports activities have been accepted as an integral part of the culture of every society in every nation.

There cannot be two opinion on the subject that sports are an integral part of people at all stages of life, as well as for all those engaged in sedantry life activities. However, people when tired of their jobs indulge in alcohol, smoking, drugs, etc. to get relief. Same problems emerge from alcohol and drugs.

Thus, sports are not merely for enjoyment of life but essential to survive. Sports does not mean to play sophisticated sports. Even simple brisks walking can be a good sport. Yog can be very good for maintaining physical and mental health.

In the new millennium we must educate the people to take interest in any kind of sport which can keep them healthy and fit. All persons of whatever age must engage in some sports which consume some energy and help you to keep fit. In this way, we can save a lot of money, spent on diseases and use that money to enjoy life.

Sports are indispensable if people want to enjoy life as sports take care of good health and health is wealth. During my visit to China in May 2007, it was amazing to see that there are gyms and gyms for people to remain fit. A large number of indoor games have been provided. Our students are finding no time for sports resulting in ailments in the early age of life, taking drugs and making life listless. Thus, regular sports can make future students and people healthy and happy.

Notes and References

1. By the Mauritius Non-Communicable disease study group, *World Health,* June 1989, p. 18.
2. F.J. Tomiche, "Sport and Health", *World Health,* November 1978, pp. 3-4.
3. Marie-Lise barguis, Eating Well to Perform Better, in *World Health,* Nov. 1978, pp. 18-21.
4. *Hindustan Times,* Oct. 9, 2007.
5. Roberto Masironi, Good for the Heart, in *World Health,* Nov. 1978.

16

CHAPTER

Urban Health: Healthy Cities

"Cities are the locus of productive economic activities and hope for the future, yet they face growing environmental problems and increasing poverty. . . It is clear that, in the short-term, the bright lights of the city have dimmed and are, for many urban households, extinguished."

—*World Bank, 1991*

In the beginning of 20th century, there was only 10 percent of the population in the world living in urban areas which increased to 80 percent, the population increased to about 50 percent. This largest movement of human beings from rural to urban area in the known history of human kind, has indeed necessitated a relook into our settlement development perspectives. To day, we have 21 mega cities with more than 10 million inhabitants in each of them. Seventeen among these are in the developing countries. The process of urbanisation appears to be irreversible at least in the near future.

V. Suresh, and P. Jayapal in their article, "Towards an inclusive city in the new Millennium" in *Shelter* rightly say:

> Today's city presents a scenario of paradoxes. On the one hand, the city exhibits considerable potential with economic vibrancy and on the other, it presents a scenario of declining opportunities for the teaming millions. Whereas this centre of prosperity is resulting in the improvement of quality of life of large population, it is also turning into an agglomeration of poverty, with even more population living in conditions which are unacceptable. While the city has created peaks of affluence, it has also created depths of poverty and despair. And, even while it acts as the centre of cultural synthesis, it also presents a scenario of 'hollow of conscience' with crimes against

CHART 16.1

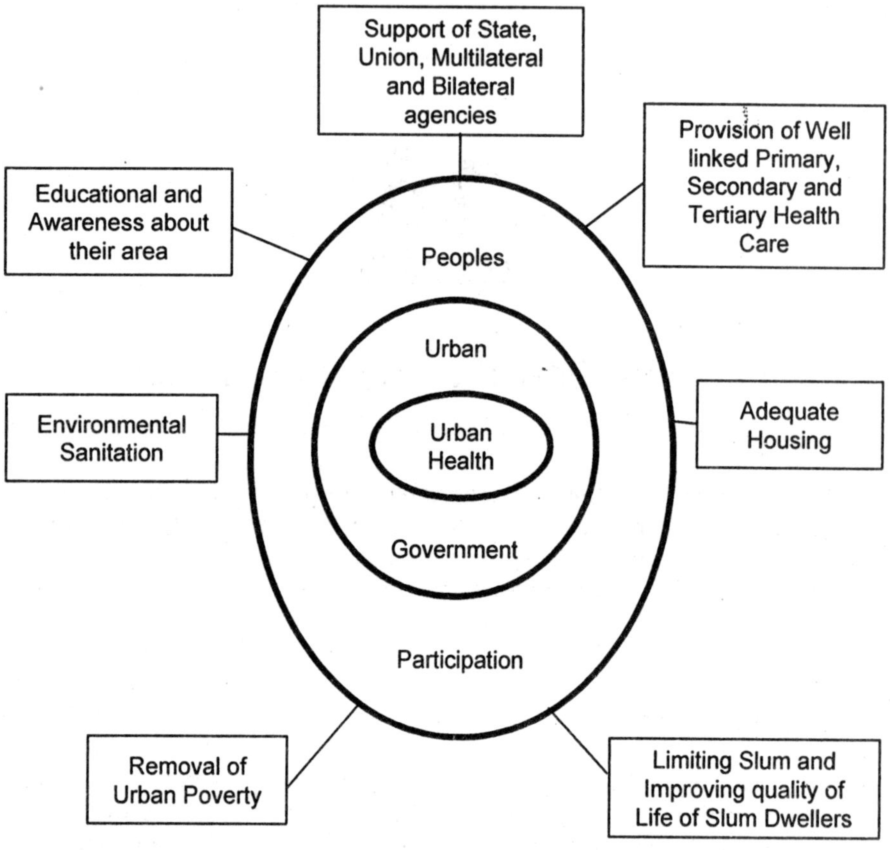

women and children to unbelievable heights. The increasing difference in the levels of income and quality of life of the people as reflected in the economic marginality, has resulted in the discernible demarcation of the 'have's and haven'ts' in terms of spatial, economic, cultural components in the city fabric.[1]

In *The Tribune*, dated 29th Nov., 2007, it was reported that women in the urban areas are at a higher risk of breast cancer. The issue was discussed by a panel of pathologists headed by Dr. Harsh Mohan, head, pathology, GMCH, on the fifth day of the annual conference of the Indian Association of Pathologists and Microbioloigists.

Surveys have revealed that there were 27 women in the urban areas, among one lakh, who are suffering from breast cancer while in the rural aras the number is as low as eight.

In *The Tribune*, dated 29th Nov. 2007, it was reported that Women in the urban areas are at a higher risk of breast cancer. The issue was discussed by a panel of pathologists headed by Dr. Harsh Mohan, head, pathology, GMCH, on the fifth day of the annual conference of the Indian Association of Pathologists and Microbiologists.

Surveys have revealed that there were 27 women in the urban areas, among one lakh, who are suffering from breast cancer while in rural areas the number is as low as eight. that Draft Status Paper-1995 of Government of Punjab, has observed that[2] Urbanisation has been considered as an index of development but in case of developing countries like India, urbanisation is not the outcome of merely the growth potential generated by urban settlements. It has been largely due to people work relationship in rural areas, in which land is the essential medium and which is right now so critically balanced that even small addition to population is pushing people out of agriculture to non-agricultural occupations. Thus, by and large, in India urbanisation is emerging as merely a process of transfer of rural poverty to urban environment which only results in concentration of Misery, this has resulted in the malfunctioning of most of the urban settlements leading to emergence of number of imbalances and problems. Thus, most of these settlements suffer from improper and haphazard development, absence of basic infrastructures and services, uncontrolled and unchecked growth of slums, lack of housing, high degree of visual and environmental degradation and uncontrolled traffic. The cumulative effect of these factors is the degradation of quality of life in urban settlements and huge amount of subsidies required to keep them going. These facts are more evident in case of larger cities especially metros and super-metros.

Urban areas in the past has not received much attention in terms of their planning, development and management despite the fact that cities and economic development are inextricably linked. Because of high productivity of urban areas, economic development activities get located in cities. Accordingly, it is desirable that human settlements are provided with necessary planning and development inputs so that their orderly growth and development is ensured. This would also be necessary for ensuring efficient functioning of human settlements for improving their productivity and for providing desirable quality of life to its residents in order to cater to their both economic and physical and metaphysical needs. The urban development strategy for any state thus assumes importance for not only its economic emancipation but also its physical well-being. All these factors and circumstances affect the health of the people.

Ninth Five Year Plan has analysed the urban health situation. To quote the plan:[3]

> Nearly 30% of India's population lives in urban areas. Urban migration over the last decade has resulted in rapid growth of people living in urban slums. The massive inflow of the population has also resulted in the deterioration of living conditions in the cities. From the data it could appear that the urban population has better health facilities and health indices than the rural population. However, in

many towns and cities the health status of urban slum-dwellers is worse than that of the rural population. The urban health facilities provide health care, especially tertiary care to both the urban and rural population. The available urban health care infrastructure is insufficient to meet the health care needs of the growing urban population. Realising this the municipalities, State Governments and the Central Government have tried to provide funds for building up urban health care. Unlike the rural health services, there have not been any well-planned and organised efforts to provide primary, secondary and tertiary care services in geographically delineated areas in urban health care. As a result, there is either non-availability or substantial under utilisation of available primary care facilities along with an over-crowding at secondary and tertiary care centers.

Urban development is accompanied by slums. Krishna Gowada and others have rightly observed that the growth and problems of slums are a consequence of city development.[4]

The growth of slums in any city is considered as a sign of environmental degradation. Yet the slums keep on proliferating as a result of the pressure of population growth and housing shortage. Slums give rise to problems relating to health, sanitation, land-use and even crime. It has been observed that the intermediary zone has the largest number of slums compared to the city centre and the periphery in Bangalore. Slums are identified in some parts of the central area. Presence of slums in the central area in Cotton belt and Kalsipalyam areas has resulted in unwholesome and improper utilization of valuable land and has added chaos to the already congested areas of the city. The slums with their associated problems like unsanitary conditions, social pathology, juvenile delinquency, etc. have become a nuisance to the smooth functioning of commercial activities. Besides these, there are a number of clusters of residential areas which may also be grouped under slums on account of overgrowing, dilapidation, lack of ventilation and which are thus detrimental to health and safety of the residents. Through the Slum Board, community toilets have been provided, but the people use them very badly. Access to toilets and availability of adequate water are the major problems. These areas have been using streets and conservancies as latrines, wastes are let out into open drains and stinking cesspools are created resulting in health hazards.

John Ashton in his Article, "Healthy Cities" defines the concept of Healthy Cities;[5] To quote:

> Defining the healthy city is not an easy task. Certainly a healthy city is more than one which simply has good health services. The idea implies that the city, as a place which allows scope for human possibility and experience, has a crucial role to play in determining the health of those living in it. Yet each city is unique and has its own life, its own soul and spirit, even its own personality.

A healthy city has been defined as one which is continually expanding and creating opportunities for people to live life to the full and to support each other. Central to such a definition is the social implication that, in a healthy city, there is some kind of common field of play and that broadly speaking the citizens are striving towards the same goal. Yet conflict and its creative resolutions are also part of a healthy city.

At its most fundamental a city is unhealthy if it cannot provide its citizens with these basic resources for health:

- safe and adequate food
- a safe water supply
- sanitation
- shelter
- freedom from poverty

However, it is clear that these alone are insufficient, and that a range of environmental prerequisites (economic, physical, social and cultural) are part of what most people expect for themselves and their families if they are to enjoy full health in the city. It has seven main elements:[6]

1. The establishment of an inter-sectoral committee for the city which brings together the key decision-makers from the different agencies and bureaucracies to take a strategic view of health in the city.
2. A parallel technical group to carry out a community diagnosis which is wide-ranging and has a particular focus on inequalities in health within the city.
3. The creation of a great debate within the city about the nature of current health problems—what can and needs to be done about them.
4. The formulation of city plans for health which are action-based and inter-sectoral in nature.
5. The development of models of good practice representing the different entry-point priorities of the different cities. These may range from major environmental action to support for better individual lifestyles or the formation of self-help groups, and will illustrate the principles of health promotion, particularly public participation.
6. Monitoring and research into the effectiveness of models of good practice on health in cities; this will involve higher educational institutions in meaningful collaboration with their host communities.
7. Mutual support, cultural exchange, collaboration and learning between cities.

Urban health studies and projects have been done by multilateral and bilateral agencies, World Bank, WHO, UNICEF, USAID, etc. have been providing great assistance to developing world to improve urban health. At present in India, World Bank is assisting 6 states of Indian Union to improve secondary health care in urban areas with a total assistance of about 3000 crores. In cities, that health system is totally disorganised as it encompasses primary, secondary and tertiary care as well as assistance by Government, Private, and Voluntary institutions. We find too many doctors, too many medicine shops and still people suffering from poor health. There is no co-ordination resulting in duplication, overlapping and wastage of resources. What can be done to make cities healthy? What can be done to keep cities clean? How can we provide good health care? How can we interlink health with other urban development services? Let us now discuss the facts and suggestions to improve health care system which can provide decent health services to all the people.

1. Need of Change of Lifestyles

People in urban areas lead sedatic life which is compounded by the habits of gambling, drinking, smoking and prostitution, etc. All these add to poor health. Since availability of transport has become easy, they easily fall prey to coronary diseases, diabetes, hypertension, etc.

Rene Dcekstra[7] has rightly said that the rapid social changes in many parts of the world especially taking the form of over-urbanisation, have brought about important changes in values, family structure and community experience, which in turn interfere with some of the important psycho-social and health needs of human beings. The shrinking of the extended family and the disintegration of communities have resulted in less effective social support networks and less likelihood of giving or receiving emotional support; in less responsibility for local affairs; in fewer opportunities for cooperative small group interaction and action; and in fewer activities in general that stimulate a sense of personal involvement, belonging, comradeship and responsibility. Gripped by a sense of isolation or alienation, young people particularly, in their search for group membership and values worth identifying with, that is, in quest of a sense of belonging and responsibility, simply cannot satisfy those needs in healthy ways. They become all the more subject to health risk behaviours like addiction, or to manipulation or abuse by political and criminal organisations. Besides there is a need to change to Active lifestyle by urban dwellers to keep metabolism active.

2. Need of Improving Environmental Sanitation and Avoid Environmental Pollution

Urban life is progressively deteriorating on account of unplanned industrialization, uncontrolled migration of population, lack of management of trade waste and human waste. Existing conditions in cities/towns are marked by congestion, overcrowding, lack of adequate drainage and poor arrangements for solid waste disposal. Various types of industries have come up in close proximity of the urban areas and within residential localities. This has resulted in discharge of obnoxious waste water on to the fields, dumping of solid industrial waste nearby and emission of poisonous fumes and smoke in the atmosphere. Housing stock which is a dominant element of physical environment, is of very poor quality.[8]

At present, there is no sanitation worth the name for 52 per cent of the urban population. The sewerage system covers only 35 per cent of the population of Class IV cities and 75 per cent of the population of Class I cities. About 34 percent of urban population does not have any arrangement even for drainage of rain water around its habitats. 60 per cent of the municipal bodies in India collect less than 40 per cent of the urban waste which is allowed to decompose and putrefy on the road side and around houses and factories. Quite a substantial portion of it goes into the drains, choking them and creating slush and stink all around, besides providing breeding ground for pests, flies and mosquitoes and cockroaches.

Urban settlements also suffer from inadequate piped water supply and underground sewerage facilities. No sewage treatment plant has been installed in most of the towns with the result that sullage is disposed of onto land or into nullahs causing land, air pollution and under ground water pollution. Storm water drainage has hardly been provided in any town. Stagnation of water along the roads and within the residential areas results in breeding of mosquitoes/flies causing nuisance and health problems. Refuse is indiscriminately thrown into lanes and backyards while squatters defecate in the open causing serious health hazards. Traffic congestion is a common problem in all-urban settlements. Due to vehicular emissions the air is also polluted. Noise pollution is constantly increasing due to heavy traffic. Recreational facilities such as parks and playgrounds are least provided in urban areas. Government is fully aware of the environmental problems and is keen to provide for good health and well-being of the citizens but action is lacking.

Health problems of big towns and cities are closely related to environmental conditions. Due to overcrowding, inadequate and poor housing, lack of adequate safe drinking water supply, lack of drainage, non-collection of waste water, and its improper disposal, untreated discharge of industrial waste discharge of smoke and toxic gases into atmosphere, etc. lead to pollution of air, water and land in urban towns and cities to a degree much greater than in rural areas. The environmental degradation leads to high prevalence of both communicable and non-communicable diseases in an urban society (Rao and Chakraborty, 1976).

In addition to above problems, the ever increasing trends of urbanization are mounting tremendous pressures on civic amenities and on health and other services. The unprecedented growth in urban population has also been witnessed by most of the urban areas which resulted in deterioration in the standard and quality of public life. In almost every urban centre, irrespective of its size and class, the availability of core civic services have been found to be scarce (NIUA, 1989).

To achieve the objective of Environmentally Sustainable Development of urban centres, it is suggested that:[9]

(i) Efforts would be made to minimise migration from rural to urban areas by creating appropriate level of infrastructure and opportunities for gainful employment in rural settlements. This would mean planned development of rural areas and promoting cottage and other industries which are agro-based.

(ii) In order to achieve maximum growth of small and medium towns and to induce desired level of population therein, it is proposed to distribute socio-economic activities in small and medium towns. More investment would be made in these towns for creating more economic opportunities for gainful employment in such centres.

(iii) It is proposed to prescribe a certain minimum limit of area to be earmarked as green cover in each human settlement, concept of city forests would be given a fair trial for ensuring appropriate level of environment.

(iv) All community open spaces would be planned, developed and managed in close cooperation with the people so as to ensure its optimum utilisation with minimum of investment.

(v) Ribbon development along important high-ways and roads would be checked in order to ensure free flow of men and material.

(vi) Planning of human settlement would be done in such a manner that it minimises the travel needs of the people living therein. Plans would encourage and give precedence to pedestrian movement, cyclists, two-wheelers and motor cars in that order of preference. Minimising travel and use of vehicle would lead to creation of human settlements which are highly energy efficient and would have minimum pollution due to reduced use of petrol driven vehicles.

(vii) Informal sector would be considered an essential part of human settlement because of its considerable contribution to city economy and capacity to provide gainful employment to its work force. Thus, informal sector would be properly planned and its requirements duly catered for in the planning and developmental process.

(viii) Burning of agro waste as an industrial fuel would be banned, so as to minimise pollution. Appropriate mechanism and safe-guards would be provided to check this growing menace.

(ix) Planting of trees on large scale along the roads, within the open spaces provided in the urban areas and around the human settlements would be undertaken to help in preserving proper environment in urban areas. People would be educated and encouraged to plant more trees in the available open spaces.

(x) Segregation of inter and intra-city traffic would be done on priority and all through traffic would be discouraged to enter urban areas. This would considerably reduce the environmental pollution and improve quality of life along the major roads.

(xi) Historical monuments and heritage buildings and areas would be properly planned, conserved and preserved by making them an integral part of city developmental process.

(xii) Tree preservation order would be made applicable in all urban areas so as to stop illegal hopping, lopping, chopping and topping of trees. All existing trees would be declared as protected trees and would not be removed without prior permission.

(xiii) Visual pollution in urban areas would be checked by using the mechanism of advertisement control.

(xiv) All future industries to be set-up in urban areas would be closely scrutinised so far as its environmental hazards are concerned and only non-polluting or industries having sufficient environmental safeguards would be permitted in urban areas.

(xv) In order to preserve the environment in residential areas all industrial areas would be sealed from residential areas by providing a green belt having trees which would minimize pollution.

(xvi) It would be made mandatory for all industrial units to use a part of their plot area for planting trees.

(xvii) Environmental Impact Assessment in case of certain categories of large industries would be carried out more scientifically.

(xviii) State would discourage the setting up of highly polluting, hazardous, chemical and other units so as to minimize adverse impact on urban environment. Eco-friendly units would be given priority and would be permitted to be set-up as part and parcel of urban settlements.

(xix) All environment-related laws would be made more simple and effective and would be strictly enforced for minimizing pollution in the state.

(xx) In order to make all urban areas environmentally sustainable, cities and towns would be planned on the basis of their holding capacity in terms of population, economic activity, etc. Growth of over-sized and metrocities would be discouraged. Emphasis would be laid on the growth and development of small and medium towns.

3. Health Promotion in Urban Areas

I. Need of Improving Health Services in Urban Areas Especially in Slums and Deprived Sections of the Urban Areas

At present, there are health facilities which are not functioning well. We find long lines and rush but no facilities. That is why private doctors are fleeing the people.

During the Ninth Plan period, efforts was directed to evolve a well structured organisation of urban primary health care to remedy the insisting situation. A health care delivery system aimed at providing basic health and family welfare services to the population. Within 1-3 kms. of their dwelling will be made available by establishing. Urban Health and Family Welfare Centres manned by Medical and para-Medical persons. These centres will have:[10]

1. adequate out-patient facility;
2. in-patient facility (at least 10 beds of which four will be for maternity care and the remaining beds will be for medical, surgical and paediatric care);
3. supportive services including laboratory and radiology facilities and pharmacy; and
4. provision for referral/transport of patients.

The essential services, to be provided, will include:

1. medical and surgical services including eye and ENT care;
2. obstetric care and new-born care and child health;
3. counselling for reproductive health and contraception;
4. dental services;
5. emergency and trauma care; and
6. prevention and control of communicable and non-communicable diseases.

For effective integration of health-related services the urban health centres will coordinate with other assigned social sector activities, Nagarpalikas especially for provision of safe drinking water and sanitation.

An overview of all the facilities available in a defined geographical area will be undertaken and appropriate linkages between primary, secondary and tertiary care centres in the area will be established so that provision of basic minimum health services and optimal utilisation of the available health care facilities for referral services will be ensured. Earmarked funds under BMS and an ACA for services will be effectively utilised to fill the critical gaps in health manpower and infrastructure in urban areas also so that the performance of both health and family welfare programmes improve.

4. Removal of Urban Poverty

Urban poverty is the root cause of all problems including health. A.K. Neog in his Article, "Urban Poverty" mentions that Urban Poverty is more visible in the slum and depressed areas where public utilities like health and sanitation services, water supply, are utterly inadequate. So on the health front also an urban areas faces hazards which affect his efficiency. In a caste-ridden, status conscious society, an urban poor is likely to face more sociological and psychological problems than a rural poor.[11]

Urban poverty is not always a by-product of rural poverty. Those urban dwellers who fail to cope with the struggle for development may also fall into poverty trap. In the areas where urbanization is more due to administrative expansion (as in North-East India) than industrialisation, many households which cannot win the race for development may have to join those below the poverty line. Displacement, land alienation, etc. aggravate the situation. Hence, the urbanization process itself may generate poverty. Thus, urban poverty can be distinct from rural poverty and presents itself as a subject of investigation and study.

Ministry of Urban Affairs and Urban Development, GOI, New Delhi, in its Annual Report, 1998-99, mentions the efforts of Government of India to alleviate urban poverty.

In a decision of far reaching consequences, the Union Cabinet on 5th August, 1997 approved the Swarna Jayanti Shahari Rozgar Yojana (SJSRY). The SJSRY has been launched as a replacement for Nehru Rozgar Yojana (NRY). Urban Basic Services for the Poor (UBSP), and Prime Ministers Integrated Urban Poverty Eradication Programme (PMI UPEP) on 1.12.97. The SJSRY seeks to provide gainful employment to the urban unemployed or underemployed poor through encouraging the setting up of self-employment ventures and provision of wage employment.

The Swarna Jayanti Shahari Rozgar Yojana is funded on a 75: 25 basis between the Centre and the States.

The Scheme consists of two special schemes, namely:

(a) The Urban Self Employment Programme (USEP).
(b) The Urban Wage Employment Programme (UWEP).

Salient Features

The Swarna Jayanti Shahari Rozgar Yojana rests on a foundation of community empowerment. This programme relies on establishing and promoting community organisations and structures to provide Supporting and facilitating mechanism for local development. Towards this end community organisations like Neighbourhood Groups (NGs), Neighbourhood Committees (NCs), and Community Development Societies (CDSs) are set-up in the target areas based on the UBSP pattern. The CDSs is the focal point for purposes of identification of beneficiaries, preparation of application, monitoring or recovery, and generally providing whatever other support is necessary to the programme. The CDSs is to identify viable projects suitable for the particular area.

The CDSs, being a federation of different community-based organisations, shall be the nodal agency for this programme. It is expected that they will lay emphasis on providing the entire gamut of social sector inputs to their areas including, but not limited to, health, welfare, education, etc. through establishing convergence between schemes being implemented by different line departments within their jurisdiction.

5. Need of Multilateral and Bilateral Assistance to Improve Urban Health

Since the resources and expertise in the developing world is limited, therefore, there is a need of support from multilateral and bilateral agencies. Forty-fourth World Health Assembly in its resolution 27 identified six imperatives for improvement of health.

The resolution specifically requested WHO to:

- strengthen its information base for the benefit of Member-states and its own work in relation to the human and environmental aspects of urban development;
- strengthen its technical cooperation with countries in order to increase awareness of the needs of the urban poor, develop national skills to meet these needs and support the extension of city networks worldwide; and
- promote regional networks and interdisciplinary panels of experts and community leaders, to advise on health aspects of urban development.

In encouraging participants to take a positive view and to identify opportunities for making a contribution to improving urban conditions and health, the Chairman of the Technical Discussions of the 44th World Health Assembly identified six personal imperatives:

1. To decentralize and put the emphasis for action at the municipal level.
2. To mobilize everyone who can help in city networks.
3. To invest in safe drinking water and waste disposal.
4. To help the poor to enhance their incomes and improve their housing.
5. To provide families with a range of sustainable health services in or near their homes with an emphasis on family planning as the centre piece.
6. To ask the poor to identify their own needs and priorities and expect surprises.

6. Need of a Well-defined Slum Policy

J.S. Sakesena and P.N. Govindarajuler in their Article, "Health Care For Urban Slums with special reference to Bangalore City" have rightly sensed the problem. To quote them:

"Slum-dwellers have the worst of both the worlds—urban and rural. On one side they suffer from economic hardships, lack of education and absence of health infrastructure like the rural population. On the other hand, they also suffer the ill-effects of overcrowding, pollution and rootlessness characteristic of large metropolitan cities."

They further add that "Most comforts and conveniences of the cities are sustained by the work done by slum-dwellers. As such, the affluent and the privileged have the moral responsibility to try to mitigate and alleviate their suffering. Rural population may be ignorant of the "goodies" they are missing, but a slum-dweller is painfully aware of the privations suffered by him due to his constantly rubbing shoulders with urban affluence and conspicuous consumption with resultant frustration and resentment.

It is reported that the Union Urban Development Ministry is finalising a draft National Slum Policy to deal with one of the most serious socio-economic problems threatening urban life in India in the form of an enormous growth of slums. Once believed to be an inevitable side effect of industrialization and the consequent migration of labour from rural areas, proliferation of slums has other causes too in India. They have grown within and on the peripheries of many towns and all the metropolitan cities, including the country's Capital.

The national policy is expected to provide a new approach to an old problem evolved in the recognition of the fact that slum residents are a major and important contributors to city resources and form an indispensable sector, providing various kinds of skilled and unskilled services to enrich city life and facilitate its functions. A draft piece of legislation is also under preparation.[12]

To improve the quality of life of these residents, slum policy should contain clauses to enhance educational, health and moral standards. This requires coordination among ministries/departments concerned.

Urban Development Strategy for Punjab suggests the following to minimise slum growth:

(i) Relaunching of the Integrated Urban Poverty Alleviation Scheme (IUPAS) which would include restructured existing urban poverty alleviation programmes providing for a package to urban poor.

(ii) Allocation and creation of a fund with annual contribution, for income generating activities and provision of infrastructure for urban poor.

(iii) Establishment of Urban Poverty Alleviation Fund in every municipality since slum-related issues are included in the Twelfth Schedule of 74th Constitutional Amendment Act, 1992.

(iv) Urban Shelter-related programmes would be community-based so as to involve the users in the programme.

(v) Close monitoring of all the programmes by State level agencies so as to ensure effective implementation.
(vi) Involvement of private sector and NGOs in the programme.
(vii) Keeping close watch on the growth and development of slums and to evolve appropriate strategies to minimize them.
(viii) To undertake shelter upgradation programmes for slums on priority basis and to link it with the issue of gainful employment.

7. Need of Mass Education and Awareness

Education seems to be an important factor in achieving better health status as also for better utilization of health facilities. Particularly, is the weaker sections treat their children as an asset for earning more, they, it seems, instigate their children to become school drop outs. Hence, in order to make them understand importance of education, adult literacy programme should be rigorously implemented. In these programmes, health education should be given due place to make them understand basic issues in health. More voluntary efforts are called for in this venture.[13]

8. Need of Linking Health with Other Sectors of Development

It is being realized widely now that the isolating therapeutic approach to civic health, hitherto in vogue, generally overlooks many critical variables determining the health of the communities and its members. The isolating approach, therefore, needs to be substituted by a broader, synchronized approach. For this, the linkages of health sector with other aspects like housing, education, income, environment, etc. are not only to be realized but also to be taken in account while ensuring an all round development. In the planning of municipal programmes, health sector should get a higher priority and larger outlay particularly to meet the requirements of the dovetailed plans.[14]

9. Need of Participation of People in Local Self-Government

Participation is essential to lubricate potential energy of the people into kinetic energy. Urban areas need the co-operation of the people to keep the city clean and healthy. K.S. Nesamani has beautifully explained the need of participation in urban development. To quote him:[15]

Participatory development is not an attempt to replace the top-down development approach with slum-dwellers/low income participation. Rather, it should stress the need for the government participation in terms of national-level economic planning and coordination of development planning and the demerits of widening disparities and worsening poverty inherent in slum-dwellers. Participatory development attempts to introduce a bottom-up style of development in order to remedy the government approach's shortcomings, specifically by focusing on qualitative improvements in slum-dwellers' participation.

Participation of slum-dwellers can reduce the cost of the social programme which government often invests. It will give an idea to the government with a great deal of information on the social and economic needs of the population. It will help the government to identify the potential leader who can assist in the development process or at least disseminate information on government goals.

10. Need of Providing Adequate Housing with All Amenities is *sine-qua-non* for Good Health

The situation of Housing is very serious as one in five families live in slums. Even those who are living in urban areas are without good facilities, half of the urban population is without sanitation facilities. The Government is making efforts but without positive results. The National Plan of Action, prepared by the Government of India for the Habitat Conference defined adequate shelter, in the Indian context as the one "which would include adequate living space with provision for incremental development and proper access to physical and social infrastructure and services including energy, fuel potable water, waste disposal and sanitation services, and education, health and recreational facilities. It must have adequate privacy and security, as also lighting and ventilation. The location of the shelter must be suitable with references turk place, markets, communication services, and social and cultural amenities. The endeavour of the government and the people of India would be to maintain the cost of such adequate shelter at an affordable level. The critical task is to ensure that access to adequate and affordable shelter is available to all, including people living in poverty, the vulnerable and the disadvantaged, either through the market or through well targetted and transparent subsidies." (pp. 99-100, India Country Report)

There is a need to take rational decisions to ensure what is contemplated. Worlds written or spoken are of no use unless put to action.

11. Need of Efficient and Dynamic Local Administration

People both elected and permanent must conduct their business in a manner which can help the urban area to enjoy quality of life. In the words of Jean Paul Jardel:[16]

"Action at the local level is also to be encouraged to the full. The Healthy Cities project is one example of the efforts being made to convince countries to put health firmly on the political agenda of communities and local governments. Once again, it's a matter of "thinking globally and acting locally." Local action is by far the most effective approach, all the more so if it takes place within a national, regional and even a world-wide framework.

The interdependence of human beings with their physical, social and economic environment must now more than ever be taken into account in health-related activities. Local power to act must therefore be reinforced, and local authorities must be convinced of the important role of health in development efforts. Furthermore, all sectors that have an influence on health must be integrated into a collaborative team. The planning and carrying out of strategies must be flexible, to take into account the wide diversity of towns, countries and situations. Enlightened leadership is called for, to encourage the participation of everyone. And, finally, it must never be forgotten that Health for All is a common, shared objective, which alone can allow us to hope for eventual justice and equity in ensuring the fundamental right of every human being: the right to health.

CONCLUSION

We may conclude in the words of Shri Jagmohan, "A World Bank Study has revealed that the polluted air in the Indian cities is causing premature death of about 40,000 persons every year. The extent of water pollution can be gauged from the state of our rivers which, for most part of the years, are hardly distinguishable from vast urban gutters. Noise is another factor that lowers the quality of life in our cities. According to the survey conducted by the National Physical Laboratory, Delhi, Mumbai and Calcutta are the noisiest cities in the world.[17]

Clearly, if the march of unhealthy new realities has to be halted and these realities have to be replaced by another set of new realities positive, productive and elevating, there has to be fundamental transformation of the institutional frame-work of urban India as well as that of the frame-work of the Indian mind and soul.

Notes and References

1. V. Suresh and P. Jayapal, Towards an inclusive city in the New Millennium, in *Shelter*, Vol. 2, Nos. 3 and 4, July-Oct., 1999, p. 9.
2. Government of Punjab Deptt. of Housing and Urban Development, Urban Development Strategy for Punjab, Draft Status Paper, 1995, pp. 5-6.
3. Government of India, Planning Commission, Ninth Five Year Plan, 1997-2002, New Delhi, p. 149.
4. Krishna Gowda, M.V. Sridhara, P. Raj Mamatha, "Planning for the 21st Century: A Case Study of Bangalore, *Shelter*, Vol. 3, No. 1, HUDO, Publication, pp. 7-8, January 2000.
5. John Ashton, Healthy Cities, in *World Health*, June 1988, pp. 9-10.
6. *Ibid.*, p. 11.
7. Rene Diekotra, City Lifestyles, in *World Health*, June 1988, p. 19.
8. Quoted in Shreekant *vs.* Khandewala, Health Administration and the Weaker Sections in an Indian Metropolies, N. Delhi, Devika, 1996, p. 4.
9. Urban Development Strategy for Punjab, *op. cit.*, pp. 37-38.
10. Ninth Five Year Plan, *op. cit.*, pp. 149-50.
11. A.K. Neog, Urban Poverty in Urbanization and Development in North East India, Ed. (J.B. Ganguly), New Delhi, Deep and Deep, 1995, p. 70.
12. S. Saraswati, Towards National Slum Policy in the *Daily Tribune*, February 1, 2000.

13. Khandevala, *op. cit.*, p. 203.
14. *Ibid.*, p. 209.
15. K.S. Nesamani, Participation of slum-dwellers in Urban Governance, in *Shelter*, A HUDCO Publication, New Delhi, Vol. 3, No. 1 (Challenge for the New Millennium)
16. Jean Paul Jardel, Health in the City, *World Health*, March-April, 1991, p. 3.
17. *The Sunday Tribune*, Specturm, June 11, 2000.

17

CHAPTER

Health and Yoga Education

Remain in bliss in this world,
Fearless, pure in heart,
Wake up in bliss every morning,
Carry out all your duties in bliss,
Remain in bliss in weal and woe,
In criticism and insult,
Remain in bliss unaffected,
Remain in bliss pardoning everybody.

—Rabindranath Tagore

Yoga encompasses all values and includes all values which sharpen the human beings in achieving their material, intellectual and spiritual goals. Yoga can promote theory and practice of all values essential for personality development. The theory and practice of yoga enrich the quality of life through the values inherent in Yoga. Yoga if followed earnestly can create happy family life, social life and peace and prosperity in the Universe.

Prof. T.R. Anandharaman, in his article, "Yoga for the Incoming Millennium " clarifies that Yoga constitutes without any doubt one of the India's many priceless gifts of perennial value to the human value. Despite being a very ancient tradition, it has all along proved ever so modern and relevant to every generation to seekers of human perfection. As the Science of Total man and Technology of Conscious Evolution, its potentialities has always been immense and its contributions manifold as well as in tune with the needs of the concerned age, whether it was the bygone age of the "Upanishads" or the present age of Science, Technology and Engineering. Infact, as this planet awaits the next millennium, Yoga seems to have approached its zenith in popularity, fascination and usefulness in more parts of the world than ever before.

CHART 17.1

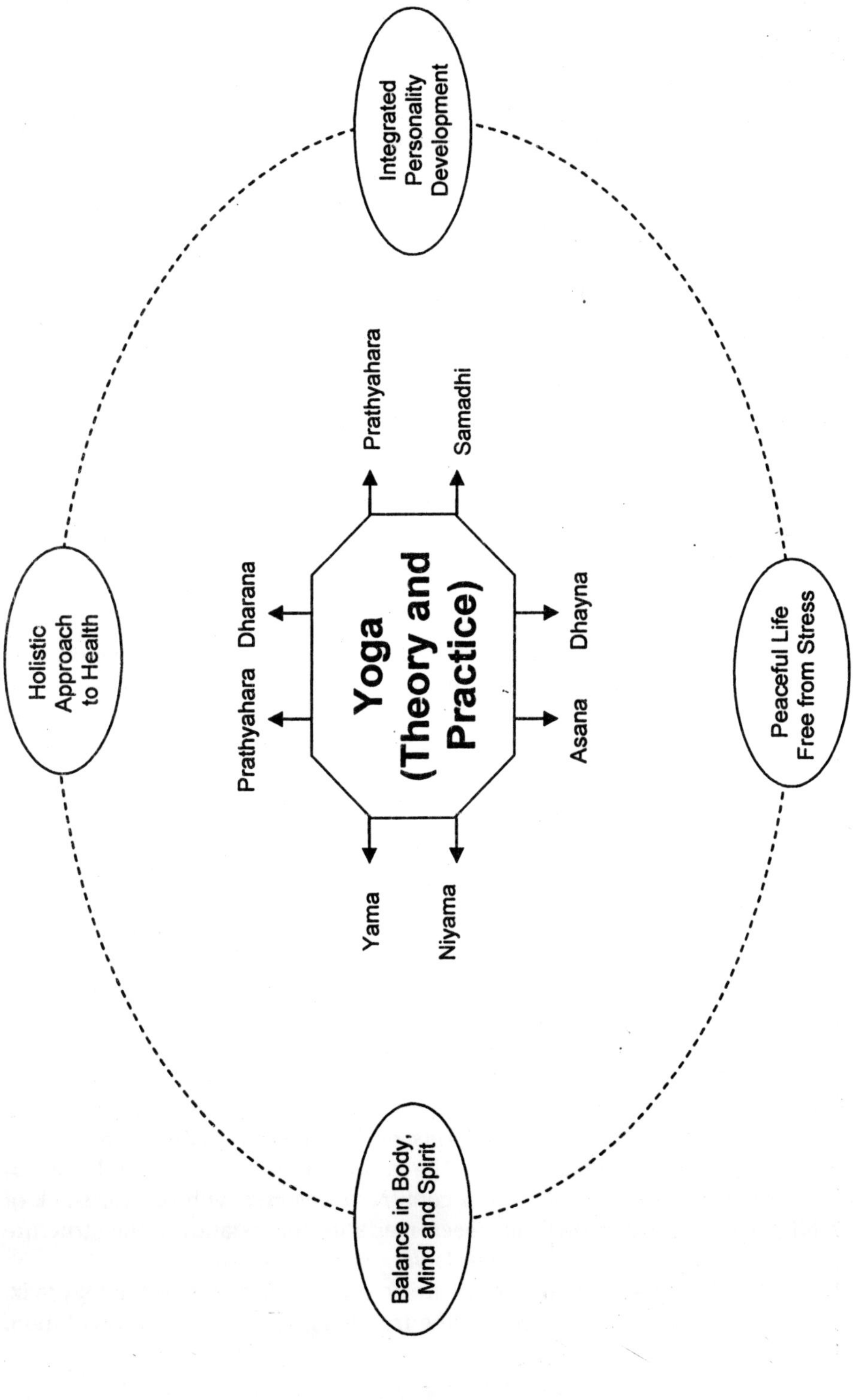
Integrated Personality Development
Holistic Approach to Health
Peaceful Life Free from Stress
Balance in Body, Mind and Spirit
Yoga (Theory and Practice)
Prathyahara
Samadhi
Prathyahara
Dharana
Dhayna
Asana
Yama
Niyama

Yoga helps in the overall development of the personality of people. The concept of positive health and lifelong learning are relatively new concepts which need to be promoted. An overall development of the individual is intended to be achieved through higher education using an affective domain in addition to cognitive skills.[1] Shri Kumar Swamiji in his book Dimension of Yoga strongly feels that Yoga aims at recreating the world. Not the acceptance of the world as it is, but to change it, to mould it in the pattern of the Divine Reality, is the main objective of Yoga. To say this, is to say that evil has no permanent place in the scheme of things. Creation is a complex movement which represents the various notes and rhythems that make up the grand harmony of the spheres. This music that moves the cosmos is magnificent and wonderful and is the glory of God manifest therein. But a doubting voice raises the question, is there not some chaos in this cosmos? Is there not a confusion in this concord? Is there not a walpurgis night in this winning light? Yes, there is. In the order of creation, first there is the consciousness and division of trenchant separation of good and evil. This is the outlook of individualized consciousness. Next, as the consciousness grows and ecompasses the whole existence, good and evil are both embraced and are found to form a secret harmony. This is the outlook of the cosmic consciousness. There is still a higher status, the status of transcendence in which evil is not simply embraced but dissolved and even transformed into supreme reality of which it is an aberration, a projection or a lower formulation. In Yoga the total eradication of evil from the world and human nature, with a remoulding of terrestrial life in the pattern of the divine Reality, is viewed not as a mere concept but as a concrete fact.

Yoga deals with the problems of human nature and human psychology through a vast repertory of practical methods which aim towards purification, regulation and awakening of human potential. At present, yoga is passing through a momentous period of growth consolidation and expansion with its rapid integration into modern society. Many institutions dealing with the theory of Yoga and its practice have come up. At many levels we can see changes and new developments as yoga is being applied in different facets of life in a variety of new ways, such as a form of therapy, a technique of health and stress management.

Modern man is all set for a revolution after nearly four centuries of continuous growth. From the era of blind faith and superstitutions he has progressed an era of rational thinking, experimentation, matter-based approach and its fascinating applications to comfort his living. The strides of this growth encompasses all facets of life including education (science and technology-orientated) and the very direction of growth of an individual (economy-based) and a country (measured with the yardstick of GNP). Tremendous growth has been made in understanding the structure of this physical universe and the laws governing them.

The two major challenges of this era of science and technology, viz. stress and pollution have become the true triggers for the new revolution.

If pollution is working at the material front to direct man towards better ecological and appropriate technology, the challenge of stress is shaking the very foundations of the matter-based objective approach of science. As we glide through the decades of transition, our understanding is bound to encompass a greater spectrum of the universe—life, mind, psyche, etc.

India, known for its wisdom has given us the Upanisads, the quintessence of the VEDAS, and a saga of knowledge. From these books of knowledge—Vedas, Upanisads, Yoga texts—are emerging new rays of hopes which are essential to face the new revolution.[2]

Scientific and technological progress all over the globe has made man highly sensitive, critical and also creative. Sharp to the core, his intellect has gained tremendous power of analysis. The left side of his brain is highly developed, helping him to unravel the subtle mysteries of nature and understand clearly the general law of nature. Technology has helped man reap the benefits of its use. Autonomation and computers have brought great speed and sophistication in all our interactions. In search of happiness we are propelled by a desire to increase our living standards by acquiring more and more comfort giving objects and experiencing sensual pleasures. To satisfy this desire we are always on the lookout to earn more and more. In the process, we have become very active and have overcome our lethargy.

Associated with this growth is the emergence of two basic challenges: pollution and stress. The challenge of pollution is being tackled effectively but not met totally. Strict pollution control measures in the industrial sectors and extensive research leading towards the use of ecologically friendly technologies, have certainly yielded dividends. But on the second front, in spite of extensive research all over the globe, a decreasing quality of life, increasing health hazards, social unrest, student unrest, etc. traits which are all different expressions of stress, have shown no trend of decrease. On the contrary, over the last two decades, it is rather on the path of ascent.

The current mechanistic world-view, the matter-based approach the increased dependence on science and technology and the associated lifestyle have to undergo basic changes towards embracing a more holistic world view and a healthier and more harmonious lifestyle. Emotion trainings and harnessing of the will-power—the growth of the right side of the brain in general—are then the associated adjuncts for such a holistic understanding and also for a healthier and harmonious living. And that is what Yoga offers.

Today, man is subjected to a large number of stressful situations in the modern fast way of life and his balance is frequently disturbed. The system is constantly kept under sympathetic stimulation without enough time for the parasympathetic to do its job. This repeated sympathetic stimulations lead to intermittent upsurges of heart rate, blood pressure, poor digestion, elevated blood glucose, etc. When this happens over a number of years it become a habit for the heart and the blood vessels to remain in stimulated state and they lose the capacity to come back to the resting levels. This is the main cause for the increasing incidence of high blood pressure and diabetes among people today.[3]

Youth in the system of higher education represents a tremendous potential for society, provided it is channeled in the right direction, the enthusiasm, initiative and idealism of young people can help others, including the elderly, the handicapped, the poor, and in so doing can create a happier and more balanced society.

Unprecedented challenges face the youth of today, said Dr. Hiroshi Nakajima, Director-General of WHO, in a message to the world assembly of Youth. And he added that young people maybe given opportunities "to demonstrate their creativity, energy and commitment to solving their own problems and helping to build a healthy future for the entire community in which they live."

Unwise lifestyles pose the biggest threats to students health. Innovative judgments, a tendency to show off, or the desire to keep up with their fellows—all these incline them towards risk-taking behaviour. This may include experimenting with dangerous substances like alcohol or drugs, driving too fast on the highway, or simply defying adult society.

In many cases, the cigarette is the very first contact young people have with the lifestyles of adulthood. This first encounter often occurs at a very early age: by the time they reach their teens, they may already be unable to break the smoking habit. It is vital that they should be aware of the short-term and long-term risks that smoking represents to their health.

The risk destroying their most important assets; the health and physical fitness through laziness and lack of exercise, rash driving and traffic accidents, suicide or attempts to suicide, slow suicide through the use of alcohol, smoking, dung abuse, excessive intake of tea and coffee, unprotected sexual encounters, sexual misadventures like rape, sexually transmitted diseases, teenager pregnancies and abortions or unwed child births. The ill-effects on their health can extend far into later life. Accidents are estimated to disable permanently three times as many as they kill, smoking and alcohol can store epidemics of respiratory diseases, liver damage and cancer. Teenager pregnancy can kill mother or child or else leave them physically and mentally handicapped. Needless to conclude that in some countries youth is the only age-group in which mortality and morbidity rate is rising, due to these ills of modern society. Alcohol and unemployment is behind alarmingly large number of deaths through accidents and suicide (Jerome, 1980).

Before a dam was constructed on Satluj River, at Bhakra, the water resource was not only wasted but it resulted in floods, leading to loss of life and property. The same is true for youth resource. The idle youth is not only a waste, but also the tide of this unutilized energy can result in negative development wasted in the field of health and economy. The youth can be our best resource if they are healthy and if their joyous energy is channelised for building a better society. The potential energy of youth has to be converted into kinetic energy with understanding, support, and technological knowledge and its use should be made to build modern India. Much needs to be done both for and by young people. It is not sufficient merely to have activities directed towards youth. If the aims and objectives of International Youth Year, 1985, and the WHO Global Strategy for Health for All by the year 2000 are to be achieved. Serious efforts of collaborative action by everyone—young and old are needed. The youngsters of today, with their capabilities, energy and commitment, represent a vital resource; they must be partners in the quest for a just future.

Life of students in higher education is becoming more and more artificial and they are travelling more and more away from natural living. In order to return to natural life, they should practice Yoga and learn to live more in consonance with nature and cosmic consciousness.

We see the disinterest and inevitable suffering among many student's. It has been realized that every individual contains hidden potential, which when developed allows him to attain pertinent bliss, inner peace and the ultimate goal of our existence.

A brief discussion with students revealed the following problems of students in the system of higher education:

(a) Lack of interest in studies
(b) Lack of vitality, enthusiasm and eagerness
(c) Enamored by affluent environment leading to alcoholism, smoking, gambling, etc.
(d) Irregular in food habits
(e) Not interested in exercises and games
(f) Drudgery in life
(g) No aim in life
(h) Lack of reading habits
(i) Not following any regular course of life
(j) Full of tensions, worries and agitations
(k) Lack of peace—restlessness
(l) Lack of concentration
(m) Problematic both at home and in a college
(n) Bad company
(o) Aimless life.

How can we overcome the problems inflicting the personality of students in higher education system? How can we channelise their potential energy into kinetic energy to make them enjoy the bliss of life? How can we stimulate students towards holistic approach? How can we make them develop their personality in totality? How can we check students from indulging in bad habits—alcoholism, smoking, gambling, etc.? How can we educate them to put them on right track? The only answer is the need of imparting yoga education which can solve all the problems simultaneously. It requires understanding and practice of science and practice of yoga. Fist let us understand the meaning of yoga.

Meaning of Yoga

Patanjali defines yoga as complete suppression of all mental modes or processes (cittavrttinirodha).[4] Vyasa defines it as absorptive concentration (samadhi). It is a universal attribute of the mind.[5] All persons can attain yoga by repeated practice (abhyasa) and detachment (vairagya).[6]

Swami Satyananda Sanswati in his book, "Asana Pranayama Mudra Bandha," (Bihar School of Yoga, Munger, Bihar, Indium, 1999) comments that, "Yoga is not an ancient myth buried in oblivion. It is the most valuable inheritance of the present. It is the essential need of today and the culture of tomorrow." The Yogic culture of tomorrow is something towards which we have to strive, we have to try to attain. Yoga has been the culture to strive, we have to try to attain. Yoga has been the culture of ancient India and the ancient civilization of the world, and it is going to be the culture of tomorrow. It is the science of today which we have to learn, which we have to accept, and which we have to understand. It is a science which deals with the developments of the human personality and which leads to the awakening of untapped energy sources within the brain and mind. The practice of yoga is not new. Ancient rishis, saints and sages have been talking about it for the last fifty thousand years. They spoke about it, not as a religion or philosophy, but as a way of life which could lead to the development and awakening of our consciousness and energy.

Yoga bestows inner strength, sharpens our intellect, teaches us to control our emotions and brings a rare concentration and efficiency into our action and work, marking one do the right thing in the right way at the right time and that is why Yoga is defined as a skill in action.

From finite to infinite it is the journey of everything in this Universe. Yoga can speed up this journey by giving a spiritual content and dimension to all human efforts. Every institutions working in the field of human upliftment—religious or secular—should understand the newly emerging—but for us, as old as our spiritual heritage—vision of Reality and adjust and adopt measures to ensure this new dimension in their growth. Scientific research, experimental verification, application in day-to-day life, ext. must strengthen the hands of Yoga practitioners so that they can take up the challenges posed by the modern age. This is Vivekānanda Kendra's approach.

The mother in her Diary for all times: The Great Adventure says "Yoga means union with the Divine, and the union is effected through offering—it is founded on the offering of yourself to the Divine."

For most people, however, yoga is simply a means of maintaining health and well-being in an increasingly stressful society. Asanas remove the physical discomfort accumulated during a day at the office sitting in a chair, hunched over a desk. Relaxation techniques help maximize the effectiveness of ever-diminishing time off. In an age of mobile phones, beepers and twenty-four hour shopping, yogic practices make great personal and even business sense.

The word yoga is derived from the Sanskrit root 'yuj' meaning 'to unite', 'to combine', and 'to integrate', which means total integration of the physical, mental, intellectual and spiritual aspects of the human personality.[7] Yoga is a way of life, propounded by Patanjali in a systematic form.

Yoga is an exact science. It aims at the harmonious development of the body, the mind and the soul. Yoga is the turning away of the senses from the objective universe and the concentrations of the mind within. Yoga is the turning away of the senses from the objective universe and the concentration of mind are eternal life in the soul of spirit. Yoga aims at controlling the mind and its modifications. The path of Yoga is an inner path whose gateway is your heart. Yoga is harmony between the individual and the cosmos, between thought and action between soul and God, between Organism and respiration.

Yoga is the discipline of a mind, senses and physical body. Yoga helps in the co-ordination and control of the subtle forces within the body. Yoga brings in perfection, peace and everlasting happiness; one can even have increased energy, vigor, vitality, longevity, resistance, calmness, and good sleep at times by the practice of Yoga. The practice of Yoga will help people to control the emotions and passions and resistance power increases and removes the disturbing elements from mind. It will enable them to keep a balanced mind and remove fatigue and get concentration, self-sufficiency, impertinence, pride, luxury, name, fame, self-assertive nature, abstinence, idea of superiority, evil company, laziness, over eating, meat eating, over work, attachments, too much talking, smoking, drinking are some of the obstacles in the path of Yoga.[8]

Swami Parmahansa Niranjanananda in his book Yoga Darshan: Vision of Yoga Upanishads (1993) Bihar observes that the aim of yoga is to take one from the impure aspect of the mind towards the pure aspect, from a state of scattered desire to a state of balanced desire, where the desire becomes positive, constructive, and self-elevating, where the desire does not limit us to the external environment only, but also encompasses the inner dimensions. By transcending the impure mind and obtaining purity of mind and by awakening the faculties of the pure mind, one attains transcendence or mukti. One must go from the impure to the pure, and awaken the faculties of the pure mind in order to attain transcendence.

Aspects of Yoga Values (See Chart 17.1)

The science of Yoga has its roots in Upanishads, Veadas, Bhagavad-Gita, Yogavashishta of Vashishta, Hathayoga Pradipika, and the Yoga Sutras of Pathanjali. However, a detailed classical work could be found in the Yoga Sutras of Pathanjali, which dates back roughly to 300 B.C. The Yoga Sutras serve as the basic text for an in-depth study on this great science. Pathanjali called it Ashtanga Yoga, i.e., science having eight limbs or constituents, viz.,

1. Yama

2. Niyama
3. Aasana
4. Praanaayaama
5. Prathyaahaara
6. dhaarana
7. Dhyaana
8. Samaadhi

यम - नियामासन - प्राणायाम - प्रत्याहार,धारणा - ध्यान - समाध्योटण्टावडगानि ।

Pantajli Yogasutra 2.2.9

(I) Yama

The first discipline of restraint (yama consists in non-injury (ahimsa), truthfulness in thought and speech (satya), non-stealing (asteya), sexual restraint (brahmacarya), and non acceptance of unnecessary gifts.[9] These are negative virtues. Non-injury (ahimsa) consists in the absence of cruelty to all creatures in all possible ways and at all times. It is tenderness, good will, and kindness for all living beings.[10]

A truthful person must have valid thoughts in his mind, speak them out correctly, excite similar thoughts in the hearer's mind, and his words must be conducive to the welfare of all creatures.

Yama is based on the principle that above all religions, human religion is the best. (Abstinences) viz., Ahimsa (Non-injury), Sathya (Non-falsehood), Astheya (Non-stealing), Aparigraha (Non-acceptance or non-hoarding of things beyond our bear necessities of life) and Brahmacharya (Non-deviation from one's on personal laws of nature).

Steady intellect is a natural and spontaneous state for a man of realization. Since he knows the truth, nothing in this world can disturb him. Even ordinary people and spiritual aspirants can derive immense benefit by cultivating a steady intellect. Intellectual, conviction about Reality may help us to develop a steady intellect to a certain extent.

He is a man of steady intellect whose mind is not disturbed by the pair of opposites, namely, happiness and misery, victory and defeat, gain and loss, praise and blame, attachment and hatred, honour and dishonour, heat and cold.[11] Sri Krishna has given a beautiful illustration in the Bhagavad Gita (2.70), of a steady intellect.

आपूर्यमाणमचलप्रतिष्ठं समुद्रमाप: प्रविशन्ति यद्वत ।

'Water enters into the sea from all directions but the sea remains full and unchanged.'

Prof. T.R. Anantharaman observes that a little reflection on the five Yamas, or restraints, will bring out, however, their enormous importance in the maintenance of what one would today refer to as external or social ecology. It is though their sustained practice that one can hope to establish a peaceful, harmonious and happy social environment, which is a *sine qua non* for real progress of any type in case of individuals or groups, who form part of a community or nation. No wonder, Patanjali calls them Saarvabhauma, supreme or universal obligatory for all and under all circumstances. It was also not a chance coincidence that Mahatma Gandhi, even though he was not a full-fledged votary of classical Yoga, included all the five Yamas in the eleven vows to be taken up seriously for practice and repeated every day in the prayers by the inmates of his Ashram.

(2) Niyama

These are the observances viz., Shoucha (Purity), Santhosha (Contentment), Tapas (Austerity), Swadyaaya (Self-Study), Eswara Pranidhaana (Total surrender to the Supreme).

Thirst for knowledge is inherent In man and no one likes to be ignorant. Knowledge alone can remove ignorance. A beautiful verse in Chanakya Niti (XVII-17) says:

ज्ञानं नराणामधिको विर्षेश: ।
ज्ञानेन हीना: पशुभि: समाना ।।

'What distinguishes a man from an animal is his capacity to acquire knowledge. Without knowledge men are equal to animals.'

Spiritual knowledge comes through direct experience of Truth, but very few can reach that state. Others have to follow the path of discrimination, using their intellect.

There is a popular saying:

स्वदेशे पूज्यते राजा विद्वान् सर्वत्र पूज्यते ।

"The king is honoured only in his kingdom whereas a learned person is honoured everywhere.[12]

This is a great psychological truth discovered by the Yoga system long ago. It is a commonplace of modern Ethics. Mackenzie says, "It is generally better to escape from our defects, not by thinking about them and trying to elude them, but by fixing our attention on the opposite excellences. It certainly seems a more effectual method as a rule to expel our evil propensities by developing good ones rather than by seeking directly to crush the evil ones.[13]

(3) Aasana

Asana means a state of being in which one can remain physically and mentally steady, calm, quiet and comfortable. In the Yoga Sutras of Patanjali there is a concise definition of yogasana:

"Sthiramsukhamaasanam", meaning that position which is comfortable and steady. So, we can see that yogasanas in this context are practiced to develop the practitioners' ability to sit comfortably in one position for an extended length of time, as in necessary during meditation.

In raja yoga, asana refers to the sitting position, but in hatha yoga it means something more. Asana are specific body position which open the energy channels and psychic centres. They are tools to higher awareness and provide the stable foundation for our exploration of the body, breath, mind and beyond. The hatha yogis also found that by developing control of the body through asana, the mind is also controlled. Therefore, the practice of asana is foremost in hatha yoga. This Involves practice of physical Postures for correcting any deformities or physical ailments. Hatha Yoga Texts claim that there are as many as 84,000,000 postures.

The third discipline is bodily posture (asana). It is a steady and pleasant posture of the body. It should not move. It should not be painful. It should not distract the mind. There are many kinds of postures, padmasana, virasana, bhadrasana, svastika, and the like. The various postures of the body are the means of controlling it and keeping it healthy and fit. They tone up the nervous system. They can be learnt from experts. The control of the body is the basis of the yoga discipline.

They are controlled by means of practice and non-attachment. Patanjli Yogasutras-12.

Practice is the repeated effort to follow the disciplines which give permanent control of the thought-waves of the mind. Yogasutra-13

Practice becomes firmly grounded when it has been cultivated for a long time, uninterruptedly, with earnest devotion. Yogasutra-14

The practice of yoga prevents psychosomatic disorders/diseases and improves individual's resistance and ability to endure stressful situations. As a primary prevention, yogic exercises should be advised to drive the benefits of prevention of diseases, promotion of health and for therapeutic purposes.[14]

(4) Praanaayaama

This limb deals with practice of breathing exercises involving rechaka, puraka, antara kumbaka and bahya kumbhaka (inhalation, exhalation, internal retention and external retention) thus exercising our lungs—the ventilators of our body.

The fourth discipline is breath control (pranayama). It consists in controlling natural breathing and subjecting it to a definite law. It consists in slow and deep inspiration (puraka), retention of breath (Kumbhaka), and slow expiration (recaka).[15] These three functions should be performed for definite periods. The time of inspiration, the time of retention of breath, and the time of expiration should be in the proportion: 1, 4 and 2.

Breath Control is conducive to concentration of mind. It removes the crust of affliction from illumination of the sattava of the mind. It removes the demerit which observes discriminative knowledge. Breath control is the supreme austerity. It purges the mind of impurities and generates illumination of knowledge.[16]

The term pranayama is derived from the Sanskrit term 'prana' which means the 'vital principal'. The vital principle permeates the brain and the nervous system of an individual. It is the source of volition, enthusiasm, spontaneity and happiness in an individual. He spreads the same in the environment which also becomes pure.[17]

Pranayama is the method of rhythmic regulation of breath. It produces stability in the body, and equanimity in the mind of an individual. The subtle physiology of an individual gets purified through regular practice of—pranayama. The body of an individual becomes free from leanness, obesity, crookedness, etc. through regular practise of pranayama. Swami Vishnu Devananda states:

Pracchardana-vidharanabhayam va pranasya

It is also achieved by the expulsion and retention of the breath.

This is a reference to the practice of pranayama as a method of purification. Regulation of the breath gives control over the thought waves, for control of breath is directly related to control of mind. There are many pranayama exercises, each of which has a special effect on the autonomic nervous system and the psyche.[18]

We do not pay any serious attention to breathing, the most important of all our bodily functions. It has never occurred to us that a great deal of our physical and mental troubles are due to the fact that we do not breathe correctly. Life and breath are synonymous. We live as long as we breathe. We start our life with the first breath and end it with the last breath. We never stop breathing whether we are awake or asleep. We can exist without food for weeks and without water for a few days but without air we cannot exist even for a few minutes. Air is the most important nourishment for our blood. All the activities of body from digestion to creative thinking depend upon the oxygen supply through breathing; yet we treat breathing with utter indifference. If there is a deficiency in the supply of oxygen, the process of ionization will be incomplete and the food is partially assimilated. Nearly 50 percent of delinquency in minors is due to oxygen starvation which is the result of shallow breathing and lack of fresh air.

The habit of shallow breathing is one of many unnatural habits that modern civilization has forced upon us. It has been proved that in the civilized world only babies can breathe in a natural way. Shallow breathing is directly or indirectly responsible for a number of physical and mental diseases ranging from nervous disorders to common colds. To function properly the brain requires three times more oxygen than the rest of the body. If it does not get its due allotment, it exacts it from the body supply. That is why brain workers often possess a poor physic and a bad health. Deep breathing not only nourishes the whole system but also cleanses it.

Prana is not mere breath but it is cosmic energy. It is a life giving principle which pervades the whole atmosphere. It is manifested in every form of existence—organic and inorganic. By breathing exercises it is possible to raise the degree of circulation of Prana in the body. The surplus of Prana is stored in the solar plexus which is the battery of human body.

5. *Prathyaahara*

If the mind is withdrawn from external sensible objects, the external senses are automatically withdrawn from them. They do not follow their objects, but they follow the mind. They are fixed on those objects only on which the mind is fixed. The restraint of the external senses depends upon the restraint of the mind. It can be acquired by repeated practice, resolute will, and sense control.[19]

The five disciplines of restrant (yama), observance (niyama), bodily posture (asana), breath-control (pranayama), and sense-control (pratyahara) are the external aids to yoga (bahirangasadhana). The last three disciplines, fixation of mind (dharana), meditation (Dhyana) and absorptive concentration or ecstasy (samadhi) are the internal aids of yoga (antarangasadhana). They directly lead to conscious ecstasy (samprajnatasamadhi).[20]

6. *Dhaarana*

This involves concentration of mind it is true that the main stumbling block in increasing our knowledge is lack of concentration. The ever-increasing aberrations in the mind with the advent of age would really worsen the situation unless the mind is cultured through yogic techniques. Everything is possible to those who can concentrate, and so we are encouraged to preserve, to break through the barriers of ordinary sense perception and to press forward fearlessly in our search for inner knowledge. The physical strength gained in a gymnasium can be used later for practical purposes. The mental strength gained through these exercises in concentration can be used for the most practical purpose of all; to unite ourselves with the Atman. विशेका वा ज्योतिटठमति ।। 36 ।।

7. *Dhyaana*

Dyaana involves relaxed dwelling of the mind for a longer duration on the object of meditation Fixation of attention on an object to the exclusion of other objects leads to meditation, if the cognition produced by it continues unbroken for a long time. There is a continuous stream of similar cognitions of the contemplated object undisturbed by dissimilar cognitions.[21]

8. *Samaadhi*

The meditation involves the continuous flowing of mind energy and steady focusing on the object of meditation effortlessly for a longer and longer time. The very essence of yoga is merger of individual soul with that of universal soul, a state of super consciousness. This essence is achieved through Samaadhi only. Fixation (dharana), meditation (dhyana) and absorptive concenration (samadhi), on the same object together are called samyama. They are the internal aids (antarangasadhana) to conscious ecstasy, while restraint, observance, bodily posture, breath control, and withdrawal of the senses from their objects are the external aids (bahirangasadhana) to it. But they are the external aids to super conscious ecstasy.[22]

Swami Sivananda in his article, "Religious Education and Practice of Yoga" mentions the causes of stresses and strains and suggest meditation as has been laid down in all our ancient Sanskrit scriptures.

"Watch your mind very carefully. Be vigilant. Be on the alert. Do not allow the waves of irritability, jealousy, hatred and lust to disturb you. These dark waves are enemies of peaceful living, meditation and wisdom. To some it is very difficult to keep the mind unruffled and pure, the causes being deep-rooted worldly Samskaras, unfavourable surroundings, and the predominance of extrovert tendencies. To some, of course, evil thoughts are not a problem at all. They appear occasionally as a passing phase without doing much havoc. The very fact that evil thoughts give you mental suffering is a sign of spiritual progress; for many do not have that much of sensitiveness."

In nutshell Meditation is the process where the mind of a person is attracted towards God without interruption and is always keen to set in prayer from the core of heart. Prayer and Japa always help in supplementing and complementing meditation.

A massive qualitative change takes place within Man along with the awakening of Prajnaa and gradually leads him on to the status of a Sthita-Prajnaa (Man of Steadfast Illumination or Wisdom), whose hallmarks are described in many old Sanskrit texts, particularly in those dozen beautiful verses towards the end of the second chapter of the Bhagvad Gita, the immortal and inspiring dialogue between Arjuna and Lord Krishna. At this stage of Man's evolution into expanded states of consciousness, words and exhortations are of only limited use. Only regular reflection and meditation under the direction of one's own pure intellect or a qualified teacher can contribute to progress in this realm, which has been differently referred to as transcendental, mystical, religious, spiritual, super-conscious, supramental, supernatural, etc. by its explorers in different parts of the world and in different ages. Whatever the name, this higher realm of consciousness is filled with Light and Joy unbounded.

Classification of Yoga

There are four yogas—Bhakti Yoga, Karma Yoga, Jnana Yoga and Raja yoga—to realize the Divine, where is the need to practise Buddhi Yoga? The answer is that even to practice the four yogas one has to take the help of Buddhi.

Shri Krishnan says in the Bhagavad Gita (18:57):

चेतना सर्वकर्माणि मयि सन्यस्य मत्पर :
बुद्धियोगमुपाश्रित्य मच्चित: सततं भव ।

"Resigning mentally all actions to Me, regarding Me as the supreme goal and resorting to Budhhi Yoga, ever fix your mind on Me.

Bhakti Yoga

Devotion mixed with discrimination is an ideal path. Without discrimination devotion ends in mere sentimentalism or emotionalism. Therefore, the place of Buddhi in Bhakti yoga is very significant. When the Lord is pleased with His devotees, he bestows His grace in the form of pure intellect. Sri Krishna himself promises in the Bhagwad Gita (10.10):

तेण सततयुक्तानां भजतां प्रीतिपूर्वकम्
ददामि बुद्धियोगं तं येन मापुयान्ति ते

"To those who are ceaselessly devoted to Me and who worship Me with immense love, I grant Buddhi yoga by which they come to Me." A concentrated mind alone is a fit instrument for prolonged and deep meditation on the Divine. Intellect alone can do this since it is superior to the mind and the senses.

Dhayana Yoga

The mind is superior to the senses and the intellect is superior to the mind. Through the constant practice of meditation, we gain control over our senses and mind, which helps us to develop the power of concentration.

शनै शनैः शनैपरमेद्बुद्धयाधृतिगृहीतया
आत्मसंस्थं मनः कृत्वा न किश्दिपि चिन्तयेत् ।।

Karma Yoga

No one can renounce work but if we learn the skill of performing work, the same work will release us from the bondage of Karma.

Sri Krishna clearly says that even to perform work in the right spirit one must exercise his intellectual faculty. Even a little work, done with the spirit of self-sacrifice and dedication, gives a sense of fulfilment. Therefore, intelligent people always choose the path of selfless work using their discriminative faculty. To work and yet to be free from the effects of work requires subtle understanding of the secret of work and such understanding comes from Buddhi. Sri Krishna says in the Bhagvad Gita (2.39)

नराणामधिको विर्षेश: ।
ज्ञानेन हीनाः पणुभिः समाना ।।

"Being endowed with such intellect you will get rid of the bondage of actions, O Pratha."

4. Jnana Yoga

Discrimination between the real and the unreal is called Viveka. Buddhi alone has the capacity to determine the real nature of an object. In the path of knowledge, the aspirant has to realize the Truth by constant reasoning and through Buddhi alone this can be done. Sankaracharya emphasizes this view in the Vivekachudamani (versa: 16):

मेधावी पुरुशे विद्वानूहपोहविचक्षण :
अधिकार्यात्मविद्यायामुक्तलक्षणलक्षित: ।।

An intelligent and learned man skilled in arguing in favour of the Scriptures. . ... is the recipient of the knowledge of the Atman."[23]

Ordinarily we speak of four Yogas, the royal roads to Reality, viz. Jnana, Bhakti, Raja and Karma Yogas. Strangely enough, the Bhagavata does not recognize Rajayoga as an independent path. It speaks of only three. Sri Krishna says to Uddava:"I have propounded three Yogas for the welfare of mankind. They are Jnana, Karma and Bhakti and there is none other anywhere. Jnana Yoga for those who are disillusioned with the world and have given up Karma ; Karmayoga for those who hanker after worldly pleasures and are attached to Karma; and Bhaktiyoga for those who happen to hear about Me and My sports and are attracted by them, yet are not totally free from worldly pursuits nor are very much attached to them." (Bh. II.10, 6.7, 8)[24]

Though the Bhagavata does not accord an independent status to Patanjali's Yoga, it recommends and incorporates all its limbs in the practice of meditation. Yama, Niyama, Asana, Pranayama and the whole host are there, may be in a slightly modified form. (Vide Bhag. 11.14. 32-35; and 11.19.33.35).[25]

According to Aurobindo's Yoga is to want to transform oneself integrally, it is to have a single aim in life, such that nothing else exists any longer, that alone exists. And so one feels it clearly in oneself whether one wants it or not; but if one doesn't one can still have a life of goodwill, a life of service, of understanding; one can labour for the work to be accomplished more easily—all that—one can do many things. But between this and doing yoga there is a great difference. And to do Yoga, you must want it consciously.

IMPACT OF YOGA ON LIFE OF PEOPLE

The ancient literature is full of philosophy, science and techniques of channelising the potential energies of people and their life long journey. But How?

The answer is compulsory education of Yoga from school to university level in graded manner. Let us mention some of the facts which can be developed by Yoga Education to improve the personality of students.

(a) Holistic Development of Personality, i.e. physical mental and spiritual

This coincides with the definition adopted by World Health Organisation. Health is a state of physical, mental and social well-being and not merely the absence of infirmily. Yoga offers us a holistic lifestyle of bliss, peace, creativeness, emotional balance and physical well being.

The concept of 'mental equanimity' is more satisfactory than the concept of mental health because the former alone can produce spiritual development in an individual. Swami Vishnu Devananda states:

नदेकवार्यमात्रानिर्भास स्वरुप्शुन्यमिव समाधि।

When consciousness of subject and object disappears and only the meaning remains, it is called samadhi. Samadhi is a merging of the mind into the essence of the object of meditation. Nothing exists but that pure awareness.[26]

Mind is the most powerful part of the human system. It is a Super Computer. Teachers in the systems of Education don't realize its potential or devise ways and means to harness this most important source. Education system can achieve excellence, provided they know the secret of tapping students mind. We generally notice that most of the students do not mentally position as one or the other problems concerning their education continuously bogs them down. Many of them become mental wrecks and a liability on the Education system. The higher education systems instead of solving their problems, cause further deterioration. 25 percent of students in every higher education system are a liability and the other 75 percent are not contributing as per their potential. Teachers should try to create positive mental attitudes among the students. Positive mental attitude is a state of mind that reflects the strength of students' belief in what they do. It generates inner and voluntary emotions which enhances motivation, resulting in positive thoughts. Positive thinking is the key to development and is result-oriented.

The ancient Indian philosophers laid stress on mental equanimity for the general well-being of individuals. The mind of an ordinary person is usually very restless. Myraids of desire produce upheavals in the mind of an individual. Over and above this, the mind of an ordinary person is afflicted by several tensions.

The ancient Indian Philosophers maintained that if the mind of an individual usually remains in a disturbed state, he is very likely to develop pathological symptoms. An individual with pathological mental symptoms quite often develop certain pathological organic symptoms because there is very close relationship between the body and the mind of an individual . The mind of an individual becomes free from anxiety and miseries, if there is peace in his mind."

The mind is a reservoir for numerous powers. By utilizing the resources which are hidden within it, one can attain any height of success in the world. If the mind is trained, made one-pointed and inward, it also has power to penetrate into the deeper levels of our being. It is the finest instrument that a human being can ever have.

Holistic approach to health represents a revisioning of the human endeavour to restore order in the organismic functioning, that has occurred in the past several centuries with the medical profession. The holistic health movement is the reflection of the growing dissatisfaction among the professional as well as lay people about the capacity of modern medicine in delivering the health care. A shortcoming of modern medicine is its failure to recognize the interactive nature of the different aspects of human existence, viz. physical, psychological social and spiritual in the etiology of illnesses and in the maintenance of health and well-being.

Since modern medicine is itself a development within the framework of science, many have argued that the change needs to be brought about in the very framework. Thus, holistic movement is viewed as a by-product and manifestation of the contemporary thrust on the revision of the scientific framework. One can find this trend in the works of behavioural, natural and social scientists which are contributing for major change in the worldview. It involves a fundamental shift in cognition leading to radical alterations in the belief and assumptions about the nature of the universe, about the human nature, about organism environment interaction, and about the nature of consciousness. The newly emerging worldview is described as holistic paradigm.

In the final analysis, the physical, social, mental and spiritual balance is the most desirable for holistic health. Unless a person is physically fit and active; he cannot perform at his best level. On the other hand, it is the mind, which accounts for 80 percent of physical and social problems. These are called psychosomatic diseases. Lastly, it is the spirit which ultimately directs the mind and through it to the body. The teachers should devise ways and means to ensure synergy of the physical, social, mental and spiritual capabilities, which would release the infinite potential powers of the students and generate efficiency and happiness in the society.

(b) Control of Negative Thought Waves in the Mind

When Patanjali speaks of "control of thought waves", he does not refer to a momentary or superficial control. Many people believe that the practice of yoga is concerned with "making your mind a blank"—a condition which could, if it were really desirable, be much more easily achieved by asking a friend to hit you over the head with a hammer. No spiritual advantage is ever gained by self-violence. We are not trying to check the thought-waves by smashing the organs which record them. We have to do something much more difficult—to unlearn the false identification of the thought waves with the ego-sense. This process of unlearning involves a complete transformation of character, "revewal of the mind", as St. Paul puts it.

(c) Creation of Positive Attitude

To attain success in life and to reach the desired goal one must have a positive attitude. Faith in oneself and in God, courage, strength and fearlessness are the characteristics of a positive intellect. For a man of intense faith nothing is impossible in this world. That person alone who is ready to undergo any amount of suffering and face any difficulty can reach the goal. One should never harbour negative thoughts, like 'I am only a householder', 'I am a sinner', 'I am good for nothing', 'I am weak'. Such negative thinking can do tremendous harm to our personality.[27] Swami Vivekananda stressed this idea again and again. He was very particular that our younger generation must cultivate positive ideas. He says, "He is an atheist who does not believe in himself. The old religion said that he was an atheist who did not believe in God. The new religion says that he is an atheist who does not believe in himself.

(d) Vast Intellect

Visala Buddhi is that characteristic of the intellect, which transcends all narrow and selfish ideas and embraces the whole world. When a person lets go his individuality and identifies himself with the whole existence, he is called a man of vast intellect. We bow down to the great sage Vyasa because he possessed this vast intelligence.

नमोस्तु ते व्यास विशलबुद्धें. . . . . (Gita Dhyana Sloka 2)

Swami Vivekananda wanted our people to develop such an intellect. In one of his lectures delivered in Madras he said, 'We want that education, by which character is formed, strength of mind is increased, the intellect is expanded and by which one can stand on one's own feet.' Further he said, 'Expansion is life, contraction is death.'

A person who is only interested in himself is like a prisoner. He remains confined within the four walls of his house, without any concern for the outside world. He is quite happy with himself and is not aware of his spiritual dimension. There is no expansion of heart. A little spiritual growth will help us to expand our intellect. The same Divine dwells in the heart of everybody and we are one spiritually. Therefore, we must change our attitude towards others.

Sri Krishna shows us how to develop this vast intellect (6.32):

ज्ञानं आत्मौपम्येन सर्वत्र समं मण्यति योऽर्जन ।
सुखं वा यदि वा दुेख स योगी परमो मत: ।।

'He who judges pleasure and pain everywhere bothersome standard as the one he applies to himself, that yogi is thought to be the highest.

The idea is, the man of vast intellect (Visala Buddhi) empathizes with the joys and sorrows of all beings as his own. He understands the sufferings and shares the happiness and miseries of others. Through this teaching Sri Krishna exhorts us, to love others as we love ourselves. Be full of kindness and compassion, identify yourself with others and partake of their joys and sorrows. Why? Because unity underlies this apparent diversity.

The man of vast intellect breaking all barriers embraces the whole world. A selfish man on the other hand feels miserable when others are happy and feels happy when others are suffering. This is called Bheda Buddhi. He always wants to preserve his separate identity. Such a man does not hesitate to harm others for selfish purposes. Because of his deluded intellect, he divides people into different categories, depending on their caste, creed, religion, sex, social status, just to exploit them for his selfish motives. What happens to such a man?[28]

All the great religions of the world have come out of one Truth. If we follow religion without practicing the Truth, it is like the blind leading the blind. Those who belong to God love all. Love is the religion of the universe. A compassionate one transcends the boundaries of religion and realizes the undivided, absolute Reality.[29]

(e) Decisions based on deep thinking

Our decisions, motives, actions should always be guided by serious and deep thinking and not by mere impulse or emotion. A calm and study mind alone is fit to discriminate between right and wrong. We find a beautiful verse in the Katha Upanishad which can guide our intellect to make the right choices (1.2.2):

श्रेयच्श्र प्रेयच्श्र मनुश्यमेत: तौ सम्परीत्य विविनक्तिधीर : ।
श्रेयो हिधीरोऽभिप्रेयसो वृणीते प्रेयो मन्दो योगक्षेमाद्वृणीते ।।

'Both the good and the pleasant present themselves to a man. The calm soul examines them well and discriminates. He prefers the good to the pleasant; but the fool chooses the pleasant out of greed and avarice.'[30]

(f) Strengthen spiritual power

Spiritual strength is the highest strength, the next being intellectual and the last, physical. Those who have made considerable progress in spiritual life alone can experience spiritual strength; till then we have to depend upon intellectual strength. Intellectual conviction is possible only through right understanding. Regular study of the scriptures, teachings of great luminaries and discussions on spiritual matters help us to develop right understanding.

The Taittiriya Upanishad says (1.19):

स्वाध्याय प्रवचनाभ्यां न प्रमदितव्यम् ।।
'Do not be careless, about learning and teaching'

Since it is difficult to keep the mind always on the spiritual plane, it is better to engage it in intellectual pursuit, lest it should go down to the physical and sensual level.

Thirst for knowledge is inherent in man and no one likes to be ignorant. Knowledge alone can remove ignorance. A beautiful verse in Chanakya Niti (XVII-17) says:

ज्ञांन नराणामधिको विशेश: ।
ज्ञानेन हीना: पणुभि: समाना: ।।

What distinguishes a man from an animal is his capacity to acquire knowledge. Without knowledge men are equal to animals;

Spiritual knowledge comes through direct experience of Truth, but very few can reach that state. Others have to follow the path of discrimination, using their intellect.

There is a popular saying:

स्वदेशे पूज्यते राजा विद्वान् सर्वत्र पूज्यते ।

The king is honoured only in his kingdom whereas a learned person is honoured everywhere.[31]

(g) Helps in sorting out psychological problems born out of tensions, conflicts, etc.[32]

What most psychologists ask their patients to do is to yield to the demands of the unconscious. In some cases this may release the inner tensions. But this may not be permanent and may even be more harmful. The super conscious is at present unknown to us, but that does not mean that it is the same as the unconscious mind of the psychologists. It can be attained through spiritual disciplines. It is the source of supreme peace and bliss. More than all, it gives man the feeling of wholeness, the feeling of supreme fulfilment.

(h) Strengthen Willpower

Development of will power is a problem that is often faced by everyone of us. If we can exercise our body and buildup its strength gradually, there is no reason why the same cannot be done with our mind! By denying ourselves small pleasures and temptations to begin with, we can gradually but surely build up our will power. The example given by the Holy Mother of the farmer who could lift a bull because he used to carry it daily since the time it was a small helpless calf, can give us much-needed encouragement here also.[33]

Fear is the greatest of all foes. It is a devil residing with. Fearlessness is the first rung on the ladder of freedom.

To cultivate the quality of humility is one step toward enlightenment.

By being humble we gain much and lose nothing. Prayer and contemplation strengthen our willpower in cultivating this inner quality.

(i) Understanding the purpose of Life

Swami Rama feels that "If a human being remains constantly aware of the purpose of his life and directs all his actions toward the fulfilment of that purpose, there remains nothing impossible for him. Those who are not aware of the purpose of life are easily caught by the whirlpool of miseries."

A human being is fully equipped with all necessary healing powers, but does not know their usage. The moment he comes in touch with the healing potentials within, he can heal himself. All the powers belong to only one God. A human being is only an instrument.

(j) Nutrition for Yogic Persons

Swami Vishnu Devananda in his book Meditation and Mantras has rightly said that, What is consumed by the human body correlates directly to the efficiency with which the brain functions. Recent studies show that certain red food colouring creates hyperactivity in children, and that refined sugar can cause emotional instability. These are just two examples of substances that are often heedlessly consumed without understanding their effect on the body and mind.

Several years ago vegetarianism was, in a sense, an under ground-practice. A person who refrained from eating meat was viewed with a certain amount of curiosity, if not suspicion. To day it is quite a different story. Health food stores and vegetarian restaurants are prevalent. There is a growing awareness that our health is directly affected by what we eat. Many diseases can be cured by a change in diet or a short period of fasting, with no medications at all. This is true not only of physical disorders, but of many mental difficulties as well. It is particularly important that pregnant mothers have this awareness; too often they do not realize the effect of their diet on the developing fetus.

There is no doubt that, "You are what you eat", a subtle part of what is consumed becomes the consciousness. Those who have changed from a meat to vegetarian diet notice a corresponding change in consciousness. There is a certain grossness that disappears, and the awareness becomes finely tuned.

In the Bhagavad-Gita three types of food have been mentioned which produce three different types of dispositions in individuals.

A person becomes healthy, moral, religious, intelligent and creative by regularly taking, sattvika food.

Sattvika spreads sattvika and the Cumulative effect is purity of environment.

आयु: सत्वबलारोग्यसुखप्रीतिविवर्धना: ।
रत्या: सिनगधा: स्थिरा हरद्या आहारा: सात्त्विकप्रिया: ।। xvii/8 Bhagavad Gita.

Foods which promote longevity, intelligence, vigour, health, happiness and cheerfulness, and which are sweet, bland, substantial and naturally agreeable, are dear to the Sattvika type of men."

कटुवम्ललवणात्युश्णतीक्षणक्षविदाहिन: ।
आहारा राजसस्येश्टा दु:खणोकामयप्रदा: ।। xvii/9 Bhagavad Gita.

Foods which are bitter, acid, salty, overhot, pungent, dry and burning, and which cause suffering, grief and sickness, are dear to the Rajasika type of men.

यातायामं गतरसं पूति पयुणितं च यत् ।
उच्छिश्टमपि चामोध्यं भोजन तामसप्रियम् ।। xvii/10 Bhagavad Gita.

Food which is half-cooked or half-ripe, insipid, putrid, stale and polluted, and which is impure too, is dear to men of a Tamasika disposition.

Research Studies about Impact of Yoga on Lives of People

P.K. Hassanagas et al in their article, Yoga in the Culture of Labour based on research have come out with the following conclusions:[34]

1. Practising yoga helps in improving the general health of the volunteers.
2. The psycho condition is reinforced and the mental capabilities are increased. The concentration and the memory are developed. Self-confidence, self-discipline and working capability are increased.
3. The capability for removing the psychophysical fatigue is increased.
4. The influence of the harmful factors from the working conditions to health is decreased because the immunity and the resistance of the body is reinforced and the participants learn how to protect themselves.
5. The number of the injuries is decreased as a result of increase of the self-consciousness, self-control of the body and the brain.
6. The number of absences due to illness is decreased.
7. The efficiency and the productivity increases leading to profits.

Nedungade V. Haridas in his article, "Physiological and Philosophical aspects of Yoga" states that:[35]

Yoga science is a well proven treasure and it is up to us to tap the yoga power to relax and rejuvenate our mind, increase our physical strength, expand our spiritual awareness, improve our concentration, help our body use oxygen and nutrients more effectively and to prevent illness and retard old age.

In conclusion, a quotation is taken from His Holiness Swamy vishnudevananda, "Health is wealth—peace of mind is happiness—yoga shows the way."

Pavlos K. Hassanages *et al.* in their article, "Yoga and Cardio Vascular Diseases state:[36]

Our results show remarkable influence of yoga on eliminating and alleviating of chronic psycho stresses, increasing of self-control, self-confidence and self discipline which help to eliminate other risk factors and to undertake responsibility for improving one's own health and the quality of living which in turn helps in preventing coronary disease.

Dr. (Mrs.) Hemalatha Murthy in his article, "Management of Respiratory Diseases by Yoga",[37] states that yoga gives us solace, confidence, redeems all our miseries, obsession, conflicts. It is suitable to all and all times. It helps the persons to change their attitude and bring a tremendous change in way of life which is simple and which is very necessary, unless, there is no true solutions to all the problems and illnesses. Right knowledge of yoga burns out the likes and dislikes, ego and ignorance and there is establishment of Pure Bliss, which is natural state of a being.

For the management of stress in order to combat the so-called stress-induced disorders all the above discussed areas should be tapped. Yoga way is more holistic, which offers the lifestyle of bliss, efficiency, emotional equipoise, mental clarity, intellectual sharpness and physical well-being.

Swami Harshananda in his article, "Attainment of Yoga" mentions that knowingly or unknowingly, all of us are struggling to get peace. As long as our mind is in pieces and the pieces are in ceaseless mutual conflict, peace eludes us. It is only when we learn to put these pieces together so as to make the mind whole and integrated that we gain the peace of Kaivalya. This is easier said than done. However, with competent guides like Patanjli who are ever eager to help out of infinite compassion, this task should not be that difficult.

Patanjli, the great master of the Yoga system, calls these pieces of the mind as vrttis, modifications, which are ever arising and never subsiding. Yoga or union of the individual self with the Supreme Self will result through Yoga or Samadhi, when these Vrttis are controlled, suppressed and eliminated, by the right kind of discipline and training. This discipline and training is also Yoga.[38]

Dr. S.C. Manchanda,[39] Professor and Head; Department of Cardiology, All India institute of Medical Sciences, New Delhi has depicted the role of Yoga lifestyle in Coronary Artery diseases in his "Research Study of Reversal of Coronary Heart Disease through Prekasha Meditation with Reference to Coronary Atherosclerotic Reversal Potential of Yoga Lifestyle Intervention." According to the study, forty-two male patients (mean age 51.0 + 9.5 range 32-72 years) with angiographically proven CAD were included. Patients in the control group (n=21) were managed on conventional medical therapy (with control of risk factors, AHA step 1 diet, moderate aerobic exertion), while those in the yoga group (n=21) were advised strict lifestyle modifications and yogic exercises as detailed below. The yogic lifestyle intervention programme consisted of:

(a) Yogic Lifestyle Methods—
   (i) Health rejuvenating exercises: a set of movements for improving the general tone of the body and to improve coordination.
   (ii) Relaxation exercise (Kayotsarg): a method of complete relaxation to prepare the body and mind for mediation.
   (iii) Breathing exercises (Pranayama).
   (iv) Yogic posters for stretch relaxation (Asanas).
   (v) Preksha meditation (preksha means seeing deeply within).
   (vi) Reflection on moral values (Anuvrat and Anupreksha.)
(b) Stress Management (relaxation, breathing exercises and Preksha meditation),
(c) Dietary control.
(d) Moderate aerobic exercises.

The change in the lesion severity was classified into regression (10% absolute reduction in diameter stenosis), no significant change « 10% change in diameter stenosis) or progression (>10% absolute increase in diameter stenosis). In the Yoga group, 3 (5%) lesions showed progression, 46 (75%) lesions showed no change while 12 (20%) lesions showed regression. In the control group 22 (37%) lesions showed progression, 36 (61%) showed no change while 1 (2%) showed regression.

Yoga lifestyle intervention is beneficial in improving the symptoms and exercise capacity, lowering weight and serum lipid levels. It also retards the progression of coronary atherosclerosis in patients with severe coronary artery diseases and reduces revasularisation procedures.

In ancient India the early Yogis were a group of mystics and scientists to whom the relationship between the mortal man and an immortal spirit was of great interest. They set about to find ways and means of uniting these two during the earthly life of man. They spent not decades but centuries in making their experiments with different methods of concentration, meditation and relaxation; with various breathing processes, postures and foods. When they finally succeeded in their experiments, they systematized the result of their findings and called it the science of Yoga. The aim of Yoga is to achieve reintegration of the individual consciousness with the cosmic consciousness.[40]

The aim of Yoga is to completely alter one's personality and outlook so that he is able to face all problems of life with equanimity, while pursuing to achieve the ideals which he cherishes. It is a complete break with normal waking consciousness. It is neither a condition of vain pursuits and frustrations of waking life, nor a condition of mere dreaming, nor even condition of absence of quality as in deep sleep, but a condition of calmness and tranquility of mind in daily pursuits. As Gita describes with an analogy, he is one into whom all desires enter as waters into these and is ever motionless though constantly being filled (11.70). He enjoys and suffers like all human beings; he has passions, fears and rages like all human beings; but unlike the ordinary human beings, he is able to maintain tranquility through them all.

Swami Lokeshwarananda feels that, "The world-wide interest which yoga has aroused is encouraging, but is not without its dangers. Already yoga centres have cropped up in many places in India and abroad, where yoga is being taught by people least qualified to do so. If yoga were only a physical exercise, no serious objection could be raised against this; but yoga is an integrated science whose sole purpose is to help to improve his spiritual life. At the moment, yoga's popularity rests on the proven physical benefit it brings. It keeps the body slim, strengthens the digestive organs, keeps off common diseases like colds, helps one preserve one's youth and beauty, and so on. The claim is also made that it can cure more serious diseases, but the claim has yet to be tested. As man's chief worry is about his body, no wonder yoga is becoming increasingly popular. More and more people are crowding round these yoga centres, hoping to push back their advancing age or retain their fast-fading beauty. That yoga has a higher purpose is hardly realized. So much fuss is made over its physical advantages that many have now come to think it is nothing but another form of physical exercise. This suits the self-styled teachers because they know little or nothing about its other advantages."

Swami Aseshananda observes that Yoga has been erroneously interpreted as crystal gazing, fortune telling, fire eating, and other types of miracle-mongering. Yoga has nothing to do with any kind of miracles or occult practices. Yoga is a rational method of self-discipline and purification of the heart. "Blessed are the pure in heart, for they shall see God", says Christ.

CONCLUSION

Systematic and regular practice of Yogic techniques viz. Postures, Pranayama, Mudras, Bandas, Shat-Kriyas, Concentration, meditation and diet regulations under experts guidance and certainly not from books alone, will go for to build up the lost muscle tone of various organs, glands, nerves, etc., mental clarity, positive attitude towards life, and in removing physical and mental restlessness and physiochemical process as the stress creates nerves disorders due to modern hectic, pressurized, frustrated living.

It has been reported in the ancient literature that Yogic practice brings change in various hormonal and physiochemical process in the human body by operating at the higher levels in the nervous system.[41]

"Yoga helps in maintaining good health
and gives resistance, stamina, vitality and vigour to the body.

Yoga is the best curative and preventive medicine
Yoga leads to chittanasa which is moksha
Yoga practitioners should not become Bhogi
If no Yoga—no health, no peace, no life."

Notes and References

1. Xth Plan of University Grants Commission, New Delhi, 2002, p. 51
2. Dr. H.R. Nagendra and Dr. R. Najarathna, News Perspectives on Stress Management, Swami Vivekananda Yoga Prakashana, Bangalore, 2003, Preface.
3. *Ibid.*, pp. 2-3. 27.
4. YB ; ii (2).
5. YS I (2).
6. YS (i) 12.
7. R.H. Singh, "Yoga and Health, Science and Philosophy of Indian Medicine", Baidyanath Bhawan, Nagpur, 1978.
8. Dr. C.H. Sudarshan, Yoga for Better Health, in *NIS Argopcar Varta*, National Institute of Naturopathy, Pune, May 2001.
9. Y.S. H. 30.
10. Y.B. R.M. ii 30.
11. Swami Srikantanada, The Intelligent Way to Yoga, Sri Rama Krishna Math, Chennai, 2001 pp. 30-31.
12. Swami Srikanthanda, *op. cit.*, p. 66
13. Manual of Ethics, 1935, p. 341.
14. Y.S. R.M. YB (i) 46.
15. YS ii 49, 50.
16. YS ii 53, UB RM ii 52.
17. Swami Sivananda, Practice of Yoga Quoted in Swami Devananda, *op. cit.*, p. 60.
18. Swami Vishnu Devananda, *op. cit.*, p. 161.
19. YS YB MP ii 54.
20. YB iii, YS, YB iii 7.
21. RM iii 2.
22. YS YB iii, 4, 7, 8.
23. Swami Siddhinathananda, Yoga in Srimod Bhagavata, Yoga and Its various Aspects, Sri Ramakrishna Math, Madras, pp. 160-61.
24. Swami Srikantanamda, *op. cit.*, pp. 7-11.
25. Swami Siddhinathananda, Yoga in Srimad Bhagavata, Yoga and Its various aspects, Sri Rama Krishna Math, Madras, pp. 160-61.
26. Swami Vishnu Devananda, *op. cit.*, p. 177.
27. Bata K. Day, Ethics: Maladies and Remedies, in *IJPA*, July-Sept. 1995, p. 46.
28. Swami Srikantananda, *op. cit.*, pp. 56-57.
29. *Ibid.*, pp. 40-41.
30. *Ibid.*, p. 17.
31. *Ibid.*, pp. 65-66.
32. Swami Yatishwarnanda, Meditation and Spiritual Life, Rama Krishna Ashram, Bangalore, 1983, pp. 17-18.
33. *Ibid.*
34. P.K. Hassanagas, "Yoga in the Culture of Labour based on Research", Arya Vidya Sala Kottakhal and University of Calicut, Holistic Life and Medicine,

Sixth World Congress on Holistic Life and Medicine held at Calicut, Kerala, 5-7 July 1996, pp. 127-28.

35. Nedungade, V. Hardias, Physiological and Philosophical Aspects of Yoga.
36. *Ibid.*, p. 150.
37. Dr. (Mrs.) Hemlatha Murly, "Management of Respiratory Disesase by Yoga." National Institute of Naturopathy, Pune, *op. cit.*, p. 12.
38. Swami Harshananda, "Attainment of Yoga: Maladies and Remedies", in *Yoga: Its various aspects*, Sri Ramakrishana Math, Madras, pp. 203-04.
39. Manchanda, S.C. *et al.*, "Research Study of Reversal of Coronary Heart Disease through Preksha Meditation with reference to coronary atherosclerotic reversal potential of yoga lifestyle intervention", A Research Study conducted by AIIMS, Deptt. of Cardiology, New Delhi, pp. 1-8.
40. Swami Prabuddhananda, Yoga in Daily Life, In *Yoga: Its various Aspects*, Shri Ramakrishna Math, Madras, pp. 121-122 and 70-71.
41. Dr. C.H. Sudarshan, *op. cit.*, p. 20.

18 CHAPTER

Urban Slums: Living Disasters

The recent report of Census of India reveals that urbanization has increased to 31.13% between 1991 and 2001 as compared to 16% in 1951 and 26% in 1991. It is expected to touch the mark of more than 40% in 2021. Thirty-five cities in the country have crossed a population of over one million. Greater Mumbai with a population of 163.38 lacs, Kolkata with a population of 132.16 lacs and Delhi with 127.91 lacs, occupy first three positions respectively in 2001. The Punjab, which is known for its villages, has 33.95% of its population living in urban areas as compared to the national average of 31.13%. Let us take the example of Punjab. The urban population in the State is distributed over 157 towns out of which 14 towns have more than one lac population in 2001 as compared to 10 in 1991. The increase in urban population has created a large number of problems for the Local Self Government, which is already under great stress and strain. The problems faced by the urban local self-government do not merely limit themselves to traditional functions of providing basic services e.g., potable water supply, sewerage, waste disposal, etc. but extend to new and emerging problems of lawlessness, prostitution, rape, distress, thefts, crimes especially against women, unemployment, shelter, etc. Thus, administration of cities has become complex; hence require the co-operation of all including adequate finance and especially the people's participation and involvement.

Provisional data relating to slums in the 2001 Census throw some interesting light on the slum population. Nearly 28 million persons lived in the slums in 1981, accounting for 17.5 per cent of the urban population. The estimates for 1991 were 45.7 million slum-dwellers accounting for 21.5 per cent of population. According to the 2001 Census, there are 40.6 million persons living in slums in 607 towns/cities, and they account for 22.8 per cent of the population of these cities. However, the latest Census data also reflect the problems inherent in not having an accepted definition of slums and absence of proper listing of slum settlements in the urban offices concerned with slum improvement and civic amenities. The practice of notifying slums under relevant laws is not being followed, especially where the land involved belongs to Government or any of its agencies. As a result of these lacunae, these data are not definitive because towns with less than 50,000 population, and slum clusters, which are not formally or informally recognized if the population was less than 300 are these excluded.

Former Hon'ble Minister for Urban Development, GOI, Jagmohan, had rightly spelled out the existing and emerging problems of Local-Self Government as follows: ('City Lights', *Hindustan Times,* December 14, 2000). "Invariably, cultural and civilization contours get imprinted on the faces of cities. The city has many facets. As an economic entity, it is a set of business and industry; as a social organisation, it is a creator of community and collective action; as a political unit, it is a centre of power and government; and as a cultural force, it is a repository of old traditions, a fountain head of new ideas, an instrument of intellectual advancement, and a moulder of attitudes and thoughts. It is a spiritual workshop of the nation, a most imposing creation of its social, economic and cultural aspirations."

Urban policies, poverty, pollution, productivity, planning and pattern, and shortages (both physical and financial) are the crucial issues around which the machinery of urban governance in India revolves. The formidable nature of these issues has thrown this machinery in deep crisis. But this crisis is not merely of governance. It extends to the governed as well. It is a crisis of character, commitment, conscience, the creative and constructive sense of the community as a whole. This crisis has been with us for quite some time. But, of late, the degree of this crisis has undergone such a change that it has virtually become a new kind of crisis. This crisis is daily weakening the structure of urban governance in India is heading to the disaster that lies ahead.

Already, in every aspect of city life-density of population, availability of land, housing, slums and squatter settlements, municipal services, open spaces, and the scale and character of migration, employment, traffic and transport, energy, communication, crime, health and environment, civic set-up and finance—the prevailing conditions present a grim picture.

Take for example, the arena of municipal services and urban infrastructure. At present, there is no sanitation worth the name for 52% of the urban population. The sewerage system covers only 35% of the population of Class IV cities and 75% of the population of Class I cities.

About 34% of urban population does not have any arrangement even for drainage of rainwater around its habitats. 60% of the municipal bodies in India collect less than 40% of the solid waste generated daily. At least 28% of the urban waste is allowed to decompose and purify on the roadside and around residential areas and factories. On an average, the slum and squatter population is increasing at more than double the general growth rate of population of the cities. At present, at least 35% of the population of our cities is living in slum settlements. Both economy and technology are changing fast. Their fallout, as well as let loose by globalization, cannot be fully anticipated and accounted for. But one thing, i.e. of fundamental importance is that the fate and future of our cities depend on the creativity and ingenuity, the vision and the will we bring to the task and the civilization and cultural underpinnings we would provide to it.

In addition the slum and squatters population is increasing at a fast rate causing a number of problems for Local-Self Government. The estimate of Census of 2001 is that about 35% of the city population lives in slums. The quality of life of the people in the city is poor. Krishan Gowda, M.V. Sridhar and Ms. Mamatha P. Raj, in their article, "Planning for the 21st Century: A Case Study of Bangalore", in *Shelter*, January 2000, draws our attention to the city of 21st century. To quote them: "We need to rethink or re-envision of city of the 21st century, i.e. one which is socially just, ecologically sustainable, politically participatory, economically viable and really capable of adaptation of future needs."

Inevitably this results in the uncontrolled physical expansion of the cities. City growth has kept far ahead of city planning and management, to the point where development of structures and activities in the city life is simply haphazard. In the older "core areas" of city slums and in the relatively new built-up areas, the scene is one of overcrowding, lack of access roads, scarcity of drinking-water, ramshackle buildings, uncollected garbage, lack of sewers, inadequate air-space, and a housing environment littered with human faces. All of these are conducive to the spread of tuberculosis, pneumonia, influenza, threadworm, cholera, dysentery and other diarrhoeal diseases. Just as intensive planning activities prevent diseases and promote health, so the lack of planning, or its inadequacy, breeds diseases and contributes significantly to a high rate of mortality, especially among children.[1]

Slums are cancerous for urban life and no effort should be spared to eradicate them. No doubt, they are manifestation of socio-economic conditions prevailing in the country, but if no heed is paid to contain them, urban life will become not only miserable but also unbearable. A serious policy of urban development, based on sound principles of town planning and efficient administration, committed to the service of the humanity with vast financial resources and authority can only successfully combat the problems of slums.[2]

Slums are a bye-product of urbanization and industrialization. Slum-dwellers are the real architect of urban facilities but their own life is endangered with poor facilities made available to them. Because of the laxity on the part of the municipal government, these slums sprang up and later on become difficult to control.

GENESIS OF SLUMS AND MAGNITUDE OF THE PROBLEM

"Slum" is defined as that area where the buildings are in any respect unfit for human habitation; or by reason of dilapidation, overcrowding, faulty arrangement of buildings, streets, lack of ventilation, light or sanitation facilities or combination of these factors, are detrimental to safety, health or morals (Slums Improvement and Clearance Act, 1956). Approximately, 68.8% of the country's slums population is concentrated in the 300 Class I cities and less than 1/3rd of this population resides in the remaining 3300 urban centers.[3]

Slums are not fit for settlement and are a danger both for residents and the urban population living nearby. Roosevelt has rightly said that poverty anywhere is a danger to prosperity. Sh. Aditya Prakash, retired Principal of the College of Architecture, Chandigarh, has termed the growth of slums in the City Beautiful of Chandigarh, as a "planning failure." He says: "The slums should not have been allowed to sprout in the first place. The need of the hour is to solve poverty and shelter problems and it can be done through proper planning."

Evolution of Slums

Urbanization has been considered as an index of development but in case of developing countries like India, urbanization is not the outcome of merely the growth potential generated by urban settlements. It has been largely due to people work relationship in rural areas, in which land is the essential medium and which is right now so critically balanced that even small addition to population is pushing people out of agriculture to non-agricultural occupations. Thus, by and large, in India urbanization is emerging as merely a process of transfer of rural poverty to urban environment, which only results in concentration of misery. This has resulted in the malfunctioning of most of the urban settlements leading to emergence of number of imbalances and problems. Thus, most of these settlements suffer from improper and haphazard development, absence of basic infrastructure and services, uncontrolled and unchecked growth of slums, lack of housing, high degree of visual and environmental degradation and uncontrolled traffic. The cumulative effect of these factors is the degradation of quality of life in urban settlements and huge amount of subsidies is required to maintain them. These facts are more evident in case of larger cities especially metros and super-metros.

Problems of Urban Areas Especially Human Settlements

Urban areas have not received much attention in terms of the planning, development and management despite the fact that cities and economic development are inextricably linked. Because of high productivity of urban areas, economic development activities get located in cities. Accordingly, it is desirable that human settlements are provided with necessary planning and development inputs so that the orderly growth and development is ensured. This would also be necessary for ensuring efficient functioning of human settlements for improving their productivity and for providing desirable quality of life to its residents in order to cater to their both economic and physical and metaphysical needs. The urban development strategy for any state thus assumes importance of not only its economic emancipation but also its physical well-being.

Concept of Slums[4]

The concept of slums and its definition vary from country to country depending upon the socio-economic conditions of each society. Irrespective of location, whether in the core of the city, in the form of old dilapidated structures or in the outskirts, in the form of squatting. Slums have often been characterized

(a) Physically, an area of the city with inadequate housing, deficient facilities, overcrowding and congestion.
(b) Socially, slum is a way of life, a special character which has its own set of norms and values reflected in poor sanitation, health values, health practices, deviant behaviour and social isolation.
(c) Legally speaking, section 3 of the Slum Areas (Improvement and Clearance) Act, 1956 defines slums as areas where buildings:
    (i) are in any respect unfit for human habitation; and
    (ii) are by reason of dilapidation, over-crowding, faulty arrangements of streets, lack of ventilation, light or sanitation facilities or any combination of these factors which are detrimental to safety, health and morals.

The slum areas are declared by a notification in the official gazette, which require:

(a) repair,
(b) stability,
(c) natural light and air,
(d) system of dump,
(e) water supply,
(f) drainage and sanitary conveniences, and
(g) facilities for storage, preparation of cooking of food and disposal of waste water, the buildings deemed to be unfit if it is so ineffective in one or more of the said matter and not found reasonably suitable for occupation in that condition.

Slums a Great Danger to the Population

Jai Saksena and P.N. Govindarajuler in their article, "Health Care For Urban Slums with special reference to Bangalore City" have rightly sensed the problem. To quote them: "Slum-dwellers have the worst of both the worlds—urban and rural. On one side they suffer from economic hardships, lack of education and absence of health infrastructure like the rural population. On the other hand, they also suffer the ill-effects of over-crowding, pollution and rootlessness characteristic of large metropolitan cities."

They further add that "Most comforts and conveniences of the cities are sustained by the work done by slum-dwellers. As such, the affluent and the privileged have the moral responsibility to try to mitigate and alleviate their suffering. Rural population may be ignorant of the "goodies" they are missing, but a slum-dweller is painfully aware of the privations suffered by him due to his constantly rubbing shoulders with urban affluence and conspicuous consumption with resultant resentment."[5]

Growth of Slums

While demographic data on slum populations and on civic amenities to slum-dwellers from the Census are still awaited, there appears to be no change in the basic level or improvement in the features of slum settlements despite several decades of programmes for the environmental improvement and upgradation of slums. There is cause to wonder whether 'Cities without Slums' is a slogan about an objective, which, however desirable, is believed to be unreachable, or whether it is a serious planning and urban development concern. Certainly the degree of effort to upgrade slums to a more habitable level does not indicate a serious effort in this direction.[6]

Slums by and large are the creation of urbanization process, which necessitates the transfer of rural poverty to urban environment. Lack of resources with the local level agencies results in non-provision of basic services and accordingly large number of slums grow in cities. Percentage of population of slums increases in direct proportion to the population and size of the city of which they form part. Larger cities have more proportion of population in slums. World Development Report of 1994 prepared by the World Bank says that growth of slums in India is primarily due to inadequate infrastructures. It further says that though proportion of population living below the poverty line has shown a decline, number of people living in slums have, however, increased. Thus, growth of slums cannot be visualized as the product of poverty alone; infact number of other factors are responsible for the growth of slums. Government of India has launched a new scheme to prevent the growth of slums in urban areas. New Scheme provides alternative sites to existing slum-dwellers/EWS Families living in cities with population ranging between 5 to 20 lacs. House sites are allotted on a graded scale of 35 sq. mts., for cities in population range between 5-10 lac, 30 sq. mts. for population ranges between 15-20 lacs. However, scheme does not provide for slums in cities-dwellers belonging to EWS category with special emphasis on people below poverty line. These schemes are operational in few selected towns.

Growths of slums have become faster over the years and this problem has spread over all the settlements. Major problem in solving shelter-related issues of EWS or shelterless is the availability of land. It is proposed to create a Land Bank for the poor in all the urban areas, which would be funded by various financial institutions like HUDCO and other State level agencies. Further addition would be made to the Land Bank through the mechanism of earmarking 5% of total land developed under any scheme for

EWS housing, which would be transferred to the Land Bank. Private colonizers would also contribute to the Land Bank. Similarly, all Town Development Schemes would earmark 5% of area for EWS housing. Thus, a large land pool would be created, which can be used for providing shelter to EWS.

The number and population of slums are always on the increase. Even many areas, in urban towns, have become so congested and short of basic services, that we can also call them slums. Life in these areas is miserable. If one has to visit old areas of Delhi, Ludhiana, Patiala, Calcutta, Bombay, for that matter, one finds that these are nothing but slums.

Life of People in Slums (See Chart 18.1)

A Survey on the health status of adolescent girls in Patiala, carried out by a team of expert lady doctors, has revealed that 92.5 per cent of girls in urban slums are anemic while the percentage of such girls in urban areas is 88.6 and 86% in rural areas. It was further found that 38.7 percent girls in urban slums were severely anemic.

Not only mental disorders but problems relating to physical abuse (15.2%), domestic violence (30.2%) and sexual abuse (10.2%) were seen in urban slums indicating poverty, illiteracy and low status of women in this category.[7] It is paradoxical situation that on the one hand they provide all services to urban population, on the other, they cannot meet their needs.

Over a period of time, slum-dwellers are beginning to see themselves as citizens contributing to the economy and, therefore, deserving their own place in the sun. It is the slum and pavement dweller, who provides the vast network of services that the middle and upper classes enjoy at cheap rates. These services include the entire food supply network (vegetables, milk, eggs, butter, bread, meat, poultry as well as restaurant services), clothing, laundry, vending and sales, transport, conservancy, communication, construction and domestic services for homes, offices. The slum-dwellers, if united, have the power to bring to a halt the entire urban system, so powerful is their role in urban economy.[8]

Most of the slum-dwellers are immigrants of villages or towns and then migrate to slums or another form of low-income urban housing. They move to the place after the migrant has established himself in the city with a job, a network of friends and some sort of understanding of the political and bureaucratic structure of the municipality. However, this pattern of movement from rural to slum is a very common one. Some move permanently. This usually happens when a migrant already has a well establishment network of relatives and friends living there. Some of migrants come not only from rural areas but also from other urban centres of the country. Others never settle permanently in the city but stay only long enough to take advantage of the economic opportunities available there before returning to their place of origin.[9]

Within the existing broad loose definition, following housing areas can be categorized as "Slum":

CHART 18.1

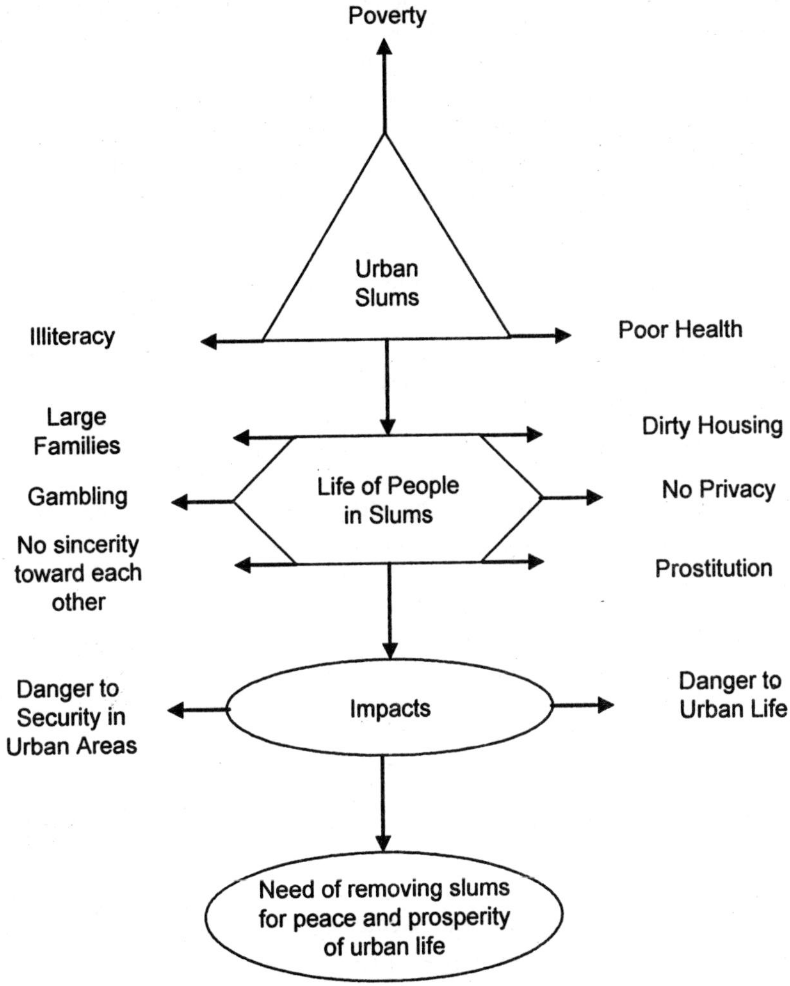

(i) Inner city blighted areas;
(ii) Squatter settlements on both private and public land;
(iii) Illegal land sub-divisions (unauthorized colonies);
(iv) Urban villages;
(v) Resettlement colonies (like those in Delhi); and
(vi) A squatter settlement improved under the environmental improvement scheme.[10]

Towards a National Slum Policy

The Draft National Slum Policy drawn up by the Department of Urban Employment Poverty Alleviation in the Ministry of Urban Development in April 1999, had been widely debated and many comments received. It needs to be finalized. A National Policy on slums is of great significance given the degree of wrong perception regarding the nature and extent of the slum problem. Such a policy can help bring an attitudinal change among the authorities and the people at large, including the urban poor and the slum-dwellers, regarding measures to improve their quality of life and make our cities free from the worst features of slums. Slums are generally treated as the inevitable outcome of continuing migration of unskilled labour, but, in fact, most slum-dwellers are permanent residents of the city. In many instances, families in slums span several generations. The main objectives of a slum policy would be:

- To create awareness of the underlying principles that guide the process of slum development and improvement and the options that are available for bringing about the integration of these settlements and the communities residing there with the urban area as a whole.
- To strengthen the legal and policy framework to facilitate the process of slum development and improvement on a sustainable basis; to ensure that the slum population are provided civic services, amenities, and economic opportunities to enable them to rise above the degrading conditions in which they live.
- To arrive at a policy of affirming the legal and tenurial rights of the slum-dwellers.
- To establish a framework for involving all stakeholders in the efficient and smooth implementation of policy objectives.

SOME CASE STUDIES IN SLUMS

In Ludhiana, a woman named Geeta about 20 years has four children. She got married at the age of 14. Her husband, a Rickshaw puller earns merely Rs. 30 per day, i.e. 600 per month, which he spends in drinking, smoking and gambling. Geeta works as maid in some houses leaving her children back, earning about 1500 per month. She has one room jhuggi with no privacy. Children are being neglected. She feels exhausted and tired of life.

In Jalandhar, a woman named Sarita about 23 years age old having three children was abandoned by her husband, as he got illicit relations with her sister who was living with them. She works as a rag picker hardly making both ends meet. She feels to commit suicide but because of children she is pulling her life.

In another case in Patiala, a woman about 25, with pale face and a mother of four children was suffering from HIV positive. Her husband alongwith his friends used to drink at night and all of them used to exploit her sexually. Her life has become miserable. She feels suffocated and cannot look after the children.

In another case in Ropar a man aged 50 has been living for the last 20 years with 3 children and his wife in small 2 rooms. Some persons in the area forced him to sell her daughters aged 13 and 15 to some persons aged 45 and 47. He resisted but could not do anything. He complained to the Police but no case was registered. He is feeling guilty and disheartened.

A Case Study of Chandigarh City Beautiful

Let us now mention about the growth of slums in the newly planned city beautiful, i.e. Chandigarh.

The city was planned on modern lines, has also been engulfed by slums, causing misery to the slum-dwellers as well as neighbouring population. Slums or so-called *bastis* are increasing at a fast rate. These *bastis* have become a danger to the inhabitants as well as to the residents of the city. Personal observations reveal the disgusting, pathetic and painful sights. Human beings are living like animals and these *bastis* are potential source of epidemics, malaria and other communicable diseases. Those responsible for creating these slums should be severely punished. If this is the state of affairs of a modern city, then what would be the condition of slums in Delhi, Bombay, Calcutta, Hyderabad and so on.

A survey was conducted by the Center for Indian Development Studies, for Municipal Corporation, Chandigarh, for the implementation of the Swaran Jayanti Shahari Rozgar Yojna (SJSRY) in the city, in 37 colonies of Chandigarh, of which 23 fall in the category of rehabilitated and 14 unauthorized ones on the government land, reveals that shortage of water, slushy conditions, lack of sanitation and drainage system, especially in unauthorized colonies, are the major problems ailing them.

We must take bold steps to save the city by providing alternate sites to the existing *bastis* and ban the creation of future slums.

An observation and case studies into the lives of people inhabiting slum areas reveal a pathetic scene, where it is difficult to watch horrible problems of people. These problems relate to the following areas:

1. Poverty.
2. Social evils like drinking, smoking, gambling, prostitution, etc.
3. Poor Health—Women mostly anemic, Children under developed, frequent pregnancies, poor health services.
4. Illiteracy—lack of education facilities, mostly illiterate.
5. Exploitation of women—Very low status of women, marriage mostly at the ages of 13-14-15, number of children high ranging from 3-5, works both for domestic services as well as maids to earn some money.
6. Poor housing causing tensions, lack of privacy, lack of safety of young girls, etc.
7. Lack of sanitation—Causing diseases and poor life.
8. Lack of potable water—They even do not get good water to drink causing many water borne diseases.
9. Poor Environment—The all around environment has been poor causing many health problems.

We have seen that people in urban areas living in slums or slums like places are faced with a large number of problems concerning their life. How to overcome them? How to provide good life to them? What should be done to provide them basic facilities needed for human beings? What has been the role of Government, NGOs and other agencies in providing them good life? The answer to these questions is simple, i.e. People living in these areas need to come together, to locate problems, find solutions and put them into action with the support of municipal bodies. This is known as urban participatory development. It is based on the premises that people both men and women and especially women, have the potentiality to solve their problems.

There is a continuous tug-of-war between city level authorities and the slum-dwellers and the battle line is continuously redrawn in the form of regularization of unauthorized colonies. This causes considerable stress on the city administration including law and order problems leading to considerable costs and inconvenience to the city population as a whole. In many cases, such unauthorized colonies are demolished or upgraded incurring huge costs. The city authorities undertake a sort of fire-fighting salvage operation from time to time incurring large expenditure. This cost is estimated to be many times more than the cost involved in habitating them by proper planning by reserving pre-planned land for this group of population. Past experience indicates that no amount of legal and regulatory mechanisms could stop movement of people in search of economic upliftment. What, therefore, is there to be done? More specifically, what our local governments do? Never in the history have there been such large urban agglomerations. Future emphasis must be on working out ways and means for interdependence between national and local units and between local governments with one another. It is realized that the solutions to slum-dwellers' problems can be found together with them.[11]

It is worthwhile to examine how our governments, specifically the urban local governments are dealing with this situation after five decades. The growth of slum population in these growing cities is so prolific that, our local governments have lost control of the deteriorating urban decay. In other words, the government organisations have generally found themselves largely ineffective to forge authentic partnership with the urban slum people in solving habitat-related issues.[12]

Role of Government in Improving Slums

Various Central Government Schemes—National Slum Development Programme (NSDP), Swarna Jayanti Shahri Rozgar Yojana (SJSRY), VAMBAY, Night Shelters, Two Million Housing Scheme, Accelerated Urban Water Supply Programme (AUWSP), Low-Cost Sanitation—provide for a wide range of services to the urban poor including slum-dwellers. They include identification of the urban poor, formation of community groups, involvement of non-government organisations (NGOs), self-help/thrift and credit activities, training for livelihood, credit and subsidy for economic activities, housing and sanitation, environmental improvement, community assets, wage employment, convergence of services, etc. What is needed is to ensure that the task of meeting the needs of the slum-dwellers is better organized and effectively administered, and duly monitored at both State and Central levels. There are also many instances of successful implementation of urban poverty alleviation/slum upgrading and services programmes in the Indian situation.

Guidelines for Special Central Assistance to States for Slum Improvement

The Government of India has introduced Special Central Assistance to States for upgradation of urban slums with the following elements:

- The scheme should be applicable to all the States and Union Territories having urban population.
- Funds are allocated to States on the basis of Urban slum population.

Components

- Physical amenities (water supply, storm water drains, street lights, etc.)
- Community Infrastructure centres for pre-school education, non-formal education, primary health care center, etc.
- Social Amenities like Pre-school education, non-formal education, adult education, maternity, child health, etc.
- Convergence between schemes being implemented by different line departments.
- Shelter upgradation or construction of new houses (including EWS) with minimum 10% of the allocation to States.
- State specific schemes for housing construction/upgradation with a mix of subsidy and loan component, sanctioned in a State-level Project Committee with one representative from the Department of UEPA, which is the nodal Department for this scheme in the GOI.

The focus is on community infrastructure, provision of shelter, and empowerment of urban poor women, training, skill upgradation and advocacy and involvement of NGOs, CBOs, Private institutions and other bodies. The scheme is applicable to all the States and Union Territories having urban population.

At the national level, Ministry of Urban Affairs and Employment is the nodal Ministry to monitor this programme. The Planning Commission in the beginning of each financial year allocates funds under this scheme and Department of Expenditure releases Additional Central Assistance to States/UTs.[13]

The Importance of Slum Upgrading

Action taken so far for slum improvement or *in-situ* upgrading is inadequate. Re-designing and re-constructing settlements with the participation of residents and assistance from public bodies is a viable option with the least amount of disturbance to the settlers or their livelihood. This method of slum improvement needs to be practised on a much wider scale. The VAMBAY Project permits *in-situ* upgradation, and it is necessary that an early decision is taken regarding land on which slums are situated in order to facilitate upgradation.[14]

Role of Urban Local Government-National Slum Policy prescribes the following role for local self-government:

Planning for Integration

(a) Modify Existing Planning Framework

All existing planning instruments such as Master Plans, Land Use Plans, etc. should be modified to ensure that slums and informal settlements can be properly integrated into the wider urban areas. In order to achieve this objective, it will be necessary to:

(i) Ensure that all Master Plans and Land Use Plans allow for high density; mixed use (for micro-enterprise) land occupation in all slums/informal settlements. This will ensure that every ULB designates sufficient and more appropriate (higher density lower cost) living and working space for the urban poor within the urban area.

(ii) Master Plans and Land Use Plans should also ensure that all new land development schemes make sufficient provision for land to house low income workers as required by such schemes.

(iii) All plans and other regulatory instruments must provide sufficient flexibility to modify layouts and building regulations in line with more realistic density/mixed use requirements.

The powers to implement such changes outlined in (i) to (iii) above should be vested in the ULBs, within parameters laid down by State governments.

(b) Integrated Municipal Development Plan (IMDP)

All ULBs should begin to work towards the formulation of an Integrated Municipal Development Plan. The principle objective of this plan is to ensure that the ULB has an adequate and sustainable level of infrastructure and services for all its residents and that such infrastructure and services are planned and delivered in an equitable manner. In order to achieve this objective it will be necessary to identify the capital and recurrent requirements and costs for the city as a whole (e.g. Bulk water supply) as well as the specific wards and neighbourhood within the city (secondary and tertiary water supply). The plan should prioritize ways and means of narrowing the gap between the better-serviced and less well serviced (slums) areas of the ULB.

(c) Convergence

The IMDP process assumes the implementation of the 74th Amendment and embodies the principle of convergence of activities and funds to achieve more efficient and equitable urban development. The IMDP will incorporate existing plans and reflect schemes and budget allocations as follows:

- Master Plans/Land Use Plans and other statutory instruments.
- Urban Development Plans and Schemes.
- Urban Poverty Alleviation Plans and Schemes.
- Department Plans and Schemes in the ULB area.

(d) Dynamic Multi-Year Planning

The IMDP, outlined in (b) above, should be undertaken as a dynamic process which will be updated and reviewed every three years. The overall plan should then be implemented through Annual Action Plans and budget allocations so that development work can be taken up in a phased manner. These Annual Action Plans should reflect plan priorities based on the level of service deprivation or service gaps pertaining in the wards and neighbourhood.

(e) Bottom-up Planning

Planning should begin at the micro-level with each urban poor area drawing up a list of existing services and identifying gaps and deficiencies. This activity should be undertaken by the community using participatory planning techniques and each plan should include a clear prioritization of needs and an indication of different stakeholder contributions towards costs. ULBs will be required to submit evidence of community participation in planning service provision.

ENVIRONMENTAL IMPROVEMENT

The provision of physical infrastructure components such as water supply, drainage, sanitation, improved access, electricity, etc. should support the ultimate objective of improved quality of life. The evidence from existing slum improvement projects clearly shows that an improved physical environment greatly facilitates the integration of the settlement in the wider urban area and at the same time, contributes to improved livelihoods and health and well-being of the community.

(a) Approach

(i) Community-based Approach

All physical upgrading and improvement in informal settlements should adopt a Community-based Approach with the active involvement of members of the community at every stage of design, implementation, and maintenance of services and assets. Community structures and systems should reflect local conditions and preferences rather than conform to any uniform pattern. Communities have an important role to play at all stages of service delivery in terms of location of the service points, day-to-day functioning of the service and guarding against its misuse. Communities should be encouraged to contribute land and resources to help establish community centres and to promote the collection of user charges to contribute to the operation of certain services.

(ii) Target Women and Children

There is a need to target women and children directly in the design and implementation of physical infrastructure and the delivery of social and economic services. Infrastructure users, especially the urban poor and women are central to the sustainability of any investment decisions related to infrastructure.

(iii) Service Delivery on Individual Household Basis

Wherever possible, the delivery of basic services such as water, sanitation and electricity should be provided on an individual household basis and may even precede the granting of full tenure rights. Individual connections will improve operations, maintenance, and facilitate recovery of user charges and thus improve the overall environment.

(iv) Contracting-out

Wherever possible works should be undertaken by communities/ CBOs under appropriate supervision of ULBs. Such works must be done according to departmental norms and procedures with proper muster rolls maintained and other stipulations to be observed. Services may also be contracted-out, where appropriate, to NGOs and other private companies. Solid waste management has already been successfully contracted-out by many ULBs. Similarly, the maintenance of pay and use toilets has also been contracted-out to NGOs and community-based organisations (CBOs). State enactments/procedures dealing with improvement works should be modified to allow the implementation of such works to be undertaken on a contract basis by the community/CBOs.

(b) Physical Infrastructure Development

The guiding principle and expected outcomes to be kept in focus while planning and implementing the following basic infrastructure and services are outlined as:

(i) Water Supply

Quantum, duration, timing and water quality are the four critical factors in planning water supply delivery. Dual and standby systems, such as piped supply supported by local hand-pumps should be considered as a means of helping to address these four factors.

Even where individual water tap connections are provided, it may be desirable to install hand-pumps or community storage facilities to offset poor frequency of supply and inadequate storage capacity at individual household level.

(ii) Sanitation

ULBs should avoid constructing community latrines within slum/informal settlements as these quickly degenerate on account of poor operations and maintenance (O & M) thus becoming counter-productive to public health. Where there is insufficient space for individual sanitation options (mostly where on-site disposal systems have to be adopted) groups or cluster latrines with clearly demarcated and agreed household responsibilities for O & M may be a suitable alternative option.

It is vital that any community-wide sanitation programme be preceded by an awareness campaign designed to raise demand for the implementation of specific sanitation options. This would greatly facilitate all subsequent O & M activities as would also assist the process of raising financial contributions. Many members of the community, especially male members, do not perceive sanitation, as a clear priority need. This needs to be addressed before embarking upon the installation of sanitation.

Considering the limitations on improving sanitation in many towns due to absence of underground drainage and sewerage systems, low cost sanitation options, particularly twin pit pour flush latrines may be a more appropriate and cost effective option for slums duly keeping environmental safeguards in mind. Efforts should be made to popularize and facilitate the introduction of such systems wherever appropriate. The tenurial status and likelihood of a settlement getting relocated at some point in the future should not deter promoting such systems since the benefits of such environmental improvement far exceed the initial investment incurred.

(iii) Pedestrian and Vehicular Access Ways

Paved access for pedestrians and/or vehicles will greatly improve overall accessibility. Paved access will encourage investment in the community and promote physical integration with neighbouring areas. It may also help to improve social integration within and between communities. Paved access will also greatly facilitate the introduction of other related infrastructure such as storm water drains, underground drainage water supply, electricity and collection/removal of garbage. Paving would also help in maintaining a clean environment and help reduce flooding and water stagnation. Paved access ways also facilitates the use of such facilities for social activity, extension of household activities and space for economic activity.

(iv) Storm Water Drains

Drains in slums serve the dual purpose of carrying sullage water from individual houses as well as draining storm water. It is crucial to integrate the outfalls of such drains with the city's main drainage system. The planning of slum drainage should be fully integrated into the planning of neighbouring systems as well as the city as a whole.

(v) Electricity

Individual house connections will greatly enhance the comfort and safety of living and working conditions for residents. The mere provision of street lighting without formal household connections leads to illegal tapping and loss of revenue and at the same time causes unplanned loading of the system and fire hazards. Community management systems for collection of user charges will facilitate improved revenue recovery and reduce revenue losses.

(vi) Solid Waste Collection

Sustained awareness campaigns and provision of waste collection receptacles will facilitate a cleaner environment. Urban Local Bodies could organize 'clean slum competitions' and institute prizes to create more awareness and encourage the community groups to maintain a clean environment within their localities. At community level, management systems that employ private sweepers by collecting monthly charges may also be adopted.

9. Improving Access to Social Services

Basic services of health, education and access to credit are crucial for human capital development and reduce the incidence of poverty. Improved access to social services would also help building up the capacities of poor and empowering them to improve their own living conditions and quality of life. Effective delivery of these services would also reduce social inequities and promote integration of people residing in slums into the social and economic networks of the city as a whole, thereby enhancing the overall productivity of the city. Various physical infrastructure components such as water supply and sanitation have a direct bearing on improving health conditions in slums. This section outlines a number of complementary services where ULBs should actively seek to improve access for the urban poor.

SUGGESTIONS

There is a continuous tug-of-war between city level authorities and the slum-dwellers and the battle line is continuously redrawn in the form of regularization of unauthorized colonies. This causes considerable stress on the city administration including law and order problems leading to considerable costs and inconvenience to the city population as a whole. In many cases, such unauthorized colonies are demolished or upgraded incurring huge costs. The city authorities undertake a sort of fire-fighting salvage operation from time to time incurring large expenditure. This cost is estimated to be many times more than the cost involved in habitating them by proper planning, by reserving pre-planned land for this group of population. Past experience indicates that no amount of legal and regulatory mechanisms could stop movement of people in search of economic upliftment. What, therefore, is there to be done? More specifically, what our local governments do? Never in the history have there been such large urban agglomerations. Future emphasis must be on working out ways and means for interdependence between national and local units and between local governments with one another. It is realized that the solutions to slum-dwellers' problems can be found together with them.[15]

It is worthwhile to examine how our governments, specifically the urban local governments are dealing with this situation after five decades. The growth of slum population in these growing cities is so prolific that, our local governments have lost control of the deteriorating urban decay. In other words, the government organisations have generally found themselves largely ineffective to forge authentic partnership with the urban slum people in solving habitat-related issues.[16]

2. Legislative Support

Legislative supports for slum improvement has been provided by the Slum Areas (Improvement and Clearance) Acts adopted by various States. The operation of the improvement schemes is made possible by statutory provisions in the Slum Act in those states, where it has been passed. The Act broadly provides the following powers:

(a) Power to the competent authority to declare an area to be slum area if the buildings in that area are unfit for human inhabitants or are detrimental to the safety of health or morals.
(b) The Act empowers the competent authority to serve notice upon the owner of a building or land in a slum area, to execute the works of improvement.
(c) Power to acquire land in a slum area to execute the improvement work.
(d) Protection to tenants in slum areas from eviction.
(e) Slum Improvement Boards were to be set-up under the Act to organize, supervise the work of slum improvement in the State.

3. Judicial Support

In a major judgment affecting at least 30 lakh people living in the Capital's slums, the Supreme Court has asked the authorities concerned to remove their shelters and stop further growth of unauthorized hutments on public land. It also asked the civic authorities to comply with the 10 directives, which are aimed at providing better hygiene, clean environment and ensuring that "the Capital of the biggest democracy in the world is not branded as being one of the most polluted cities in the World."

Passing strictures on the civic authorities, the court said: "Tolerating filth, while not taking action against the lethargic and inefficient work force for fear of annoying them, is un-understandable and impermissible." "The employees", the judges said, "were perhaps sanguine in their belief that non-performance is not frowned upon by the government or by the head of organisation and no harm will befall them."

On the mushrooming growth of the slums, the court said, "establishment or creating of slums, it seems, appears to be good business and is well organized. Large areas of public land, in this way, are usurped for private use free of cost. It is difficult to believe that this can happen in the Capital without passive or active connivance of the land-owning agencies and/or the municipal authorities."

4. People's Participation

Participatory development is not an attempt to replace the top-down development approach with slum-dwellers/low income participation. Rather, it should stress the need for the government participation in terms of national-level economic planning and coordination of development planning and the demerits of widening disparities and worsening poverty inherent in slum-dwellers. Participatory development attempts to introduce a bottom-up style of development in order to remedy the government approach's shortcomings, specifically by focusing on qualitative improvements in slum-dweller's participation.[17]

5. Taxing the Beneficiaries

Most of the Services in urban slums are free of cost. The slum dwellers can contribute in a small way, which should be tapped. This would add to the resources to make slum life better as well as create interest among slum-dwellers, when they spend their own money.

The environmental improvement scheme is based on total subsidy from the Central Government. The promise of public grants, which is a corollary to the declaration of an area "as slum often encourages the inclusion of settlements belonging to middle income households also." In some cases private land has been illegally sub-divided and sold by owners to circumvent the Urban Land Ceiling Act, they managed to get the area declared as slum. The area was subsequently improved at Government cost. In such cases beneficiaries of government subsidy are certainly not the "Urban Poor." Even in square settlements, there are significant number of households, who can afford and are willing to pay for improvements, which they want. The study of popular settlements in Bhopal confirms this (Risbud, Neelima, 1987).

Resource mobilization from beneficiaries has not at all been explored and Slum Improvement Programme is offered as a welfare action. This has gradually shaped people's attitude of expecting everything free of cost from

Government. This is further strengthened, when the politicians condone the recoveries. Credit available for improvement from Housing and Urban Development Corporation (HUDCO) and World Bank requires recovery and minimization of subsidy. In some cities all the three programmes are implemented simultaneously in different settlements (e.g. in Indore, the Environmental Improvement Schemes, the HUDCO aided schemes and World Bank- aided schemes, all are operative).[18]

CONCLUSION

We have to cease presenting slum-dwellers and squatters as a total liability to the city. In most of today's mushrooming cities, the work force living in peripheral areas has become an essential and irreplaceable component of the urban economy.[19]

Urban slums are a slur on the face of the modern civilization. There is a need to help the slum-dwellers to lead a decent life since they are doing a lot for the development of the city.

Notes and References

1. WHO: Dr. Layi Egunjobi, Tackling Africa's Slums, *World Health*, March-April, 1991, p. 14.
2. Puri, K.K., "Urbanization and Slums: A Dimensional Analysis", in "Revamping Urban Governments in India", edited by Dr. Pardeep Sachdeva, New Delhi, Kitab Mahal, p. 43.
3. Sanganal, Ashok, "Participation of Slum-Dwellers in Urban Governance", *Shelter*, Vol. III, No. 1, p. 35.
4. Gurumukhi, K.T., "Slum-Related Policies and Programmes", *Shelter*, Vol. 3, No. 2, April 2000, pp. 57-58.
5. Goel, S.L., "Planning and Administration of Urban Basic Services: A Case Study of Una (H.P.)" in "Development Planning and Administration", Ed. S. Bhatnagar and S.L. Goel, pp. 167-68.
6. Government of India, Planning Commission, "Tenth Five Year Plan (2002-07", Volume II, Sectoral Policies and Programmes, pp. 627-28.
7. *The Hindustan Times*, 24 December, 1999.
8. *Shelter*, Vol. III, No. 1, p. 35.
9. *Ibid.*, p. 42.
10. Risbud, Neelima, "Slum Improvement in India—Some Issues", *Delhi Vikas Patra*, p. 27.
11. *Shelter*, Vol. VIII, No. 1, pp. 36-37.
12. *Ibid.*, p. 36.
13. Annual Report, 2002-03, Ministry of Urban Affairs and Employment, Government of India.
14. *Shelter*, Vol. VIII, No. 1, pp. 36-37.
15. *Shelter*, Vol. VIII, No. 1, pp. 36-27.
16. *Ibid.* p. 36
17. WHO: Dr. John Clements and Dr. Diana Silimperi, Immunizing the Children of Poverty, *World Health*, March-April, pp. 18-20.
18. *Shelter*, Vol. III, No. 1, p. 43.
19. Risbud, Neelima, Delhi Vikas Patra, p. 28.

19

CHAPTER

Population Explosion Disaster

The growing imbalance between the available resources and accelerating pace of population growth is frightening. As per United Nations projection, the world population by 2025 AD will cross 850 crore and a major chunk of this growth will be recorded in the countries of Africa and South Asia. It should be a matter of concern for us that India, occupying a meagre 2.4 per cent of its population and with each passing year a staggering 1.8 crore people are being added to our already bloated population base. At this rate of adding one Australia to our population each year, India is surely going to overtake China by 2040 AD.[1]

The existing and growing population is disturbing the population equilibrium, as the existing earth cannot accommodate the growing numbers resulting in large number of environment problems leading to disaster.

PROBLEM OF NUMBERS

Centre can't Abdicate its Responsibility

The Planning Commission's observations against the Union Ministry of Health and Family Welfare for its failure to implement various projects and initiatives for population control are alarming. In a paper, *Yojna Bhavan* has voiced concern on the increasing population growth and feared that the situation would worsen by 2015 if remedial steps were not taken. Clearly, the Union Ministry's lackadaisical attitude is deplorable because it is expected to play a leadership role in executing various birth control schemes. If it does not take the initiative, show dynamism and direction, how would it convince the states about the crucial need for population control?[2]

Genesis of Population Growth in India

Socio-Economic Implications of Population Explosion

The growth rate in population absorbs the national income and lowers the standard of living. The world population conference indicated in the population plans of action that population growth and population policy must be viewed not in isolation, but in the context of development. It was mentioned by the Secretary-General that "Current and potential worldwide population trends evidently cannot continue for as long as even one century without causing serious dislocations and crises in many areas."[3]

Myrdal in his book, "Asian Drama" gave a stern warning to the world in regard to population explosion when he said, "Demographers are of the view that if fertility does not decrease, a time will come when mortality will lose its relative independence of levels of living and begin to rise again."[4]

Family planning programmes have led to a considerable decrease in average family size in developing countries: from 6.1 children per woman in the early 1960s to 3.9 today. Yet this is still far higher than the average of 2.1 children per woman at which level the population would stop growing. Actual numbers continue to increase. The population of developing countries has doubled in the same period, reaching 4100 million in 1990. It is predicted to rise to 5000 million by 2000, out of an optimistic forecast of a world total of 6300 million.

This poses enormous challenges in terms of providing the food, water, energy and services required to support such numbers, let alone improve their quality of life. For the health sector, the sheer numbers magnify the burden of disease. More training, facilities and funding will be needed for all services, including family planning.[5]

In view of this alarming situation, an urgent call was made by the representatives of the national academies of science throughout the world at an unprecedented "Science Summit" on World Population in New Delhi, India, on 24-27 October 1993. The participants, in a joint statement, asked for immediate action by governments and decision-makers to adopt an integrated policy on population and sustainable development on a global scale. They hoped that the Statement would reach the attention of governments and peoples of all countries and contribute to further discourse and appropriate policy decisions on these complex but critically important matters, and provide scientific input into preparations for the International Conference on Population and Development.

The Statement declared: "Humanity is approaching a crisis point with respect to the interlocking issues of population, environment, and development. Scientists today have the opportunity and responsibility to mount a concerted effort to confront our human predicament. But science and technology can only provide tools and blueprints for action and social change. It is the governments and international decision-makers, including those meeting in Cairo in September 1994 at the United Nations International Conference on Population and Development, who hold the key to our future.

> "We urge them to take incisive action now and to adopt an integrated policy on population and sustainable development on a global scale. With each year's delay the problems become more acute. Let 1994 be remembered as the year when the people of the world decided to act together for the benefit of future generations."

Signed by representatives of 58 academies, the Statement reflects continued concern about the intertwined problems of rapid population growth, wasteful resource consumption, environmental degradation and poverty. The academies believe that ultimate success in dealing with global social, economic and environmental problems cannot be achieved without a stable world population. The Statement underscored the goal of reaching zero population growth within the lifetime of our children.

One of the main conclusions reached was that sustainability of the natural world is everyone's responsibility, including individuals, communities, private institutions, governments, non-governmental organisations and the international community.

Among the major recommendations are:

- Equal opportunities for women and men in sexual, social and economic life so they can make individual choices about family size;
- Universal access to convenient family planning and health services, and a wide variety of safe and affordable contraceptive options; and
- Encouragement of voluntary approaches to family planning, and elimination of unsafe and coercive practices.

The Statement ended by declaring: "Action is needed Now."[6]

Thus, there is a great need of stabilising population. According to Frank W. Notestein:

> "The ultimate goal of the worlds population policy must be to achieve an equilibrium based on low birth and death rates that can be sustained throughout a distant future for the world and its several parts."[7]

As long as the birth rate is not restricted in these countries, it would not be possible to bring about improvements in the living standard of the people.

In a 'capital poor' and technologically backward country, growth of population diminished the rate of capital accumulation, increases the amount of disguised unemployment and lowers the standards of living of the people, i.e., resources go to the formation of population, not capital. According to Prof. A.W. Singir, population growth has a negative effect on the rate of economic development. According to him:

$$D = SP - r$$

where D = rate of economic development,
S = rate of net savings,
P = productivity of new investment, and
r = rate of increase in population.

In the above equation, r appears as a negative factor with a minus sign.

"Population growth is an important variable determining the rate of improvement in per capita income."[8] P.B. Desai analysis this problem in its broader context. To quote him, "We must, however, emphasize that the impact of rapid population increase is not limited to the enlargement of the denominator of the ratio of national product and national population. It is much more pervasive. It is quite plausible that its absence would have made a positive contribution to the growth of national product. Besides, creating the imperative of demographic investment required to prevent deterioration in the levels of living, it has served to increase the dependency load, tended to undermine the achievement of predetermined composition of the national product, hampered the path of changes in the structure of its economy warranted by development, and led in all probability, to accentuation of the imbalances in the regional as well as in the rural-urban distribution of population. Implications of rapid population growth should thus appear to be more serious.[9]

Let us examine the impact of population growth on the socio-economic development.

I. Offset Economic Growth

Thomas Mathur has rightly mentioned that population explosion offsets economic growth. To quote him:

> "The increasing population has been eating into the gains of economic growth. While the net national product at constant prices increased by 165 per cent, the per capita income went up by only 45 per cent. That this Yawning chasm between the growth of national product and per capita income is the direct result of the prolific increase in population needs no elaboration."[10]

The population growth requires more investment while the population rise reduces the capacity of the people to save. This creates a serious gap between investment requirements and the availability of investible funds resulting in the low rate of growth of an economy.

CHART 19.1

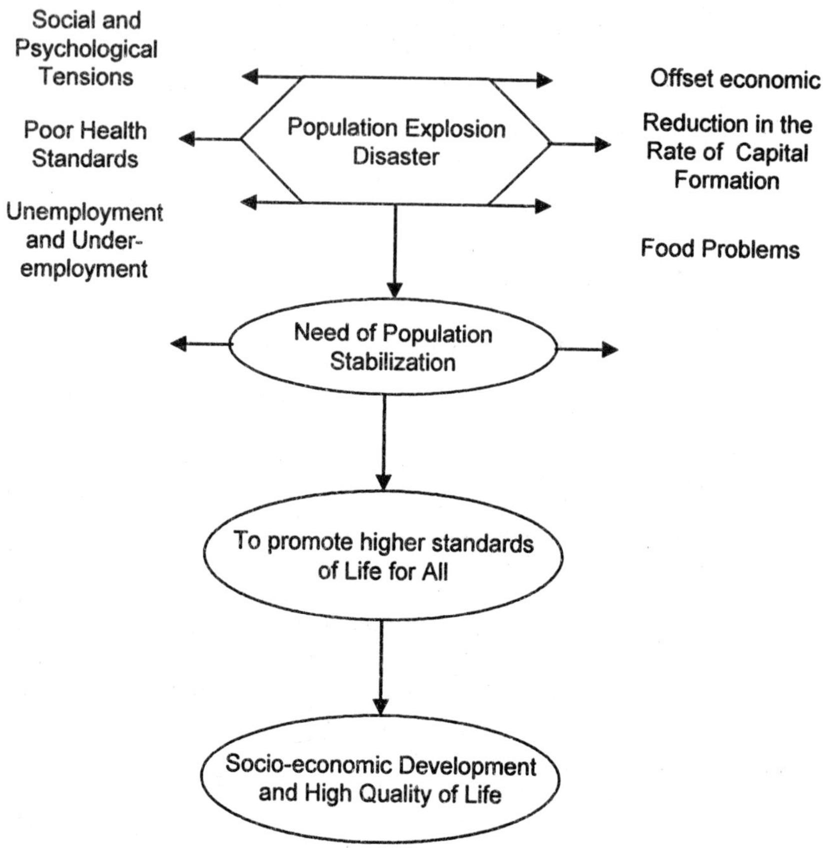

According to Coale and Hoover, "The significant feature of population as such is that a higher rate of population growth implies a higher level of needed investment to achieve a given per capita output; while there is nothing about faster growth that generates a great supply of investible resources."[11]

2. Reduction in the Rate of Capital Formation

The composition of the people in underdeveloped countries (40-50 per cent of the population in unproductive age-group) is such that it reduces the capacity of the people to save which affects the rate of capital formation. According to Prof. Meier, "This high dependency requires the economy to divert a considerable part of its resources, that might otherwise go into capital formation, to the maintenance of high percentage of dependents who may never become producers or, if so, only for relatively short working life."[12] Recognizing this, the Third Plan States:

"In an underdeveloped economy with very little capital per person, a high rate of population growth makes it even more difficult to step up the rate of saving which, in turn, largely determines the possibility of achieving higher productivity and incomes. Moreover, for a given investment, a larger proportion will need to be devoted to the reduction of essential consumer goods at the expense of investment goods industries thereby still further slowing down the potential rate of growth."[13]

3. Food Problem

Food is an essential item of consumption for human survival. The demand of food is rising faster than the production of food. In a study carried out by Food and Agricultural Organisation, it was found that the failure of food production to keep up with population growth was especially pronounced in the case of the developing countries. Out of the total of 106 countries studied, 72 were classified as developing; but in 24 of these (or one-third) food production lagged behind the growth of population. In the more recent period, it was mentioned; the situation was even less favourable. In India, Food Production increased from 51 million tones to 151 million tones between 1950-51 and 1983-84 giving an increase of three times. During the same period, the population has doubled. However, per capita availability of food grains has not increased much.

4. Unemployment and Underemployment

The result of more population would affect the employment situation as there is already a back-log of unemployment and underemployment in these countries. The growing unemployment of these countries is not only an economic but it is also a social evil.

5. Poor Health Standards

Family Planning and Health are intimately-related. Family planning can promote women's health through the prevention of unwanted pregnancies, limiting number of births, and proper spacing, timing of births and foetal health. Family planning also promotes the health of the child through the reduction of child mortality, and promotion of the child development. Maryellen Fullam stresses the importance of family planning as instrument for the promotion of health. He says:

"Uncontrolled fertility directly threatens the health of mothers and infants and may undermine the health of other family members. Today, no health programme can be considered complete unless it offers ready access to the appropriate family planning measures for all potential parents."[15]

Angile Petros-Barvazian in his Article, "Family Planning a Preventive Health Measure" in *World Health* (June 1984) has rightly mentioned that the effects of unregulated fertility of births to women who are too young or too old, of closely spaced births and of high parity births—make themselves felt very early in life, often even before birth, in high foetal and neonatal death rates. In many developing countries, deaths in the first months of life make up the major portion of infant mortality. The indirect effects of unregulated fertility—through infection and malnutrition—tend to make themselves felt later. Family Planning has an important contribution to make in reducing all the above mentioned risks. . . . Pregnancy makes heavy demands on a woman and too closely spaced pregnancies that do not allow enough time for her body to recover may lead to maternal depletion. This is particularly marked under conditions of deprivation and shows itself in fatigue, depression and a general lowering of health status which may result in higher reproductive risk. Many chronic hygaecological conditions which cause long-term ill-health and suffering increase with the number of pregnancies that the woman has. Debilitating conditions such as prolapsed uterus add to the burden of women with large families. Reductions in the number of high-risk pregnancies, brought about largely through family planning, have substantially lowered mortality in many countries, compared with about 10 in the U.S. and U.K. Family Planning can prevent maternal mortality because it can help couples a void high-risk pregnancies.

Professor Fraser Brockington has rightly said that over-population affects the health of the community, physically and mentally. It undermines physical health by increasing the risks of infection and by the most subtle, but more powerful influence of malnutrition; by shortening life; by disrupting the family through deaths of its younger members; by damaging the health of the child bearing population through frequent pregnancies without corresponding gain; by denying the community many of the essentials of health. Mental health suffers because of the hopelessness of life in circumstances where there exist neither house-room, food, well-being, nor any of the essentials which make a life of fulfilment and purpose possible."[16]

A recent UN report on World Population Trends, Vol. I (1983) has rightly concluded that in many developing countries, rapid population growth is considered to be a matter of great concern and programmes to reduce fertility have been given high priority. Furthermore, it is now well documented that family planning can favourably influence the health, development and well-being of the family, particularly mothers and children.

In a population Report, it has been rightly said that family planning is an effective way to prevent maternal and infant mortality because family planning can help couples avoid high risk pregnancies. Evidence from around the world shows that the risk of maternal or infant illness and death is highest in four specific types of pregnancy:

(a) Pregnancies before age 18,
(b) Pregnancies after age 35,

(c) Pregnancies after four births, and
(d) Pregnancies less than two years apart.

In developing countries, about 6.6 million infant deaths and 200,000 maternal deaths could be avoided if women choose to have their children within the safest years. This amount to about half of the estimated 10.5 million infant deaths and 450,000 maternal deaths now occurring.

6. Social and Psychological Tensions

Rapid population growth leads to social and psychological tensions, and breakdown of a distribution system. Civil amenities such as water and power supply, housing, transport and social utilities like schooling, educational, health and medical services fall much short of demand inspite of their constant expansion. Besides, it leads to political and social corruption and accentuates economic disparities. The frequency of communal riots or clashes has increased. There has always been a clash between landowning class and landless labourers resulting sometimes into armed struggle. Because of competition in urban life, people fall to many social risks like gambling, prostitution, etc.

Thus, we can say that the problem of growing population has reached such menacing proportions that it has become a real threat to the socio-economic stability of the country. The excessive growth in population does not affect the stability of the national economy alone, it disturbs the stability of the entire body politic. It poses a colossal threat to our social structure. In our fight against poverty, disease, hunger, malnutrition and unemployment, checking the rapid growth of population is as raising production in the farms and factories and provision of social services. Population control is one of the chief issues which the country has to resolve and accord top priority in its march towards social and economic development.

The programme of family planning is of vital importance for our country. It is a positive and constructive approach to the betterment of the quality of life of the community. Thus, it is evident that the key to India's economic future based on social justice lies in the immediate and effective implementation of a nation-wide population programme.

The experiences and lessons gained from Indian Planning suggests that effective population control, designed to restore the balance between vital rates by reducing the level of fertility, has a positive influence on the process of economic development and modernization. An eminent scholar has rightly mentioned that "A reduction infertility would make the process of modernization more rapid and more certain. It would accelerate the growth of income, provide more rapidly the possibility of productive employment of all adults who need jobs, make the attainment of universal education easier and it would have the obvious and immediate effect of providing the women of low income countries some relief from constant pregnancy, porturition and infant care."[17]

L.R. Brown in his book on "Twenty-two Dimensions of the Population Problem", Washington, D.C., 1976 "has given twenty-two dimensions" of the population problem which underlines the need for the control of population growth. Important of them are:

(i) Hunger
(ii) Housing
(iii) Crowding
(iv) Environmental Illness
(v) Income
(vi) Urbanization
(vii) Political Conflict
(viii) Health Services
(ix) Water
(x) Unemployment
(xi) Energy
(xii) Individual Freedom
(xiii) Literacy
(xiv) Natural Recreation Areas
(xv) Pollution
(xvi) Inflation

With a population of about one billion, India has achieved many dubious distinctions. Now India is a country with largest number of unemployed youth, handicapped people, beggars, slum-dwellers and illiterates in the world. The population of illiterates in India is larger than the total population of any country in the world except for People's Republic of China. Every third illiterate in the world is an Indian. It is irony that in all these areas India, come what may, will lead the world for many more years to come. It is pity indeed that in near future we will be able to achieve a few more dubious demographic distinctions.[18]

What has happened elsewhere can happen in India too provided there is a massive campaign to educate eligible couples, particularly in villages, about the benefits of limiting the size of the family. This point has of course been emphasized innumerable times and at different places but it has never been sincerely implemented. Rural people, steeped in ignorance and obsolete religious belief, still do not know the harm that big family size brings to them and consider every child as a gift of God. This notion must be altered if family planning is to succeed. However, the education campaign must always be backed by easy availability of modern contraceptive measures that can enable people to plan their families. One of the reasons why family planning measures have not yielded the desired results is that it has not been honestly implemented. The unmet need for family planning has been reported to be quite high. According to the National Family Health Survey 2, the current unmet need for family planning is 16 per cent and it is higher in rural areas than in urban areas.[19]

If the country opts for a natural course of demographic transition, then it will have to pay a heavy price in the form of unmanageable unemployment, rampant poverty, political chaos leading to ethnic violence and even dismemberment of the country in the long-run. In fact, the whole South Asia would have no encounter a similar experience and would take the shape of Africa or Europe in terms of number of independent nations fighting among themselves. Here the process have already set in, as the population bomb has already exploded. It is altogether a different matter that some of us at the helm of affairs deliberately tend to camouflage the reality or do not want to recognize it. Some of them even ignore the description of dismal demographic scenario of India by branding it a pure academic exercise. Even many Indian social scientists seem blissfully unaware of how rising population of India threatens its future, while the population issues have already started dominating India's future. One simply wonders whether new advancements in science and technology will really do any magic to save India from impending disaster following population explosion.[20]

Before, we discuss the genesis and growth of Family Planning Programme in India let us understand the meaning of Family Planning Programme.

Meaning

Family Planning Programme makes a planned and scientific approach to the issues and problems of family life and attempts to solve them to make the family lie happier, harmonious and fruitful. Family planning was though of as a public health problem. It was stated in the First Five Year Plan.

It is apparent that population at a level consistent with the requirement of national economy should be established. This can be secured only by the realization of the need for family limitation on a wide scale by the people. The main appeal for planning is based on considerations of health and welfare of the family. Family limitation or spacing of the children is necessary and desirable in order to secure better health of the mothers, and better care and upbringing of children. The measures described to this end should, therefore, form part of the public health programme.

A distinction must be made between population control and family planning. Population control is influenced and determined by a government policy motivated by socio-economic considerations. Family planning, on the other hand is a responsibility of the family. Who has given various definitions of family planning.

An Expert Committee (1971)[21] of the WHO defined family planning as "a way of thinking and living that is adopted voluntarily upon the basis of knowledge, attitudes and responsible decisions by individuals and couples, in order to promote the health and welfare of the family group and thus contribute effectively to the social development of the country."

Mr. Ramkrishna Mukherjee has defined family planning in broader and narrower context. In broader context, he says that:

(i) It is not matter of mere biological arrangement between a man and woman, albeit in the "social" setting of a family.
(ii) It is not exclusively a "cultural" issue: culture defined as an aggregate of what a person or group of persons desires and detests in every-day life, the aggregate being formed, from the past upto date in the course of socialization and, thus, provides the person or the group with a matrix of perception of life itself.
(iii) It is a matter of systematic understanding of the human kind with reference to the world as a whole and not merely one of its sectors: The Third World.

In the narrower sense, he says, that family planning is regarded as a managerial issues particularly relevant to the Third World. It involves the following measures:

(a) Propagation of appropriate slogans for a "small family";
(b) Funding family planning centres for sterilization; and
(c) Distribution of contraceptives and education of the people to use them for their own good.

Another Expert Committee (1971)[22] defined and described family planning as follows: "Family Planning refers to practices that help individuals or couples to attain certain objectives:

(a) to avoid unwanted births;
(b) to bring about wanted births;
(c) to regulate the intervals between pregnancies;
(d) to control the time at which births occur in relation to the age of the parents; and
(e) to determine the number of children in the family."

The following definition of reproductive health, approved last April by the WHO Global Policy Council, provides the basis for action in this field:

- "Within the framework of WHO's definition of health as a state of complete physical, mental and social well-being, and not merely the absence of disease or infirmity, reproductive health addresses the reproductive processes, functions and system at all stages of life."
- "Reproductive health implies that people are able to have a responsible, satisfying and safe sex life and that they have the capability to reproduce and the freedom to decide if, when and

how often to do so. Implicit in this last condition are the right of men and women to be informed of and to have access to safe, effective, affordable and acceptable methods of fertility regulation of their choice, and the right of access to appropriate health care services that will enable women to go safely through pregnancy and childbirth and provide couples with the best chance of having a healthy infant."

Reproductive health must address, as its basic elements, sexual behaviour, family planning, maternal care and safe motherhood, abortion, reproductive tract infections (including sexually transmitted diseases and HIV/AIDS), and certain reproductive tract malignancies such as cervical cancer.[23]

Dr. H. Mahler, ex-Director General of WHO has rightly said in *World Health* (June 1984) that in all societies, the family in one form or another is the Central nucleus for people, for their lives, their loves, their dreams and their health. So the people must be helped to understand that it is in their own interest to plan their families. And when they want to plan their family, appropriate information and services must be available in a context that provides confidence and security. Clearly what most parents want are healthy children who will grow upto become healthy adults. Today, it is possible for families through the use of technically and culturally appropriate contraceptive means to choose the timing and spacing of their children, and thus to complement other traditionally accepted means of child spacing such as breast-feeding. And quite apart from the positive health effects of family planning, the ability of couples to control their own fertility has opened the way for women to achieve the full and equitable participation in social and economic development that is their due.

There is an urgent need to increase the available financial resources and to change family planning policies:

- By incorporating the awareness that the sexual relationship is one that empowers people at different levels. Everything suggests that the most effective solution is to increase the negotiating power of women.
- By re-evaluating family planning methods on a basis of the risks of HIV infection, either because the methods do not prevent it or because they increase the risks. For example, the IUD presents a risk by facilitating pelvic infections. In Brazil, the high rate of tubal ligations makes women more vulnerable, since they find it harder to insist on a barrier method when there is no longer any need for contraception.

It is vitally urgent to give priority to methods that combine contraception with prevention of sexually transmitted disease. Barrier methods, which help to prevent an unwanted pregnancy as well as these diseases and cervical cancer, must be given priority if we are committed to the sexual and reproductive health of women—indeed of the whole human race.

A healthy reproductive life is essential to attain the goals set for infant and child survival. Reproductive health specifically implies that people have the ability to reproduce, to regulate their fertility and to practise and enjoy sexual relationships. Greater spacing of births would substantially reduce worldwide child mortality, while the increased chances of newborn babies surviving will eventually influence couples to reduce the size of the family, and this will contribute to lower population growth.

To provision of information, guidance and support to enable people to enjoy a healthy, safe and fulfiled sexuality is a fundamental responsibility of any truly comprehensive health care system. Equipping individuals with the knowledge and ability to protect themselves, their partner or their family from the potential hazards of unsafe sexuality has always been important, but with increasing exposure to sexually transmitted diseases, especially among young adults, and the spread of HIV/AIDS, the need to promote healthy sexuality has become urgent.

In addition, the loosening of traditional constraints on sexual behaviour as a result of chaotic urban growth, migration, conflicts, disasters or social and economic degradation make it all the more vital for health policies to take steps to promote healthy sexuality to prevent the spread of disease. Health and population policies must respond to the needs of individuals and communities for information, support, and counselling on sexuality, as these are all integral components of ensuring the health of individuals and families.[24]

In *World Health* (June 1984), it is correctly stated that healthy families do not just happen they are planned. The birth of a healthy wanted child is a joyous occasion. A child is chance of being born healthy, of surviving the first few years of life and growing well are enhanced if parents plan their children, so that they are born not before the mother is 18 or after she is 35—at least 2 years apart. Family improves the health of women by helping them avoid high-risk pregnancies."

The current high population growth rate in some parts of the country is due to:

- The large size of population in the reproductive age group (estimated contribution 60%).
- Higher fertility due to unmet need for contraception (estimated contribution 20%).
- High wanted fertility due to prevailing high infant mortality rate (IMR) (estimated contribution about 20%).

A look at the census figures of the last four decades indicates a perceptible decline in recent years, in the growth rate of the country's population. However, it is very high as compared to the countries of the world.

Deep-rooted customs, traditions and socio-cultural beliefs favour large family size in many parts of the country and impede the process of change which would accelerate the willing adoption of the small family norm. As per National Family Health Survey-II, 72% of couples with two children and 84% of couples with three children are either sterilized or do not want more children. Socio-economic factors such as female literacy, age at marriage of girls, status of women, strong son preference and position of employment of women have a crucial bearing on the fertility behaviour of the people.[25]

As per Census-2001 Report, the growth in indices of GDP and food production has been more than the growth in population as shown in the Chart 19.1.

Initially, planners placed greater thrust on population control measure but later, the significance of addressing issues pertaining to Child and Mother Health was recognized. During the Sixth Five Year Plan (1980-85), Government of India adopted a National Health Policy with the aim of achieving "Health For All by year 2000" and undertook to develop a primary health care system as an integral part of this strategy. Universal Immunization Programme (UIP), Oral Rehydration Therapy (ORT) and safe motherhood programme were introduced nationwide during the Seventh Five Year Plan (1985-90). Under the Eighth Five Year Plan, achieving a slower rate of population growth was considered as one of the most important priorities facing the nation. During Ninth Five Year Plan, focus was on reduction in the population growth, mortality and achieving desired level of fertility. During the Tenth Five Year Plan (2002-07), the main approach of the family welfare programme will be to provide need-based, client centered and demand driven RCH care; to strengthen the infrastructure for service delivery and bridging the gap in essential infrastructure and manpower; providing additional assistance to poorly performing districts identified on the basis of the 1991 census and RCH Surveys and ensuring uninterrupted supply of essential drugs and contraceptives; and promoting male participation in the planned Parenthood.

The Tenth Five Year Plan has identified the following monitorable targets relating to the Department of Family Welfare for the Plan (2002-07) and beyond:

- Reduction in the decadal rate of population growth between 2001 and 2011 to 16.2%.
- Reduction in Infant Mortality Rate (IMR) to 45 per thousand live birth by 2007 and 28 by 2012.
- Reduction in Maternal Mortality Ratio (MMR) to 2 per thousand live births by 2007 and 1 by 2012.

The Current Scenario in respect of these targets is as follows:

- The decadal growth rate of population has declined from 23.86% during 1981-91 to 21.34% during the decade 1991-2001.
- Infant Mortality Rate, which has been stagnant at a level of 70 during the 90s, has started showing a decline and currently it has been estimated to be 68 (SRS, 2000).
- Maternal Mortality Ratio has been stagnant during the 90s and the current estimate of this indicator is 407 per 100,000 live births (SRS, 1998).

To assessing the sources of pollution in this subcontinent, the principal factor appears to be overpopulation. Due to the monstrous rate of increase in population, there has been a heavy demand on natural resources including the soil, air and water; the floral and faunal wealth, resulting in a serious disbalance in the ecological system. Deforestation—a major factor for pollution—is the direct result of the demand on natural resources. The mechanics for the production of energy has been responsible for the discharge of by-products, affecting simultaneously human health and environment, in all the principal cities and industrial centres of India, the air is contaminated with a high level of chemical pollutants. The problems of sanitation, impurities in water and food grain, affecting human health due to chronic exposure are some of the major contributors to environmental pollution. The saying that "God helps those who rise early", is undoubtedly applicable to our urban population since the availability of pure air is restricted mostly to the early morning hours.[26]

NATIONAL POPULATION POLICY

India adopted a comprehensive and holistic National Population Policy (NPP), 2000 with clearly articulated objectives, strategic themes and operational strategies. The Policy enumerates certain socio-demographic goals to be achieved by 2010, which will lead to achieving population stabilization by 2045. The Policy also prescribes an Action Plan for implementing the strategic themes listed in the Policy.

The National Population Policy, 2000 has identified the immediate objectives as meeting the unmet needs for contraception, health care infrastructure and trained health personnel and to provide integrated service delivery, with the following interventions: (i) Strengthen community health centres, primary health centres and sub-centres; (ii) Augment skills of health personnel and health care providers; (iii) Bring about convergence in the implementation of related social sector programme so that the Family Welfare Programme becomes a peoples' programme; (iv) Integrate package of essential services at village and household level through mobile clinics and counselling services; and (v) Explore the possibility of accrediting private medical practitioners and revive the system of licensed medical practitioners, who could provide specified clinical services.

S.P. Singh in his Article, "Problems of Population and Sustainable Development in India" in *IJPA*, January-March 2003, observed that, with a population of about one billion, India has achieved many dubious distinctions. Now India is a country with largest number of unemployed youth, handicapped people, beggars, slum-dwellers and illiterates in the world. The population of illiterates in India is larger than the total population of any country in the world except for People's Republic of China. Every third illiterate in the world is an Indian. It is irony that in all these areas India, come what may, will lead the world for many more years to come. It is pity indeed that in near future we will be able to achieve a few more dubious demographic distinction.

To quote S.P. Singh again, "According to the provisional results of the 2001 Census, India's population stood 1,027 million on March 1, 2001, comprising 531 million males and 496 million females. From 361 million at the time of Independence the population reached one billion in 2001, registering an increase of nearly three times. All this had happened when the country is not in a position to guarantee adequate nutrition, health-care and education to the burgeoning population. At the same time, it is also true that all this has happened because of mass poverty in the country. Indifferent governance is also partly responsible for the current demographic and health scenario. Every year about 18 million people were added to India's population during 1991-2001 as against 16 million annually during 1981-91. In other words, each year India's population increases by the equivalents of the number of inhabitants of Ghana, Australia, Mozambique or Saudi Arabia."

NOTES AND REFERENCES

1. Seema Sengupta, *The Sunday Tribune*, Chandigarh, November 7, 2004.
2. *The Tribune*, Chandigarh, Thursday, July 15, 2004.
3. UN: E.F.s. 75, XIII, 4, p. 76.
4. Gunnar Myrdal, Asian Drama: An Inquiry into the Poverty of Nations, Vol. III, London, 1968, p. 154.
5. WHO: Alexander Kessler, Family Planning and the Role of WHO, *World Health*, May-June, 1994, p. 5.
6. WHO: Leila Mehra, *World Health*, May-June, 1994, p. 7.
7. Frank Notestein, W., "Population Policy and Development, a Summary View", *Population Debate*, Vol. I, Part Four, Para 5.
8. Fourth Five Year Plan, *op. cit.*, p. 31.
9. P.B. Desai, "Economic Development and Population Control" in *Aspects of Population Policy in India*, Council for Social Development, New Delhi, 1969, p. 11.
10. Thomas Mathur: "India's Population: The Worsening Senario" in *Yojna*, Vol. 30, No. 19, Oct. 16-31, 1986, p. 4.
11. Coale and Hoover, Population Growth and Economic Development in Low Income Countries, 1958, p. 19.
12. Geral Meier, Leading Issues in Economic Development, OUP, 1975, p. 591.

13. GOI Planning Commission, Third Five Year Plan, p. 22.
14. FAO: Population, Food Supply and Agricultural Development, *Population Debate*, Vol. I, Part Four, para 8.
15. *Maryellen Fullan in People*—a Journal of the Internationals Planned Parenthood Federation, Vol. 5, Number 4, 1978, p. 27.
16. P.F. Brockington: "The Health of the Developing World", The Buh Guild Limited, Lewes, 1985, p. 94.
17. Ansley J. Coale, "Population and Economic Development", in Philip M. Hauser (ed.): *The Population Dilemma*, p. 69.
18. *Indian Journal of Public Administration*, Vol. XLIX, No. 1, January-March 2003, p. 88.
19. For detailed information on this issue see the findings of the National Family Health Surveys I and II, India: Introductory Report, Mumbai, International Institute for Population Science, 1994 and 2000.
20. *Indian Journal of Public Administration*, Vol. XLIX, No. 1, January-March 2003, p. 94.
21. WHO, (1971) Techn. Rep. Ser., No. 483.
22. WHO, (1971) Techn. Rep. Ser., No. 476.
23. WHO, Reproductive Health, *World Health*, May-June 1994, p. 30.
24. WHO, 47th Year, No. 3, May-June 1994, pp. 15 and 17.
25. WHO, 47th Year, No. 3, May-June 1994, p. 36.
26. Indian Science Congress Presidential Addresses, Vol. II: 1948-81, p. 1232.

BOOKS BY THE SAME AUTHOR

1. International Administration: WHO South East-Asia Regional Office (New Delhi, 1977), Sterling Publishers
2. Principles, Problems and Prospects of Co-operative Administration (New Delhi, 1979), Sterling Publishers (Co-Author Dr. B.B. Goel)
3. Administration of Personnel in Co-operative (New Delhi, 1979), Sterling Publishers (Co-Author Dr. B.B. Goel)
4. Health Care Administration: Ecology, Principles and Modern Trends (New Delhi, 1980), Sterling Publishers
5. Health Care Administration: Policy-making and Planning (New Delhi, 1980), Sterling Publishers
6. Health Care Administration: Levels and Aspects (New Delhi, 1980), Sterling Publishers
7. International Civil Service: Principles, Problems and Prospects (New Delhi, 1984), Sterling Publishers
8. Public Health Administration (New Delhi, 1984), Sterling Publishers
9. Public Personnel Administration (New Delhi, 1984), Reprint 1987, Sterling Publishers
10. International Civil Services—Principles, Problems and Prospectives (New Delhi, 1984), Sterling Publishers.
11. Social Welfare Administration: Theory and Practice (Vols. I and II) (New Delhi, 1988), Deep & Deep Publications Pvt. Ltd.
12. Hospital Administration and Management (ed.) Co-Author Dr. R. Kumar in 3 volumes (New Delhi, 1989), Deep & Deep Publications Pvt. Ltd.
13. Policy and Administration: Family Planning & Beyond (New Delhi, 1990), Deep & Deep Publications Pvt. Ltd.
14. Modern Management Techniques (Revised and Reprinted) (New Delhi, 1990), Deep & Deep Publications Pvt. Ltd.
15. Development Planning and Administration (ed.) S. Bhatnagar (Co-editor) (New Delhi, 1992), Deep & Deep Publications Pvt. Ltd.
16. Financial Administration and Management (New Delhi, 1993), Sterling Publishers
17. Advanced Public Administration (New Delhi, 1993), Sterling Publishers

18. Personnel Administration and Management
(New Delhi, 1994), Deep & Deep Publications Pvt. Ltd.
19. Educational Policy and Administration
(New Delhi, 1994), Deep & Deep Publications Pvt. Ltd.
20. Slum Improvement Through Participatory Urban Based Community Structures
(New Delhi, 1999), Deep & Deep Publications Pvt. Ltd.
21. Distance Education in 21st Century
(New Delhi, 2000), Deep & Deep Publications Pvt. Ltd.
22. Health Care System and Management: Organization and Structure
(New Delhi, 2000), Deep & Deep Publications Pvt. Ltd.
23. Health Care System and Management: Policies and Programmes
(New Delhi, 2000), Deep & Deep Publications Pvt. Ltd.
24. Health Care System and Management: Management and Administration
(New Delhi, 2000), Deep & Deep Publications Pvt. Ltd.
25. Heath Care System and Management: Primary Health Care Management
(New Delhi, 2000), Deep & Deep Publications Pvt. Ltd.
26. Management Techniques: Principles and Practices
(New Delhi, 2001), Deep & Deep Publications Pvt. Ltd.
27. Encyclopaedia of Disaster Management in 3 Volumes
(New Delhi, 2001), Deep & Deep Publications Pvt. Ltd.
28. Management of Hospitals: Hospital Core Services
(New Delhi, 2002), Deep & Deep Publications Pvt. Ltd.
29. Management of Hospitals: Hospital Supportive Services
(New Delhi, 2002), Deep & Deep Publications Pvt. Ltd.
30. Management of Hospitals: Hospital Preventive and Promotive Services
(New Delhi, 2002), Deep & Deep Publications Pvt. Ltd.
31. Management of Hospitals: Hospital Managerial Services
(New Delhi, 2002), Deep & Deep Publications Pvt. Ltd.
32. Public Personal Administration
(New Delhi, 2002), Deep & Deep Publications Pvt. Ltd.
33. Public Financial Administration
(New Delhi, 2002), Deep & Deep Publications Pvt. Ltd.
34. Urban Development and Management
(New Delhi, 2002), Deep & Deep Publications Pvt. Ltd.
35. Public Administration: Theory and Practices
(New Delhi, 2003), Deep & Deep Publications Pvt. Ltd.
36. Advanced Public Administration (Revised and Enlarged Edition)
(New Delhi, 2003), Deep & Deep Publications Pvt. Ltd.

37. Panchayati Raj in India
(New Delhi, 2003), Deep & Deep Publications Pvt. Ltd.
38. Encyclopedia of Higher Education in 21st Century: Organisation and Structure
(New Delhi, 2004), Deep & Deep Publications Pvt. Ltd.
39. Encyclopaedia of Higher Education in 21st Century: Quality and Excellence
(New Delhi, 2004), Deep & Deep Publications Pvt. Ltd.
40. Encyclopedia of Higher Education in 21st Century, Extension Education Services
(New Delhi, 2004), Deep & Deep Publications Pvt. Ltd.
41. Stress Management and Education: An Indian Perspective
(New Delhi, 2004), Deep & Deep Publications Pvt. Ltd.
42. Human Values and Education:
(New Delhi, 2004), Deep & Deep Publications Pvt. Ltd.
43. Public Health Policy and Administration
(New Delhi, 2004), Deep & Deep Publications Pvt. Ltd.
44. Administration and Management of NGO's: Text and Case Studies
(New Delhi, 2004), Deep & Deep Publications Pvt. Ltd.
45. Nursing Services: Management and Administration
(New Delhi, 2005), Deep & Deep Publications Pvt. Ltd.
46. Population Policy and Family Welfare Administration
(New Delhi, 2005), Deep & Deep Publications Pvt. Ltd.
47. Human Resource Development in 21st Century
(New Delhi, 2005), Deep & Deep Publications Pvt. Ltd.
48. Encyclopaedia of Disaster Management (3 Volumes)
(New Delhi, 2006) Deep & Deep Publications Pvt. Ltd.
49. School Health Education
(New Delhi, 2007), Deep & Deep Publications Pvt. Ltd.
50. Health Education: Theory and Practices
(New Delhi, 2007), Deep & Deep Publications Pvt. Ltd.
51. Good Governance: An Integral Views
(New Delhi, 2007), Deep & Deep Publications Pvt. Ltd.
52. Right to Information and Good Governance
(New Delhi, 2007), Deep & Deep Publications Pvt. Ltd.
53. Disaster Management: Text and Case Studies
(New Delhi, 2007), Deep & Deep Publications Pvt. Ltd.
54. Hospital Administration: Theory and Practices
(New Delhi, 2007), Deep & Deep Publications Pvt. Ltd.
55. Environmental Health Values and Education,
(New Delhi, 2008), Deep & Deep Publications Pvt. Ltd.

56. Administrative and Management Thinkers: Revelvance in New Millennium
(New Delhi, 2008), Deep & Deep Publications Pvt. Ltd.
57. Principles and Practices of Human Values
(New Delhi, 2008), Deep & Deep Publications Pvt. Ltd.
58. Distance Education: Principles, Potentialities and Perspectives
(New Delhi, 2008), Deep & Deep Publications Pvt. Ltd.
59. Educational Administration and Management: An Integral View
(New Delhi, 2008), Deep & Deep Publications Pvt. Ltd.
60. Women Health Education
(New Delhi, 2008), Deep & Deep Publications Pvt. Ltd.
61. Health Care System and Hospital Administration
Vol. 1 (Organizational Structure)
(New Delhi, 2008), Deep & Deep Publications Pvt. Ltd.
62. Health Care System and Hospital Administration
Vol. 2 (Resources: Human, Finance and Material)
(New Delhi, 2008), Deep & Deep Publications Pvt. Ltd.
63. Health Care System and Hospital Administration
Vol. 3 (Policy-making and Programmes)
(New Delhi, 2008), Deep & Deep Publications Pvt. Ltd.
64. Health Care System and Hospital Administration
Vol. 4 (Emerging and Thrust Areas)
(New Delhi, 2008), Deep & Deep Publications Pvt. Ltd.
65. Health Care System and Hospital Administration
Vol. 5 (Primary/Rural Health Care)
(New Delhi, 2008), Deep & Deep Publications Pvt. Ltd.
66. Health Care System and Hospital Administration
Vol. 6 (Secondary and Tertiary Health Care)
(New Delhi, 2008), Deep & Deep Publications Pvt. Ltd.
67. Health Care System and Hospital Administration
Vol. 7 (Management Techniques and Good Governance)
(New Delhi, 2008), Deep & Deep Publications Pvt. Ltd.
68. Education of Lifestyle and Lifetime Diseases
(Deep & Deep Publications Pvt. Ltd.)
69. Health Education Administration—From International Level to Village Level
(Deep & Deep Publications Pvt. Ltd.)
70. Education for Healthy Urban Cities
(Deep & Deep Publications Pvt. Ltd.)
71. Rural Health Education
(Deep & Deep Publications Pvt. Ltd.)

Bibliography

Acton Society Trust, Hospitals and the State: Hospital Organisation and Administration under the National Health Service Series, London: Action Society Trust, 1956, 54p.

Acton Society Trust, Hospitals and the State: Hospital Organisation and Administration under the National Health Service, London: The Trust, 1959, iii, 80p.

Andhra Pradesh, Health and Local Administration Department Panchayats Executive Officers Regulations relating to Recruitment, etc., Hyderabad: The Author, 1956, l6p.

Bannington, B.G., English Public Health Administration, 2nd ed., London: P.S. King, 1929, 325p.

Berkov, Robert, The World Health Organisation: A Study in Decentralized International Administration, Geneva Droz, 1957, 173p.

Better Health by Community Projects Administration, Planning Commission, New Delhi: Community Projects, Planning Commission, n.d., 32p.

Blum, Henrik L., Public Administration: A Public Health Viewpoint, N.Y.: Macmillan, 1963, 532p.

Hugh Flanagan and Peter Spurgeon, Public Sector Managerial Effectiveness: Theory and Practice in the National Health Service, Buckingham: Open Univ. Press, 1996, 128p.

Freeman, Ruth B., Administration of Public Health Services and Edward M. Holmes, Philadelphia: Saunders, 1960, 507p.

Goddard, H.A., Principles of Administration Applied to Nursing Service by H.A. Goddard, Geneva: World Health Organisation, 1958, 106p.

Goel, Rajneesh, Community Health Care, New Delhi: Deep & Deep Publications Pvt. Ltd., 2004, 403p.

Goel, S.L., Health and Care Administration: Policy-making and Planning, Delhi: Sterling, 1980, 288p.

Goel, S.L, Health Care Administration: Ecology, Principles and Modern Trends, Delhi: Sterling, 1980, 233p.

Goel, S.L., Health Care Administration: Levels and Aspects, Delhi: Sterling, 1980, 245p.

Goel, S.L., Health Care System and Management, New Delhi: Deep & Deep Publications Pvt. Ltd., 2004, 4 Vols.

Goel, S.L., International Administration: WHO South-East Asia Regional Office, Delhi: Sterling, 1977, 344p.

Goel, S.L., Population Policy and Family Welfare: Reproductive and Child Health Administration, New Delhi: Deep & Deep Publications Pvt. Ltd., 2005, 526p.

Goel, S.L., Public Health Administration, Delhi: Sterling, 1984, 472p.

Goel, S.L, Public Health Policy and Administration, New Delhi: Deep & Deep Publications Pvt. Ltd., 2005, 651p.

Graduate Study in Public Administration: A Guide to Graduate Programs by Office of Education, Department of Health, Education and Welfare, Washington: United States Government Printing Office, 1961, 158+p.

Greenfield, Margert, State-Local Service for Mental Health, Bureau of Public Administration, Berkeley: The Bureau, 1955, 93p.

Guangde, Sun, Health Care Administration in China, Westport: Greenport, 1993, pp. 53-62.

Handbook on Human Services Administration, edited by Jack Rabin and Marcia B. Steinhauer, New York: Marcel Dekker, 1988, 604p.

Health Policy Research in South Asia: Building Capacity for Reform, edited by Abdo S. Yazbeck and David H. Peters, Washington, D.C.: World Bank, 2003, 428p.

Heaver, Richard, Managing Primary Health Care: Implications of the Health Transition, Washington, D.C.: World Bank, 1995, 41p.

Health Status of the Underprivileged, New Delhi: Centre for Urban Studies, Indian Institute of Public Administration, 1991, 225p.

Indian Institute of Public Administration, Centre for Urban Studies, Urban Health System, edited by P.K. Umashankar and Girish K. Misra, New Delhi: Reliance and IIPA, 1993, 259p.

Institute for Training in Municipal Administration, Administration of Community Health Services, Chicago: ICMA, 1961, 560p.

Johnston, Timothy, Investing in Health: Development Effectiveness in the Health, Nutrition, and Population Sector, Washington, D.C.: World Bank, 1999, 69p.

Khandewale, Shreekant V., Health Administration and the Weaker Sections in an Indian Metropolis, Delhi: Devika, 1996, 231p.

Klinoubol, Kriengkrai, Public Health Development and Administration: A Study of Developing Economy, Delhi: Deep & Deep Publications Pvt. Ltd., 1989. 436p.

Local Self-Government Administration in States of India, 1956, New Delhi: Ministry of Health, 1956, 149p.

Local Self-government Administration in States of India, 1962, Ministry of Health, Delhi: The Manager of Publications, 1962, 161+p.

Legislature Committee on Local Administration by Health, Education and Local Administration Department, Madras, Madras: Health, Education and Local Administration Department, 1958, 5 Parts.

Morden, Margaret Gorsuch, Cooperative Health Administration in Metropolitan, Los Angeles: The Bureau, 1949, 52p.

Panchayat Manual, Madras: Health, Education and Local Administration Department, 1956, 368+p.

Papers in Public Administration, No. 6, Ann Arbor: The Bureau, 1950, 85p.

Public Services M.B.A. Induction Module: India-U.K. context (August-September, 1999: Indian Institute of Public Administration, New Delhi), Gender-related Issues (course material), New Delhi: Indian Institute of Public Administration, 1999, vp.

Report of the Regional Training Seminar on Social Security Administration, New Delhi: Regional Office for Asia and Oceania, 1979, 75p.

Rowbottom, R., Hospital Organisation: A Progress Report on the Brunel Health Services Project, London: Heinemann, 1973, 314p.

Survey of Research in Public Administration, 1980-90, edited by V.A. Pai Panandiker, Delhi: Konark, 1997, 631p.

Tebow, Hilda P., Staff-Development as an Integral Part of Administration, Washington, D.C.: Department of Health, Education and Welfare, 1959, 33+p.

The Indo-US Symposium on Community Mental Health at National Institute of Mental Health and Neuro Sciences, Bangalore: National Institute of Mental Health and Neuro Sciences, 1992, 520p.

Weaver, Jerry L., Conflict and Control in Health Care Administration, Beverly Hills: n.p., 1975, 197p.

Welfare Administration and Social Welfare Around the World, by Department of Health, Education and Welfare, United States, Washington: Government Printing Office, 1963, 9p.

Wishwakarma, R.K., Health Status of the Underprivileged, New Delhi: Centre for Urban Studies, Indian Institute of Public Administration, 1993, 283p.

Index